Public Health in Asia and the Pacific

The Asia-Pacific region has not only the greatest concentration of population but is also, arguably, the future economic centre of the world. Epidemiological transition in the region is occurring much faster than it did in the West and many countries in the region face the emerging problem of chronic diseases at the same time as they continue to grapple with communicable diseases.

This book explores how disease patterns and health problems in Asia and the Pacific, and collective responses to them, have been shaped over time by cultural, economic, social, demographic, environmental and political factors. With 14 chapters, each devoted to a country in the region, the authors take a comparative and historical approach to the evolution of public health and preventive medicine, and offer a broader understanding of the links in a globalizing world between health on the one hand and culture, economy, polity and society on the other.

Public Health in Asia and the Pacific presents the importance of the non-medical context in the history of human disease, as well as the significance of disease in the larger histories of the region. It will appeal to scholars and policy makers in the fields of public health, the history of medicine and those with a wider interest in the Asia-Pacific region.

Milton J. Lewis, a historian of medicine and public health, was a Senior Research Fellow in the School of Public Health, 1989–2006 and is now at the Australian Health Policy Institute, University of Sydney.

Kerrie L. MacPherson, a historian of public health and diseases of China and Hong Kong, is an Associate Professor in the Centre of Urban Planning and Environmental Management, the University of Hong Kong.

Routledge Advances in Asia-Pacific Studies

1 **Environment, Education and Society in the Asia-Pacific**
Local traditions and global discourses
David Yencken, John Fien and Helen Sykes

2 **Ageing in the Asia-Pacific Region**
David R. Phillips

3 **Caring for the Elderly in Japan and the US**
Practices and policies
Susan Orpett Long

4 **Human Rights and Gender Politics**
Asia Pacific perspectives
Edited by Anne Marie Hilsdon, Martha Macintyre, Vera Mackie and Maila Stivens

5 **Human Rights in Japan, South Korea and Taiwan**
Ian Neary

6 **Cultural Politics and Asian Values**
The tepid war
Michael D. Barr

7 **Social Policy in East and Southeast Asia**
Education, health, housing and income maintenance
M. Ramesh

8 **Sino-Japanese Relations**
Facing the past, looking to the future?
Caroline Rose

9 **Directors of Urban Change in Asia**
Edited by Peter J.M. Nas

10 **Education Reform and Education Policy in East Asia**
Ka Ho Mok

11 **Public Health in Asia and the Pacific**
Historical and comparative perspectives
Edited by Milton J. Lewis and Kerrie L. MacPherson

Public Health in Asia and the Pacific

Historical and comparative perspectives

Edited by
Milton J. Lewis and
Kerrie L. MacPherson

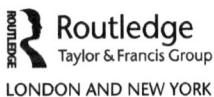

First published 2008
by Routledge
2 Park Square, Milton Park, Abingdon, Oxon, OX14 4RN

Simultaneously published in the USA and Canada
by Routledge
711 Third Avenue, New York, NY 10017

*Routledge is an imprint of the Taylor & Francis Group,
an informa business*

First issued in paperback 2011

© 2008 Milton J. Lewis and Kerrie L. MacPherson, selection and
editorial matter; the contributors, their own chapters

Typeset in Times New Roman by
Newgen Imaging Systems (P) Ltd, Chennai, India

All rights reserved. No part of this book may be reprinted or
reproduced or utilised in any form or by any electronic,
mechanical, or other means, now known or hereafter
invented, including photocopying and recording, or in any
information storage or retrieval system, without permission in
writing from the publishers.

British Library Cataloguing in Publication Data
A catalogue record for this book is available
from the British Library

Library of Congress Cataloging in Publication Data
A catalog record for this book has been requested

ISBN10: 0–415–35962–7 (hbk)
ISBN10: 0–415–66649–X (pbk)
ISBN10: 0–203–00756–5 (ebk)

ISBN13: 978–0–415–35962–7 (hbk)
ISBN13: 978–0–415–66649–7 (pbk)
ISBN13: 978–0–203–00756–3 (ebk)

Contents

List of illustrations vii
Notes on contributors ix

Public health in Asia and the Pacific: an introduction 1
MILTON J. LEWIS AND KERRIE L. MacPHERSON

1 Invisible borders: Hong Kong, China and
   the imperatives of public health 10
   KERRIE L. MacPHERSON

2 History of public health in modern Japan:
   the road to becoming the healthiest
   nation in the world 55
   MASAHIRA ANESAKI

3 A history of public health in Korea 73
   IN-SOK YEO

4 History of public health in modern India: 1857–2005 87
   RADHIKA RAMASUBBAN

5 Public health in Thailand: changing
   medical paradigms and disease patterns
   in political and economic context 106
   PAUL T. COHEN

6 'Could confinement be humanised'? A modern
   history of leprosy in Vietnam 122
   LAURENCE MONNAIS

7 Conflict and collaboration in public health:
   the Rockefeller Foundation and the Dutch
   colonial government in Indonesia   139
   TERENCE H. HULL

8 The political determinants of public
   health in Timor-Leste: foreign domination
   and the path to independence   153
   SUE INGRAM

9 From colonial economy to social equity: history
   of public health in Malaysia   170
   KAI HONG PHUA AND MARY LAI LIN WONG

10 From colony to global city: public health
   strategies and the control of disease in Singapore   188
   BRENDA S. A. YEOH, KAI HONG PHUA AND KELLY FU

11 Public health and the clash of cultures:
   the Philippine cholera epidemics   206
   WILLIE T. ONG

12 Public health in Australia from the nineteenth
   to the twenty-first century   222
   MILTON J. LEWIS

13 Papua New Guinea: epidemiological transition,
   public health and the Pacific   250
   VICKI LUKER

14 History of public health in Pacific Island countries 276
   RICHARD TAYLOR

   Index   308

Illustrations

Figures

2.1	Infant mortality rates in selected countries (1947–2004)	70
2.2	Infant mortality rates by age in selected countries	70
2.3	Perinatal mortality rates in selected countries	71
14.1	Life expectancy and infant mortality in Pacific Island states $c.2000$ in relation to GDP per capita	298
14.2	Life expectancy in Pacific Island states in 1980 and 2000 in relation to GDP per capita	299
14.3	Life expectancy in Pacific Island states in 1980 and 2000 in relation to proportional mortality from cardiovascular disease (CVD) and infection	300

Tables

2.1	Number of hospitals by owners in the Meiji period	58
2.2	Number of hospitals in the Meiji period	59
3.1	Life expectancy of Koreans (in years)	84
9.1	Public investment for social services 1956–1960	175
9.2	Annual budget allocation for Ministry of Health 1970–2000 in Malaysian ringgit	180
9.3	Vital statistics of Malaysia 1957–2000	181
9.4	Population annual growth and vital rates, Malaysia 1970–2000	182
13.1	Country data: Melanesia, Micronesia and Polynesia	252

Contributors

Masahira Anesaki has a BSc in Physics and a BA and MA in Sociology from the Tokyo Metropolitan University, and a Diploma in Social Administration from the University of Manchester. He was Professor of Sociology at Nihon University School of Medicine, 1968–2002 and is now Professor of Sociology at Daiichi Welfare University, Japan. He has published extensively on health services in Japan.

Paul T. Cohen PhD (London) is Associate Professor and Senior Research Fellow, Department of Anthropology, Division of Society, Culture, Media and Philosophy, Macquarie University, Sydney. There he has taught courses on medical anthropology, the cultural dimensions of drugs, and health and development in the Third World. He has done fieldwork in Thailand and Laos over several decades. He is co-editor with John Purcal of two books on public health: *The Political Economy of Primary Health Care in Southeast Asia* (1989) and *Health and Development in Southeast Asia* (1995).

Kelly Fu is a PhD student in Sociology at Goldsmiths College, University of London. Her major areas of interest include post-colonialism, feminist thought and popular culture.

Terence H. Hull holds Chairs in Demography in the Research School of Social Science and in Population, Health and Development in the National Centre for Epidemiology and Population Health at the Australian National University. Born in the United States and educated in both Australia and America, he has spent 35 years working on issues of health and population in Asia, with particular concentration on Indonesia.

Sue Ingram is currently Senior Adviser on Machinery of Government in the Regional Assistance Mission to the Solomon Islands, established in 2003 under the auspices of the Pacific Islands Forum to assist in the restoration of security and economic stability following a protracted period of conflict. She has previously worked in senior posts in government and the United Nations, including 16 years as a senior executive with the Australian Government, latterly in the Department of Health and Ageing. She joined the UN peacekeeping mission in East Timor in 2000 where she served in several posts including Director of

Transition Planning in the lead-up to independence and Chief of Staff in the post-independence mission. Her association with Timor goes back to 1974 where she undertook research for a year until her fieldwork was brought to an end by the political upheaval in August 1975.

Milton J. Lewis, an historian of medicine and public health, was a Senior Research Fellow in the School of Public Health, 1989–2006 and is now at the Australian Health Policy Institute, University of Sydney. His most recent authored books are: *The People's Health. Public Health in Australia, 1788–1950* (2003); *The People's Health. Public Health in Australia, 1950 to the Present* (2003); and *Medicine and Care of the Dying. A Modern History* (2007). He has edited a number of books including *Sex, Disease, and Society. A Comparative History of Sexually Transmitted Diseases and HIV/AIDS in Asia and the Pacific* (1997) and *Histories of Sexually Transmitted Diseases and HIV/AIDS in Sub-Saharan Africa* (1999).

Vicki Luker is Executive Editor of *The Journal of Pacific History* and Visiting Fellow in the State, Society and Governance in Melanesia Project, both of which are located in the Research School of Pacific and Asian Studies, Australian National University, Canberra. She works on the history of medicine and health in the Pacific and in particular HIV/AIDS.

Kerrie L. MacPherson is an Associate Professor of History in the Centre of Urban Planning and Environmental Management, the University of Hong Kong. Her research and publications focus on the history of diseases and urban public health in China and Hong Kong. She served on the Care and Prevention Committee of the Hong Kong AIDS Advisory Council.

Laurence Monnais is an Associate Professor at the Université de Montréal (Department of History – Center for East Asian Studies, CETASE), Canada. She is a specialist in the history of medicine in French Indochina and modern Vietnam. She is the author of *Médecine et colonisation. L'Aventure indochinoise, 1860–1939* (Paris 1999). She is currently working on two projects: one on the social life of medicines and the other a general history of medicine in Southeast Asia.

Willie T. Ong is Medical Director, Pasay Filipino-Chinese Charity Health Center, Manila. He has a Master of Public Health, Public Health Administration and Health Policy Tracking, University of the Philippines, Manila and in 2000 held a History of Medicine and Public Health Post-Doctoral Fellowship at the University of Wisconsin-Madison. Since 2003 he has been chairman of the Society of Philippine Health History.

Kai Hong Phua has joint appointments in Health Policy and Management at the Yong Loo Lin School of Medicine and the Lee Kuan Yew School of Public Policy, National University of Singapore. He is a graduate of the Harvard School of Public Health and holds a PhD in Social Administration (Health Economics) from the London School of Economics and Political Science.

Contributors xi

Radhika Ramasubban is a sociologist and social historian whose work focuses on India. In recent years her research has addressed issues of public health policy, urban health, women's reproductive health and HIV/AIDS. She is currently Director, Centre for Social and Technological Change, an independent research institute in Mumbai.

Richard Taylor is Professor of International Health and Head of the International and Indigenous Division in the School of Public Health, University of Queensland, Brisbane. He has had long-term involvement in the Asia Pacific region, particularly the Pacific Islands, and works not only in the epidemiology and disease control aspects of the health transition, especially in relation to cardiovascular diseases, diabetes and cancer, but also communicable and vector-borne diseases.

Mary Lai Lin Wong has just completed her PhD at the National University of Singapore and is now working as the Principal Assistant Director, Corporate Policy and Health Industry Division, Malaysia Ministry of Health. She graduated in History from the University of Malaya and holds a Master's degree in Health Services Management from the University of Manchester.

In-sok Yeo is Assistant Professor of the History of Medicine at Yonsei University in Seoul. He has published widely on the history of medicine in Korea and on ancient Greek medicine.

Brenda S. A. Yeoh is a Professor in the Department of Geography and Head of the Southeast Asian Studies Programme, National University of Singapore. She is also Research Leader of the Asian Migration Research Cluster at the University's Asia Research Institute. Her research interests include the politics of space in colonial and post-colonial cities; and gender, migration and transnational communities.

Public health in Asia and the Pacific
An introduction

Milton J. Lewis and Kerrie L. MacPherson

This volume explores how disease patterns and health problems in different Asian countries, and the collective responses to them, have been shaped over time by cultural, economic, social, demographic, environmental and political factors. With 14 chapters, each devoted to a country in the Asia-Pacific region – East Asia represented by China and Hong Kong, Japan and Korea; South and Southeast Asia by India, Thailand, Vietnam, Indonesia, East Timor, Malaysia, Singapore and the Philippines; and Pacific Island nations by Australia, Papua New Guinea, Polynesia, Melanesia and Micronesia – the authors take a comparative and historical approach to the evolution of public health and preventive medicine, and offer a broader understanding of the links in a globalizing world between health on the one hand and culture, economy, polity and society on the other; that is, the authors show how the non-medical context is important in the history of human disease, as well as how significant disease is in the larger histories of the region.

The comparative history of public health in the Western world has been ably explored from a diversity of perspectives. The transference of Western or scientific medical practices to many parts of the world through the expansionist phase of European history has also been examined.[1] Broad delineation of the development of public health and preventive medicine identifies three so-called revolutions in public health strategies, though each should be viewed as a complex set of reciprocal relationships that overlap and inform one another, not as discrete breaks with the past. The first 'revolution' in the nineteenth century was the sanitary and hygiene movements, fundamentally environmental in perspective, the provision of pure water supplies and the scientific techniques to understand the aetiology of diseases and their population impacts, linked to infectious diseases control. By the early twentieth century the definition of public health expanded beyond environmental concerns and scientific–technological advances to an inclusive recognition of the role of individual behaviours and societal (and political) responsibility for health status. This constitutes the second 'revolution' and is best summed up by Charles-Edward Amory Winslow in 1920.[2] He wrote that public health should be defined as:

> the science and the art of preventing disease, prolonging life and promoting physical health and efficiency through organized community efforts for the sanitation of the environment, the control of community infections, the

education of the individual in principles of personal hygiene, the organization of medical and nursing service for the early diagnosis and preventive treatment of disease, and the development of the machinery which will ensure to every individual in the community a standard of living adequate for the maintenance of health.

(Winslow 1920: 30)

The third 'revolution' arose from the internationalization of public health policies, subsequent to the founding of the World Health Organization in 1948, contributing to what has been called a 'new public health' strategy in the 1980s based on the Alma-Ata Declaration (1978), the World Health Organization's (WHO) 'Health for All' philosophy (1984) and the Ottawa Charter for Health Promotion (1986). Essentially, the goals and objectives of the new public health strategies target issues of equity tied to social and economic reform, governance and capacity-building, 'a shift in perspective from input to outcomes: governments were to be held accountable for the *health* of their populations, not just for the health services they provided' (Kickbusch 2003: 383). Public health and public policy are conjoined, not just at the local, regional or national levels but internationally, through global health initiatives and international donor and aid agencies as well as non-governmental organizations (NGOs).

The building of what has been called 'social capital' is a model of public health based on social structures and community-focused interventions rather than a focus on individual risk factors and discretionary treatment modalities (Lomas 1998: 1181). For developing economies in Asia and elsewhere the financial implications of adopting such a broadly based health developmental policy will be significant and most likely be politically contentious. As the *Millennium Ecosystem Assessment Report* underscores, there is a continuing failure in many parts of the world – including half the urban population in parts of Asia – to achieve acceptable levels of potable water, sanitation and hygiene – what passed in the nineteenth century as the fundamentals of public health.[3] The historic links between health and the environment remain central to the promotion of a community's well-being despite the rapid advances in the medical sciences and technology in the last 50 years. New or newly emerging infectious diseases in Asia such as H5N1 (bird flu) are clearly linked to environmental factors. Environment and social factors contributed to the emergence and spread of SARS (severe acute respiratory syndrome) and drug-resistant tuberculosis and malaria, all of which highlights the continuing struggle to deliver effective primary health care in the region as well as to restructure public health systems to be more responsive to challenges posed by the internationalization of new, or re-emerging, infectious diseases. A comparative and historical approach to the evolution of public health and preventive medicine in the region may offer specific insights and lessons as well as a broader understanding of the linkages between health and society in a globalizing world.

A comparative study of the development of public health in Asia and the Pacific, with its very different cultural and political heritage and economic history and its experience of Western and Japanese colonialism, can contribute to an understanding of the issues facing non-Western nations. Furthermore, the comparative approach usefully delineates the commonalities and the differences in the disease experience of the countries of the region as well as between them and the rest of the world.

The history of European expansion into Asia is well known. Briefly reviewed, it reveals that from about 1500, European maritime nations sought the spices, silk and tea of the fabled Orient, importantly fomenting a commercial revolution and abetted by opportunities to introduce Christianity. In this trade-based, first wave of colonialism, the Europeans focused their efforts on port cities like Kolkata, or Macau on the periphery of China. In the second and larger wave in the nineteenth century, industrializing Europe's desire to exchange manufactures for raw materials, and the imperial rivalries of the European powers, led them to assume control over much larger areas of Asia and the Pacific (Lewis and Bamber 1997: 4). In the nineteenth century, moreover, there was large-scale emigration from Europe to Australia and New Zealand (just as there was to other parts of Europe overseas like the United States and Canada). In these settler colonies, transplanted European culture and institutions overwhelmed indigenous, small-scale, tribal societies. However, in the non-settler, economic colonies, while Western political and economic ideas and institutions (including public health) had a significant, long-term impact, the ancient cultures of Asia emerged mainly intact in the era of decolonization in the first two decades or so after World War II. Recently, globalization and the speed of Asian economic development have made more urgent the need for viable public health services as Asian nations encounter all at once old and new public health problems from malaria and contaminated drinking water to smoking-related, chronic disease and air pollution.

One recurrent theme stands out from this historical research which is as relevant today as it was in the past, regardless of geography. Preventive and environmental medicine and public health since the nineteenth century, where developed, introduced, adapted and extended, has transformed societies and the quality of life. Perhaps the most transformative factor has been the remarkable increase in human life expectancy, the by-product of economic development and improved nutrition, but also due to preventive health measures, the eradication and control of infectious diseases (particularly childhood diseases), access to safe water supplies, sanitation and health-care delivery, all of which directly bear on mortality rates. As Hull argues in Chapter 8 on Indonesia, in the debates over what causal factors have shaped the modern mortality decline, advances in medical technologies and biomedicine or sanitary–environmental and economic–nutritional advancements, this 'framing of dichotomies' detracts from the interdependent and supportive role both have played in the remarkable improvement of a community's health.

To give some Asian and Pacific examples, China, in the nineteenth century, was reckoned to have an average life expectancy in the total population of 33 years, rising only to 35 years in the first half of the twentieth century. By 2004 it was estimated to be 71.96 years. Japan experienced significant gains in life expectancy, from 44 years in 1900 to 81.04 in 2004. Hong Kong, a British crown colony from 1841 to 1997 (now a Special Administrative Region of the People's Republic of China (PRC) under the one country, two systems concept), rose from a base estimate the same as China's to one slightly exceeding Japan's, estimated to be 81.5 years in 2004, despite waves of immigration from China prior to and after World War II. South Korea's gains are equally impressive, rising from 51.1 years (male) and 53.7 (female) in 1960 to an estimated 75.58 years in the total population in 2004. Singapore and Malaysia followed similar trajectories, with Vietnam, Thailand and the Philippines close behind. Indonesia and India, with large and diverse populations, lag behind, followed by Papua New Guinea and East Timor. Australia's life expectancy, on the other hand, very quickly exceeded that of the 'mother country' (see Chapter 12 by Milton J. Lewis).

No matter how heartening such statistics may be, health and preventive strategies need to respond swiftly to changing conditions. Epidemiological transitions have been noted in all these countries following similar trends in the United States, Europe and Australia, a shift from infectious diseases as the source of the highest cause-specific mortality to heart disease, cancers and cerebrovascular and other chronic diseases related to aging populations and changes in lifestyles. Another caveat is that gains in life expectancy can quickly recede in the face of adverse economic, political and social conditions, all of which affect the health-care system. In May of 2001, North Korean officials admitted to a decline in life expectancy from 73.2 years in 1993 to 66.8 in 1999. Malnutrition, lack of medicines and shortages in hospitals were identified as serious problems. Childhood vaccination coverage for measles and polio fell from 90% of the population to 50% in 1997. Even more worrying is that access to safe drinking water for the population declined between 1994 and 1996 from 86% to 50% (*The New York Times* 16 May 2001).

The chapters do not constitute a comprehensive survey of public health in Asia and the Pacific. Rather, they are linked together in significant ways by the thematic continuity of interacting histories, cultures, environments, disease patterns, inter-regional population migrations and medical practices. Despite identifiable differences that exist between these countries as well as between regions, a more integrated view of public health and preventive medicine in the region that takes into account the various factors that gave rise to these developments will hopefully take shape. Although in South, Southeast and East Asia as well as Australia, New Guinea and a number of Pacific Island nations, public health services and institutions were founded on the same principles as their Western predecessors, they diverge from that model in important ways. The introduction of Western sanitary science, preventive medicine and the mechanisms to ensure their effectiveness – arising as they did from the particular economic, social, political and scientific development of the West – made the transplantation of the Western model in Asia (perhaps with the exception of Australia) culturally specific. Therefore the contributors have approached their subject from a variety of perspectives and emphases, though each was asked by the editors to consider how any or all of the following concerns apply in the history in his or her country:

1   How social, cultural, political, economic, demographic and environmental factors have influenced historical disease patterns and the development of policies and practices to advance the health of the people. Two key historical phenomena have been colonization and mass poverty.

2   Double health burdens: The demographic and epidemiological transitions from communicable to non-communicable diseases (especially cardiovascular diseases, cancers and diabetes) as leading causes of death and illness. But, at the same time, the emergence (or re-emergence) of infections like HIV/AIDS, drug-resistant TB and SARS as threats to health.
3   Ethnic, economic and gender inequalities which promote health problems within countries.
4   The human impact on the natural environment producing changes like global warming and deforestation which directly or indirectly affect the health of large numbers of people.
5   The double-edged effects of globalization: on the one hand, promoting the spread of infectious disease, but, on the other, offering a more rapid exchange of the information and expertise needed to contain disease outbreaks.
6   The influence of international bodies like the World Health Organization on national public health policy and practice; for example, WHO endorsement, in the 1970s, of primary health care and Health for All by the Year 2000.
7   Modern public health was born in Europe in the nineteenth century as a response to the mass health problems created by large-scale urbanization and industrialization in a capitalist mode. The state played a central role in developing public health policy and services (preventive and directed at the population as a whole, not curative and directed at the individual, as in clinical medicine). The market economy not only created conditions in which diseases and deaths increased but in the longer term it produced the additional wealth that the state used to fund the new sanitary infrastructure and health services, and allowed poorer wage-earning individuals to improve their own standard of living (especially their nutrition). The nature of the state and the economy has also been important in the history of public health in Asia and the Pacific; for example, some Pacific nations with weak state structures lack the political as well as the economic resources to provide adequate primary health care for all their people; and as it has moved towards a market economy, China has shifted from the 'barefoot doctor' model of delivering primary health care to a fee-for-service model.
8   Urbanization, in the colonial and post-independence periods, has been a significant source of health problems. Closely associated has been the phenomenon of internal (rural-to-urban) migration of labour as well as immigration from external sources. A notable example of the latter is the immigration of Chinese and Indian labourers into Southeast Asian and Pacific countries in the nineteenth and early twentieth centuries. This profoundly influenced the ethnic, cultural, economic and political environments as well as disease patterns.
9   War in the region has been a source of additional health problems (apart from direct military and civilian casualties) and a barrier to improving services. Thus, the health needs of the colonial military forces came before those of the indigenous population in the Western imperial era; and warlordism in the 1920s and war with Japan in the 1930s contributed to famines and the spread of infections in China.

All the contributors grapple with the role of medicine focused on the individual and the state (community-based medical interventions) in developing a scheme of public health. Historically, in monarchical states such as India, China, Japan, Korea and Thailand, elite medicine and health care centred on the monarch and the continuation of the imperial lineage although grassroots medical and curative practices – homeopathy and cultural prescriptions existed in all the countries under examination. Great pre-modern medical theories and practices (Arab-Islamic, Ayurvedic and Chinese) circulated around the region by trade and migration, and were adopted by elites and commoners alike, framing the context within which Western or scientific medicine and public health measures were introduced, adapted or resisted. If, as in Thailand (see Chapter 5), scientific medicine tended to marginalize indigenous medicine, in Hong Kong a dual system of medicine was officially countenanced and in China traditional medicine was actively promoted as a national cultural treasure that in turn was reinvigorated and 'scientized,' a process also seen in Korea and Japan. In Vietnam (see Chapter 6 and also Chapters 1, 2, 3 and 4 on China, Japan, Korea and India), pre-colonial perceptions and control of leprosy had an influence on the subsequent schemes of containment and exclusion under French colonial rule as well as that of a modern unified Vietnam. However, in all the countries under examination, recognition existed that the application of modern medicine and preventive health care, no matter how selective, was contingent on societal change.

Perhaps no greater test of the efficacy of governance (pre- and post-colonial and national), medicine and public health approaches to disease control was the toll exacted on human life from epidemic and pandemic infectious diseases. As Pollitzer stated in his classic study of cholera for the WHO, 'it was through cholera, and the fear to which its pandemic sweeps gave rise, that international solidarity in matters of health were born' (Pollitzer 1959: 7). The incidence and more rapid dissemination of infectious diseases was abetted by the expanding and interlocking trade networks throughout the region and the world via the growing port cities as the nodes of contact. The geopathology of disease patterns was intensified or shifted due to settlement, war, revolution or conflicts; for example, the introduction of leprosy and tuberculosis in East Timor (see Chapter 8) by soldiers imported from Africa, or the high incidence of tuberculosis in the Straits Settlements (see Chapters 9 and 10) among Chinese immigrants working in the mines and plantations. Hong Kong as a colony experienced the resurgence of epidemics of smallpox, cholera, plague, malaria and tuberculosis when masses of refugees fled to the colony due to unsettled conditions in China. 'Tropical diseases' became a new field of clinical investigations arising from medical research in colonial possessions – the 'laboratories' of 'exotic' diseases (see the Chapter 4 on India). During World War II, military operations in Asia and the Pacific exposed the dearth of knowledge of these diseases and their treatment, which affected troops returning to Europe, Australia, the United States and Japan. With the prospect of expanding political, commercial and cultural relations with peoples in the region after the war, 'health security' from the 'potential world threats' of these diseases called for a new approach concerned not only with specific diseases (or parasites) but with their ecological niches and their regional peculiarities (Dieuaide 1945: 656–658).

The emphasis here is upon preventive approaches and all they entailed; that is, a scheme of public health represented a departure from the quarantine mentality that had been reinforced from the late eighteenth century throughout the world by the deadly onslaughts of smallpox, cholera, plague and influenza, as well as tuberculosis and venereal diseases. Other infectious diseases such as measles had devastating effects on populations in the Pacific islands (see Chapters 13 and 14) where no natural immunity existed. Hostile political and social environments magnified a public health crisis in the Philippines (see Chapter 11) initiated by American interventions to control cholera epidemics in the early twentieth century. Drastic plague control measures by colonial officials in Hong Kong were also resisted by local populations as were Japanese methods of policing and the isolation of patients in Korea during their occupation of that country. The slow process of public acquiescence in the possibility of disease control as a public responsibility was precipitated in China by the massive outbreaks of pneumonic plague in Manchuria, helping to create a national health ministry. In Malaysia (see Chapter 9), the expansion of health services was seen as a way to win over indigenous peoples and Chinese settlers during the Communist insurgency.

International cooperation in matters of public health and the sharing of disease intelligence was abetted by the above factors, and in the case of the British empire (which included many of the countries in this volume) by the establishment of medical schools, teaching hospitals and public health and sanitary departments, as well as the production of colonial medical and sanitary reports and then medical research reports 'in the colonies, protectorates and mandated territories' for official use only (and put to good use by researchers in this volume). Medical missionaries of various religious denominations and nationalities circulated around the region establishing clinics and hospitals, and who in turn produced an appreciable body of medical literature by sharing disease intelligence with their religious compatriots in the region and at 'home.' The word 'health' as the Rockefeller Foundation learned, 'is a talisman which can successfully unlock many a foreign door' (Balfour 1926: 462). The ubiquitous activities of this philanthropic organization in Asia and the Pacific are well noted in this book. The League of Nations and its health branch founded after World War I (sometimes viewed as a competitor of the Rockefeller Foundation) enhanced the acceptance of and support for international assistance in matters of health even as national interests pulled in other directions. The founding of the World Health Organization after World War II helped standardize disease surveillance reporting and the development of analytical tools like DALYs (Disability Adjusted Life Years), introduced in 1999, helped refine health indices ('quality of life' indicators), thereby making comparisons of disease and health burdens and strategies of prevention within and between nations, more meaningful.

The historic links between health and the environment remain central to the promotion of a community's well-being despite the rapid advances in medical sciences and technology in the last 50 years. In Asia, new or re-emerging infectious diseases like SARS and H5N1 are clearly linked to environmental factors. Along with re-emerging contagions such as multi-drug-resistant tuberculosis, they have the potential to devastate populations massed in large urban agglomerations. Since the nineteenth century, rapid and sustained urbanization in Asia and the Pacific, rural-to-urban migration, poverty and disease patterns historically linked the evolution of public health and urban planning in the region, and the planning of the 'sanitary city' challenged governments on all fronts. The interconnectedness of human health and well-being with the built environment has again generated a great deal of interest among health-care professionals, government officials, environmentalists, architects, engineers and town planners. With the rapid growth of cities, increasing environmental degradation and the threat of continued adverse effects to living conditions have elicited a global effort to address the factors in the environment that affect current health and the health of future generations. In advanced nations, the problems of poorly designed cities produce excessive consumption of water and energy resources as well as unnecessary waste and pollutants, all of which diminish the health of communities. There are lasting biological effects on human health from exposure to environmental influences pre-natal or in infancy which takes full cognizance of the social origins of health and disease. In developing nations which are experiencing the most rapid urbanization in world history, the situation is acute. China's response to unprecedented urban and economic growth coupled with an equally impressive environmental decline affects not just Hong Kong but also the region as a whole. All the contributors to this volume have attempted in one way or another to identify the lessons of the past that may help to place the future in perspective, as regards to the priorities of governments and the communities which they serve.

The growing disparity of rich and poor countries in the Asia-Pacific region (and marked socio-economic inequalities within individual countries) has highlighted the fact that the provision of basic aspects of public health for half of the world's population lags well behind the rest of the world, as well as the accelerating human impact on the ecosystem due to the growing demand for resources. Economic development has without question contributed to human health, but the degradation of the environment, especially air, water and food quality, unless rectified, will negatively impact on these gains. Public health and preventive medicine must continue to respond to these challenges and public and private initiatives, sustained by growing material resources, must work in parallel to promote what is at once the noblest and most practical of objectives – the enhancement of life.

Notes

1 For a few salient examples of the development of public health in the West, see: Rosen (1958), Duffy (1968), Porter (1994, 1999), Porter (1997), Hamlin (1998) and Lewis (2003). For the impact of western public health on non-western communities see: Ramasubban (1982), MacPherson (1987), Phua (1987), MacLeod and Lewis (1988), Arnold (1993), Harrison (1994) and Manderson (1996).
2 C-E. A. Winslow (1877–1957) was regarded internationally as the elder statesman of the public health movement. He served for 30 years as the Anna R. Lauder professor

of public health at Yale University School of Medicine, was president of the American Public Health Association and editor of the *American Journal of Public Health*, the *Journal of Bacteriology* as well as author of more than 600 books and articles concerned with the advancement of the field (Fulton 1957: 1236). Winslow noted in 1920 that the rapid expansion of the public health movement meant that 'The New Public Health' heralded 15 years earlier was of only 'conventional' interest to present-day concerns (Winslow 1920: 23).

3 *Millennium Ecosystem Assessment Synthesis Report* 30 March 2005, p. 25.

References

Arnotd, D. (1993) *Colonizing the Body: State Medicine and Epidemic Diseases in Nineteenth-Century India*, Berkeley: University of California Press.
Balfour, A. (1926) 'Hygiene as a World Force', *Science*, 64(1663): 459–466.
Dieuaide, F. R. (1945) 'Tropical Diseases and Geopathology', *Science*, 102(2661): 656–658.
Duffy, J. (1968) *A History of Public Health in New York*, New York: Russell Sage Foundation.
Fulton, J. (1957) 'C-E. A. Winslow, Leader in Public Health', *Science*, 125(3260): 1236.
Hamlin, C. (1998) *Public Health and Social Justice in the Ages of Chadwick: Britain, 1800–1854*, Cambridge Mass.: Harvard University Press.
Harrison, M. (1994) *Public Health in British India: Anglo-India Preventive Medicine, 1859–1914*, Cambridge: Cambridge University Press.
Kickbusch, I. (2003) 'The Contribution of the World Health Organization to a New Public Health and Health Promotion', *American Journal of Public Health*, 93(3): 383–388.
Lewis, M. J. (2003) *The People's Health. Public Health in Australia, 1788–1950*, Vol 1; *Public Health in Australia, 1950 to the Present*, Vol 2, Westport CT and London: Praeger Press.
Lewis, M. and Bamber, S. (1997) 'Introduction', in M. Lewis, S. Bamber and M. Waugh (eds) *Sex, Disease and Society: A Comparative History of Sexually Transmitted Diseases and HIV/AIDS in Asia and the Pacific*, Westport CT and London: Greenwood Press.
Lomas, J. (1998) 'Social Capital and Health: Implications for Public Health and Epidemiology', *Social Science and Medicine*, 47(9): 1181–1188.
MacLeod, R. and Lewis, M. (1988) *Disease, Medicine and Empire: Perspectives on Western Medicine and the Experience of European Expansion*, London: Routledge.
MacPherson, K. L. (1987) *A Wilderness of Marshes: The Origins of Public Health in Shanghai, 1843–1893*, London, New York and Hong Kong: Oxford University Press.
Manderson, L. (1996) *Sickness and the State: Health and Illness in Colnied Malaya*, Cambridge: Cambridge University Press.
Phua, K. H. (1987) 'The Development of Health Services in Malaya and Singapore 1867–1960', unpublished thesis, London School of Economics and Political Science.
Pollitzer, R. (1959) *Cholera*, Geneva: WHO.
Porter, D. (ed.) (1994) *The History of Public Health and the Modern State*, Amsterdam: Rodopi.
Porter, D. (1999) *Health, Civilization and the State: A History of Public Health from Ancient to Modern Time*, London: Routledge.
Porter, R. (1997) *The Greatest Benefit to Mankind: A Medical History of Humanity*, New York: W. W. Norton.
Ramasubban, R. (1982) *Public Health and Medical Research in India: Their Origins Under the Impact of British Colonial Policy*, Stockholm: SAERC.
Rosen, G. (1958) *A History of Public Health*, New York: MD publications.
Winslow, C-E. A. (1920) 'The Untilled Fields of Public Health', *Science*, 51(1306): 23–33.

1 Invisible borders
Hong Kong, China and the imperatives of public health

Kerrie L. MacPherson

Introduction

Hong Kong and China have experienced profound changes and developed in ways unperceived when Hong Kong was seized during the Opium War of 1841–1842 and incorporated as a crown colony (and free port) into the British empire. Territorial expansion on the Chinese mainland with the cession of Kowloon (1860), and the leasing of the New Territories (1898), subsequently created an integrated and highly urbanized area of 398.25 square miles, the majority of the population drawn from Guangdong province contiguous with the territory. The anticipated expiry of the New Territories lease (in 1997) opened negotiations between Britain and China over Hong Kong's future. Despite Britain's misgivings about the political, economic and developmental differences (including medical and public health standards) with China, a communist state since 1949, the Sino-British Joint Declaration (1984) returned Hong Kong to Chinese sovereignty in 1997. This was achieved partly due to China's guarantee that Hong Kong would 'retain its capitalist system and lifestyle' for fifty years under the 'one country, two systems' concept. It was also a clear recognition by Britain of the human and geographical interdependence of Hong Kong and south China, despite the maintenance and surveillance of a political border (on both sides of the boundary) throughout the colonial period, and continuing today.

This chapter will examine the factors that influence the epidemiology and control of diseases in Hong Kong over the past century and a half and the evolution of the public health system in relationship to its human and ecological interdependence with southern China. We will examine this interdependence in matters affecting the health of the population, major disease patterns (both endemic and epidemic) and environmental factors that historically have given impetus to significant developments in public health as well as refined assessments of its shortcomings. Furthermore within this context we will explore the application of the 'one country, two systems' concept embodied in the Basic Law of Hong Kong. With the rise of newly emerging epidemic diseases such as H5N1 (bird flu) and more recently SARS (severe acute respiratory syndrome), both of which presented themselves in south China prior to the Hong Kong outbreaks, we will evaluate the utility of the concept in relation to the future of public health initiatives.

International transfer of modern medicine and public health

Public health as a scientific movement was introduced to China first in the treaty port enclaves and concessions opened to foreign trade and residence such as the Shanghai International Settlements and the French Concession, and in colonial outposts like Hong Kong, areas where foreigners could exert control under their treaty rights. Since these areas were overwhelming populated by Chinese it necessitated an accommodation to Chinese customs and traditional medical practices. Hong Kong's colonial administrators, for example, guaranteed that the Chinese population, although under British rule, would be 'governed according to the laws, customs and usages of the Chinese' (Endicott 1964: 27). This naturally included Chinese traditional medicine (TCM) and health care. They understood that China, like other ancient cultures, had developed principles for the preservation of health (*weisheng*), a distinctive medical system and an impressive pharmacopoeia, a system that had widespread influence throughout Asia. However, even at its traditional best, Chinese medical theory and its quasi-empirical underpinnings, free of quantitative implications, was primarily inductive and synthetic rather than causal and analytic. Medicines were individually concocted and experiences uncollated and there was little knowledge of the pathology of diseases and their impact on populations. Epidemics were recorded in Chinese local histories with some regularity, but there was little attempt to map these diseases by place, population, incidence, standardized types and effects or aetiology – a biometrical perspective that underpins the practice of preventive medicine and public health. Indeed, there was no standardized Chinese medical education system leading to professional qualifications and registration for practitioners (with the exception of various sectarian schools and the imperial college in Beijing that trained doctors for treating the imperial family), despite the production over the centuries of a body of medical literature that potentially could have fostered one. It constituted an entirely different system than the evolving science of medicine in the West (MacPherson 1987: 12–14).

This encouraged foreign medical doctors and sanitarians in Hong Kong and China to put in place their own systems for the control and abolition of deadly diseases; the need for sanitary reform of their environment and the means to ensure its effectiveness; and the nurturing of personal and professional initiatives and institutions supportive of civic or public health. Self-governance in colonial administrations such as Hong Kong or in the municipal governments formed in the treaty ports such as the Shanghai settlements was integral to the creation and implementation of public health systems, and, as had been the experience in major Western cities, urban government was preponderantly the consequence of the drive for better health. In traditional China, urban and rural administration was indistinguishable and there was no 'municipal' government or central self-governing body in the cities required to register its needs, oversee its activities, or obliged to respond to the effects of rapid change communally and plan for the future (MacPherson 1987: vii–ix). By the 1890s and the first decade of the twentieth century, Chinese reformers and modernizers were vigorously discussing prospects for establishing their own municipal governments based on Western models and were quick to grasp the importance of the connection between self-governance and public health. Indeed it was in Guangzhou (Canton), the capital of Guangdong province that the first Chinese municipal government was founded in 1921 (Keith 1922: 101; Rogaski 2000: 30–46; Sun 1919: 1–17).

Public health in Hong Kong, 1842–1941

The assumption that underlay the British acquisition of Hong Kong in 1841–1842 was that it would serve as an entrepôt and naval and military station between the vast markets of India and China. The colony's subsequent growth as a free port and in matters affecting the health of the community was dependent on several factors: the interconnectedness of the population with the Pearl River delta, political and economic conditions in China which became increasingly unstable throughout the century and Sino-British relations. The Chinese population of approximately 7,450 in 1841 grew to 22,860 (excluding 957 Europeans and Indians) in 1847, and increased to 280,564 (excluding 20,096 non-Chinese) by the end of the nineteenth century. Over 70% of the population, Chinese or foreign, was predominately male and 55.9% were between the ages of 20 and 45 years, Chinese families remaining in the towns and villages of south China (*Hong Kong Government Gazette* 11 June 1898: 532).

High mortality from fevers (malaria) and dysentery amongst the military and civilian populations in the early years gave the colony a reputation for unhealthiness. In 1843, a committee of public health was created after 24% of the troops and 10% of the civilian population died of fever between May and October of that year. The first law relating to public health was passed in 1844 and amended as the Good Order and Cleanliness Ordinance No. 14 of 1845, superseded in 1856 by an ordinance modelled on the principles established by the London Board of Health, adapted to local conditions (Hooper 1908: 158). A colonial surgeon and a surveyor general (responsible for sanitary matters) were appointed in 1843 but the construction of a civilian hospital would have to wait until the 1850s when the revenue was deemed 'sufficient' by the Home government, although the governor secured a house for that purpose in 1848 because of the 'unhealthy state of the colony' (Endicott 1964: 69, 85). In the interim, a seaman's hospital was built by private subscription in 1843 (eventually taken over by the British Admiralty and reopened as the Royal Naval Hospital, eventually closing in 1941) and in 1844 a military hospital. The first charitable hospital for Chinese using Western medicine was supported by the London Medical Missionary Society of Guangzhou, opening in 1843 and closing in 1853, when they transferred their work back to China. In 1887, the Alice Memorial Hospital carried on its work by expanding to four hospitals that were merged into one in 1954 and which is still operational today.

Arguably the most important charitable and welfare institution was the Tung Wah Chinese hospital opened in 1872 for 'the care and treatment of indigent sick'. It was financed by local subscription organized by leading Chinese merchants and a government grant of land and funds (Lethbridge 1971: 147). The Tung Wah expanded its services in clinics and dispensaries as well as establishing a hospital in Kowloon (Kwong Wah, opened in 1911) and eastern Hong Kong Island (Tung Wah Eastern Hospital, opened in 1929). All three hospitals were amalgamated in 1931 as the Tung Wah Group of Hospitals (Hong Kong Museum of Medical Sciences Society 2006: 91–99). The Tung Wah, whose directors functioned as an unofficial channel of communication and advisory body to Chinese officials on the mainland, offered exclusively traditional Chinese medical treatment. Although Western medical doctors may have grasped the principles of TCM, they discounted its effectiveness and eschewed it in their practice. But non-interference with Chinese practices seemed prudent since the colony and south China benefited from the Tung Wah's travelling smallpox vaccinators. Governor Hennessy noted with some satisfaction that the 'amount of professional life amongst the Chinese' could be seen by the increase of traditional Chinese doctors from 198 in 1876 to 333 in 1881, and herbalists from 164 to 243 (Hennessy 1881: 3).

However, the two systems came into conflict over the control and treatment of bubonic plague introduced into the colony from Guangzhou – a city that was initially compared favourably with Hong Kong by medical missionaries in the 1880s (Kerr 1888: 134–138). Although neither medical system could 'cure' the disease until the pathogen was identified, its aetiology investigated and a vaccine had been produced, methods of control did affect its prevalence. Western medical understanding of contagions (from the 1870s to 1890s many of the causal agents of important contagious diseases had been identified) dictated a very different course of action than those practiced by TCM practitioners. In the aftermath of the 1896 epidemic, an official inquiry recommended that a Chinese doctor trained in Western medicine be appointed to the Tung Wah hospital and treatment, whether Chinese or Western, be provided on a voluntary basis (Whitehead 1896: 18).

Fortuitously, finding qualified candidates was possible as the Hong Kong College of Medicine for Chinese, founded in 1887 (Dr Patrick Manson, the 'father of tropical medicine', was the first dean), had graduated its first two students in 1892, including Sun Yat-sen who would become the 'father of the Chinese revolution'. In 1912, the college became the medical faculty of the newly opened University of Hong Kong and in the following year its medical degrees were fully recognized by the United Kingdom General Medical Council. Yet a dual system of medicine was countenanced; Chinese medicine and traditional practitioners however were basically unregulated (Western-trained medical practitioners were first registered in 1884) and the acceptance of Western (scientific) medical and sanitary practices faced keen competition, thereby complicating the ability of colonial administrators or medical practitioners to deal effectively with the rise of contagious and epidemic diseases due to the rapid influx of mainland Chinese and exacerbated by poverty and overcrowding.

Demographics and public health

The demographic character of Hong Kong's foreign and Chinese population, and its role as a major port of call for merchant shipping, foreign troops and navies, attracted large numbers of prostitutes from south China. This affected the incidence of venereal diseases; the British admiralty attributing 50% of all sickness of the force to enthetic diseases. In 1857, the colonial government passed Ordinance 12 of 1857 for checking the spread of venereal diseases. The scheme of control entailed the licensing of brothels and restricting them to certain portions of the town, as well as enforcing the medical inspection of prostitutes and their detention in Lock hospital until 'cured'. The brothels were taxed to support medical treatment. Keepers of licensed boarding houses for seamen were responsible for reporting sickness among the men and seamen could be fined or imprisoned for not complying with the regulations. In 1867, the Hong Kong government was instructed by London to replace this with the Contagious Diseases Ordinance modelled on the British law. Whether the ordinance had any significant effect on the spread of these diseases is difficult to ascertain from the reported statistics, although the Inspector General of Her Majesty's Naval Hospital declared that venereal diseases had 'all but disappeared from the colony' (*Medical Times and Gazette* 24 June 1871: 717). Opposition to the acts in England due to the compulsory powers of the state led to their repeal in 1886 and in Hong Kong three years later, although Hong Kong continued to license brothels and provide medical examinations for prostitutes. Brothels exclusively for Chinese continued to be exempt from medical inspection (MacPherson 1997: 85–112; Miners 1988: 191–199).

The male predominance in the population began slowly to diminish and an increase in 'family life' was noted in the early twentieth century, partly attributed to the sanitary reforms undertaken in the preceding decades, although epidemics of smallpox (1887–1888), cholera (1890) and plague (first notified in 1894) continued to take their toll along with fevers, malaria, dysentery, typhus and so on. Statistics, such as they were, also revealed the crude death rate among Chinese of 24.18 per 1,000 (underestimated) and 18.2 for non-Chinese which, the registrar general opined in 1891, compared favourably with the annual death rate in England and Wales of 26.2 per 1,000 (Registrar General 1892: 233). Yet the registrar general also knew that Chinese deaths went unrecorded and bodies were shipped back to China for burial (a service provide by the Tung Wah) and many of the seriously ill returned to their home villages to expire, evasions purportedly obviate Ordinance No. 7 of 1872, copied from British law and requiring the registration of births and deaths. The birth rate also exposed serious issues of under-reporting, particularly of female births which were usually one-third less than male births. The Chinese infant mortality rate (below five years of age) accounted for nearly half of the number of total deaths registered in the general population (Registrar General 1894: 148).

Provisions were made for the registration of persons in 1844, and for purposes of ensuring the health and safety of ships carrying Chinese in 1856, but immigration into the colony was basically unrestricted (Registrations of Persons No. 18 of 1844; Chinese Passengers Act of 1855). The annual movement across the border – arrivals and departures – ranged from 73,767 arrivals and 51,247 departures in 1884 to a high of 1,436,710 arrivals and 1,425,897 departures in 1924 (Medical and Sanitary Reports 1924: 38). Furthermore, the colony functioned as a transhipment point for Chinese emigration, not only to the Straits

Settlements but also many places throughout the world. Some attempt was made at medical inspection in 1867, specifically for 'securing the Health of Emigrants... clearing through Hong Kong' (Ordinance No. 6 of 1867). Diseases, endemic or epidemic, could be imported or exported as readily as opium or tea and had an impact on disease patterns in the region. Rapid migration into and out of the colony accompanied major disturbances on the mainland, a pattern that would continue throughout the colonial period, straining resources and creating serious conditions of overcrowding in the urban areas.

Sanitary reform

Official cognizance of the insanitary state of the colony in the 1870s and threats to the general health of the community from deaths due to 'filth poison' can be attributed to several vectors: the governor's enlightenment over the contamination of his water supply at his residence on the Peak due to the dumping of rubbish and night soil on the slopes overhanging the reservoir; the annual reports of the colonial surgeon condemning housing, drainage, water supplies and sanitation; and 'constant representations' by the officer in command of the troops to the secretary of state for the colonies as to the insalubrious condition of the town and the affects on the health of his men (Colonial Surgeon 1879: 1–45). The upshot was an invitation to Osbert Chadwick C.M.G., a former royal engineer and son of the great British sanitarian Sir Edwin Chadwick, to visit Hong Kong and report on the sanitary conditions of the city and to recommend a course of reform which was submitted to the government in 1882. Chadwick was also invited to Guangzhou, the provincial capital of Guangdong province, to advise on water supplies, no doubt reflecting the interest in these developments in the Shanghai International Settlements which opened the first modern waterworks in Asia in 1883 after a ten-year struggle to map out the medical topography and sanitary reforms requisite to the growth and prosperity of the port (MacPherson 1987: 83–122). The Chadwick report was a tour de force and laid bare deficiencies in drainage, water supply, sanitation, particularly defective housing construction and design, all of which were compounded by overcrowding in the urban areas. Extensive recommendations were made affecting all aspects of environmental hygiene, town planning and public works by creating a partially elected Sanitary Board in 1883 (replaced by the Urban Council in 1935) as well as the reorganization of the medical department (Chadwick 1882: 1–15).

Implementation of the proposed Public Health Ordinance was stalled due to controversy over the clauses requiring landlords (the majority of whom were Chinese) to provide open spaces in the rear of their properties thereby diminishing their rental income, clauses that were deleted before the passage of the ordinance in 1887. Dr Kai Ho Kai (later Sir Kai), a Hong Kong-born, British-trained medical doctor and barrister who served on the Legislative Council, the Sanitary Board as well as founding the Alice Memorial Hospital (named after his deceased wife), led the opposition unexpectedly on the basis that Chinese should not be treated like Europeans and forced to comply with sanitary measures or 'improvements' they did not want (Choa 1981: 71–90); surprisingly too, since sanitary reform in Shanghai and proposals for a pure water supply in Guangzhou were generally known (MacPherson 1987: 68–82; Sun 1957: 1020–1023). Although the ordinance based on Chadwick's report was the most important piece of public health legislation in the colony, in practice it would not come into full force until the arrival of bubonic plague in May 1894.

Bubonic plague and public health

Bubonic plague, an annual visitor, became resident in Hong Kong from 1894 to 1924 with high mortality rate – 93.7% of the 21,867 reported cases. Most authorities identify its importation (not origin as Yunnan province and northern Vietnam were historically reservoirs for the disease) from Guangzhou and the Pearl River delta communities where regular connections by steamer and junks to Hong Kong moved goods and people around the region rendering quarantine measures difficult to enforce. Plague was reported in Guangzhou several months prior to the Hong Kong outbreak with 60,000 deaths in March alone (Yersin 1894: 662–667). Further complicating the epidemiological picture was the fact that the Hong Kong government acquiesced, against medical advice, to aggressive demands from the Chinese community who distrusted Western medicine, hospitals and plague prevention measures to allow the removal of the infected, the dying and the dead to China, no doubt sustaining the epidemic (Atkinson 1896: 289–306).

The aetiology of bubonic plague was settled by Dr Alexandre Yersin and Dr Shibasaburo Kitasato who both discovered the bacillus in Hong Kong in June of 1894. They established that it was primarily a disease of rodents and vectored by infected fleas (Soloman 1997: 59–62). Amid conflicting views over its aetiology and prevention and control was the stark realization that the resolution of conflicts between divergent perspectives, that is, the acceptance of Western medical and sanitary practices by the local inhabitants, could not be achieved without stringent application of existing legislation as well as education supportive of public health. This was particularly important as 'malicious placards and rumours' concerning measures taken in Hong Kong to control plague had proliferated in Guangzhou abetted by anti-foreign elements (sharpened by Hong Kong's economic rivalry with the city) and Chinese officials, leading to an official protest by the British Minister in Beijing to the Zongli Yamen (office of foreign affairs) (Colonial Office (CO) 129/263, 1894: 187–193; 548–564).

Public health and the built environment

Plague prevention measures – the cleansing and disinfection of houses (about 7,000 people were removed from infected dwellings), burning of contaminated clothes and household articles, and the removal of infected persons to hospital, that had angered the population as an intrusion on their privacy, would be followed by even more uncompromising measures. The Tai Ping Shan district, a focus of the epidemic, was condemned, resumed and rebuilt (Hong Kong Museum of Medical Sciences Society 2006: 26–38; 153–156; Platt et al. 1998: 47–67). The controversial handling of the epidemic came to a head with an official inquiry into the deficiencies of the medical department in 1895, which recommended the reorganization of the department and the abolition of the title of the 'Colonial Surgeon as a misnomer' and its replacement with a 'Principal Medical Officer' a clear indication that the notion of 'public' had expanded beyond the so-called colonizer to the colonized. Dispensaries were established providing free or nominally priced medicines staffed by licentiates of the medical college who could serve as a grassroots disease surveillance system and could spread knowledge of Western medicine and medical practices (Medical Committee Report 1895: v–vi; 23–24; 41–46). Ten new ordinances were enacted from 1894–1901 to improve the sanitation of the colony and Osbert Chadwick was invited back with Dr W. J. Simpson in 1901–1902 to point the way forward. Simpson's memoranda on the plague incorporated the new medical understanding of the disease and the 'machinery for the early discovery of human and rat plague' recommending a cross-border 'weekly bulletin' functioning as an early warning system for pandemics (Simpson 1902: 421–435).

Chadwick's report of 10 April 1902 covered water supply, sewerage, scavenging and removal of excreta, house construction and overcrowding. He served as an expert witness to the official inquiry into the public works department, leading to its reorganization. A report was also commissioned on the housing of the population and the 'cubicle question', that is, overcrowding in two senses – the close proximity of housing (thereby preventing ventilation and scavenging and rat control); and the subdivision of floors into small 'cabins' (without windows) to squeeze as many people as possible into one building. The commission's view was that Chinese tenement houses in Hong Kong differed from European working-class housing or ordinary Chinese housing in Guangzhou because 'by some gradual process of evolution they have taken the worst features of both kinds of houses and none of the best' (Chadwick and Simpson 1902: 635). Another factor that contributed to overcrowding in the urban areas of Hong Kong Island and Kowloon was the hilly physical topography that precluded building without major engineering works. Land was increased by reclamations in the coastal areas in the 1880s, and was a major source of government revenue, a process that continues today. Although the leasing of the New Territories should have alleviated land-use pressure, development of the leased area awaited the major transport infrastructure needed to link it to the urban areas. Nonetheless, the groundwork was laid for the consolidation of all public health and buildings ordinances by the enactment of the Public Health and Buildings Ordinance No. 1 of 1903 – this constituted landmark legislation with greater powers linking public health to the built environment.

Incremental improvements to the environment were viewed cautiously as having a 'slow but effective influence' on the crude death rate which declined from 21.89 per 1,000 in 1895 to 18.29 per 1,000 in 1904 (including plague deaths). However the crude death rate between 1904 and 1914 stayed within the rage of 21.16 to 25.67 per 1,000. Infant mortality appeared alarmingly high with more than two-thirds of Chinese children born in the colony dying in infancy (Medical and Sanitary Reports 1914: 19). Figures for infant births and deaths remained problematical until after World War II because of the Chinese custom of not registering a birth unless the child survived for a month. Female births were often not registered at all. Furthermore it was thought that since infant deaths exceeded registered births, many children were brought into the colony from the mainland of China (Medical and Sanitary Reports 1915: 18).

Growing political unrest in China (particularly in the south) due to external threats and internal rebellion from 1895–1910, culminating in the revolution of 1911 that overthrew the Qing dynasty and established a republic in 1912, meant the 'conversion of Hong Kong into a refugee camp'. Some 40,000–50,000 people poured into the colony in 1911, with another 50,000–60,000 in 1913. There was a slight respite in 1914, when 60,000 people 'hastily' returned to the mainland because of fear that the colony would be bombarded due to the outbreak of the European war, but the population continued to increase by 37% from 1911 to 1921, making a total of 625,166. Yet fewer than 2000 houses were built to accommodate the additional 150,000 people (Medical and Sanitary Reports 1914: 9; Miners 1988: 10). Conditions of overcrowding and poor nutrition influenced the incidence of tuberculosis, responsible for 12% of all deaths recorded in 1912 (rising to 30% in 1928); respiratory diseases, beriberi (a disease originally thought to be infectious but later proved to be a vitamin deficiency disease prevalent in those whose staple diet is polished rice), malaria, dysentery, typhoid and continuing epidemics of smallpox (despite the compulsory vaccination of infants since 1888, a law amended in 1923 to extend vaccination coverage to all who entered the colony). In late 1917, a high incidence of influenza – as yet not a notifiable disease – was observed, but it coincided with an outbreak of cerebrospinal meningitis (over 1,235 cases) that had been ravaging the China ports. This prompted the government to seek advice from experts working in the Rockefeller Institute for Medical Research in New York for the production of serum at the government's Bacteriological Institute, established in 1906 (Medical and Sanitary Reports 1918: 4).

The interwar years

Public health measures and infrastructure continued to expand exponentially and in consonance with scientific developments in medicine. Provision of health services was abetted by international organizations like the League of Nations (particularly in epidemiology, child labour and industrial health and safety), the Rockefeller Foundation (which funded three chairs in the faculty of medicine at the university in 1922), the Red Cross Society, the St John Ambulance Brigade (founded in 1916) and a host of other non-governmental health supportive organizations like the Y.M.C.A. and Y.W.C.A (Medical Report 1922: 18). Empire-wide associations like the British National Council for Combatting Venereal Diseases visited in 1921, promoting social hygiene education and writing an excoriating report on the health conditions in the colony, particularly the need for greater health protection and care for women and children

(MacPherson 2001: 173–190). The Eugenics League organized in 1934, with ties to the British National Birth Control Association, provided birth control linked to infant and maternal welfare, changing its name to the Family Planning Association in 1939. The Association also sent birth control devices to China after supplies were cut off during the early years of the Japanese occupation. The League's work was considered vital since the infant mortality rate was 345 per 1,000 living births, the 'cumulative effect of malnutrition, bad housing and overcrowding and insanitary environment' (Director of Medical Services 1939: 18).

Important environmental and social investigations into sanitation, water supplies, nutrition, labour and housing conditions were commissioned, the latter an intractable problem with densities reckoned to be on average 1,000 people per acre in the built-up areas (Housing Commission 1938: 279). Tenements designed for housing (usually three to four storeys) were converted into factories thus worsening the acute housing shortage and contributing to environmental degradation. A Town Planning Committee was formed in 1939, after which all government buildings needed the approval of the deputy director of health services before construction – an authorization recommended to be extended to the private sector. Other reports concentrated on specific diseases like venereal diseases, malaria and the need to reorganize the medical and sanitary branches of government and the hospital and clinical facilities (Director of Medical Services 1939: 26; Selwyn-Clarke 1939: 1–92).

Hospitals, specialized clinics and dispensaries – public, subvented and private – numbered over 47, plus 74 maternity homes with new or extended facilities planned in all parts of the territory (Selwyn-Clarke 1939: 10–18). Public health expenditure in 1939 consumed 14.59% of the general revenue, but was still inadequate to cope with the problems aggravated by the rapid influx of population from mainland China as a result of the Sino-Japanese hostilities in 1932, the invasion of China in 1937 and the capture of Guangzhou and Guangdong province in 1938. The population doubled between 1937 and June of 1939 and was estimated at 2 million people (revised to 1.7 million), all of whom needed to be cared for. Although a small percentage of the refugees was financially secure or had transferred their commercial or manufacturing interests to the colony for safety, the majority were unskilled rural or urban workers, often destitute and malnourished. The government set up three semi-permanent urban camps and five rural refugee camps near the border and encouraged many to return to unoccupied China. However, mat-shed hovels or squatter areas materialized without any sanitary arrangements and presented a major health danger, somewhat alleviated when the government set aside sites providing water, drainage and sanitation for temporary mat-shed camps.

Epidemic diseases – smallpox, cholera, cerebrospinal meningitis and, most importantly, tuberculosis (the highest cause of death) – became rife. More than 1 million people received smallpox vaccinations in 1939 alone and 320,748 anti-cholera inoculations were carried out. Propaganda posters were distributed for the first time, drawn by local artists because of the high rate of illiteracy among the refugees. Anti-tuberculosis campaigns used the press and radio to educate the public on preventative measures. An increase in lepers was noted among the refugee population as many came to Hong Kong from Guangdong and other southern provinces, some walking over 20 days to reach the colony. The Tung Wah Smallpox Hospital was purchased and turned into a settlement, but the government continued its policy of sending lepers back to China and maintaining them at government expense in hospitals on the mainland. Because of limited facilities in the colony, a similar policy was in force for psychiatric patients: Chinese nationals were sent to Guangzhou (where the first mental hospital was started by the medical missionary, John C. Kerr, in 1898) and Europeans back to their home countries (Director of Medical Services 1939: 54). Inspection of food supplies and disinfection of markets increased since inadequate sewage and refuse disposal, particularly night soil, was linked to the increase of helminthic diseases. Port health services and quarantine measures were stepped up but hundreds of miles of coastline and land connections made effective monitoring of the border impossible. With the outbreak of the European war on 3 September 1939, a scheme for the 'medical defence of the Colony' was updated and preparations made in case of war with Japan (Director of Medical Services 1939: 17).

Hong Kong was attacked by Japan on 8 December 1941, and occupied for three years and eight months. The Japanese forced over 1 million people back to China, reducing the population to around 600,000 people, interned national enemies and appropriated civil and private hospitals for their own use (with the exception of the Chinese hospitals). The population that remained 'was systematically starved' and suffered from malnutrition, beriberi, pellagra and an upsurge of contagious and communicable diseases – malaria, tuberculosis and venereal diseases – since medicines were scarce, and sewerage and purification of water supplies neglected. The Director of Medical Services, Dr P. S. Selwyn-Clarke, was allowed to keep a small staff to attend to the medical and health needs of the community until his arrest and imprisonment in 1943, and his brief report on the health conditions of the colony published in 1946 was a dismal record of Japanese ruthlessness (Selwyn-Clarke 1946: 18). The Chinese members of the health department who had stayed at their posts instead of fleeing to unoccupied China were credited with the swift recovery of medical services within weeks of Japan's surrender in 1945 (Selwyn-Clarke 1975: 101–103). General rehabilitation of the colony and its health services from 1945–1949, intelligently planned and vigorously implemented, faced once again the mass influx of 1,760,000 people from the mainland, some returning but many fleeing the outbreak of civil war between the Nationalists (Guomindang) and the Communists, prior to the Communist victory in October 1949 and the establishment of the People's Republic of China (PRC). On 14 October, the through trains to Guangzhou ceased and border control on both sides was enforced.

Hong Kong's epidemiological transition, 1949–1997

Ironically, the closed-door policies of the PRC from 1949 to 1978 helped to accelerate Hong Kong's economic development from entrepôt trade in the pre-war period to industrialization, manufacturing and its restructuring as a high-end financial and services economy. After the war, plans for decolonization were considered but indefinitely suspended because of the civil war in China and the establishment of a communist state across the border, although Great Britain did recognize the new regime. Steps were taken to register the entire resident population and to require each individual to carry an identity card. After 1949, the labour, entrepreneurial skills and capital from Shanghai and Guangzhou that accompanied the massive influx of people fleeing the anti-capitalist policies of the new regime, helped to create a sizable local market and to supply goods, especially textiles and clothing, for an international market. The Korean conflict and the UN embargo restricted imports to China (Hong Kong's traditional entrepôt role), and cheap labour, low-taxes and the laissez-faire policies of the government helped attract an inflow of capital and investments from foreign sources. Hong Kong's trade would exceed Shanghai's by 1958. The Hong Kong government's policy until the 1970s of continuing to accept refugees from China rather than force repatriation or third-country resettlement – all three possible solutions recommended by a special commission of the United Nations – and the natural population increase determined its public health priorities if the territory was to prosper.

Demographic transition 1949–1967

The population more than doubled from 1,857,000 in 1949–1950 to 3,692,200 in 1966–1967, while the crude death rate dropped from 8.8 per 1,000 in 1949 to 5.1 per 1,000 in 1966–1967, with 85% of the population continuing to be concentrated in the urban areas of Hong Kong Island and Kowloon. Although in 1967, 40% of the population was under the age of 15 years and only 6% over 60 years, for the first time in Hong Kong's history, the leading cause of death was not infectious, respiratory or intestinal diseases but cancer, heart diseases and cerebrovascular lesions: the diseases of aging – a disease pattern that would continue as longevity increased and fertility declined in the coming decades (Director of Medical and Health Services 1950: 6–7; 1967–1968: 2–4).

This 'demographic transition' owed much to the expansion of maternal and child health-care services, 'the single most impressive feature of Hong Kong's epidemiological change' (Phillips 1988: 37). Infant mortality declined from 99.4 per 1,000 live births in 1949 to 37.7 in 1961; neonatal mortality declined from 29.4 per 1,000 live births to 21.0; and maternal mortality declined from 2.12 per 1,000 live births to 0.45 (Director of Medical and Health Services 1950: 10–13; 1961–1962: 14–15). Partly, this decline was attributable to the expansion of maternal and infant health services as well as the 'remarkable appreciation' of these services by the population – 97.8 % of all births were attended by a medical doctor or qualified midwife (Director of Medical and Health Services 1950: 36). Reduced infant and neonatal mortality are good indicators of the general health and longevity of the population, and the elimination of vaccine-preventable diseases in children was of the highest priority, as was controlling tuberculosis, 'the major health problem of Hong Kong', if that end was to be achieved (Director of Medical and Health Services 1966–1967: 10).

Tuberculosis

In 1948, the non-governmental Anti-tuberculosis Association was formed. It was spearheaded by Jehangir Hormusjee Ruttonjee, who also donated funds to build the Ruttonjee Sanatorium (and later the Grantham Hospital) which opened in 1949 and which was staffed by the St Columban sisters, an Irish order that had served in China and which was dedicated to the treatment of tuberculosis (Humphries 1996: 23–43). The government began BCG vaccinations for infants in 1952, with blanket coverage helped by the increase in birth registrations – 'approaching the 100% mark' – among the population partly because of the fear of being forced back to China (Director of Medical Service 1950: 6). Deaths from tuberculosis below the age of five years declined from 34.3% of the total deaths from tuberculosis in 1952 to 5.74% in 1962, and infant mortality from tuberculosis would disappear by 1976. However, new acute infections continued to rise because of medical 'tourists' from China seeking low- or zero-cost treatment in government hospitals and clinics and the influx of 140,000 refugees in 1962 (fleeing the famine caused by Mao's Great Leap Forward campaign).

In that cohort, 68,000 were diagnosed with acute tuberculosis and 81% were drug resistant (Director of Medical and Health Services 1961–1962: 2, 27). Hong Kong had one of the most unenviable records of having 'the highest level of drug resistance in the world' with '40% resistance to one or more of the first-line drugs' (Director of Medical and Health Services 1967: 14). However, the death rate from tuberculosis continued to decline from 158.8 per 100,000 population in 1952 to 55.5% in 1962, although it still accounted for 74.8% of all deaths from communicable diseases (Director of Medical and Health Services 1962–1963: 27).

The intractable problem of tuberculosis was tackled by international cooperation in curative and health outreach services. In 1957, Hong Kong (as well as China) participated in the founding of the Eastern Tuberculosis Committee in New Delhi as part of the International Union against Tuberculosis headquartered in Paris (*Science* 15 February 1957: 276). F. R. G. Heaf (advisor to the colonial office) and Dr Wallace Fox from the British Medical Research Council (BMRC) visited Hong Kong in 1962 to provide long-term planning and research capacity for controlling the disease. In 1967, a twenty-year collaborative research agreement was signed with the BMRC. The World Health Organization (WHO) assisted these efforts with advice systematizing the reporting and recording of the disease (Hong Kong Museum of Medical Sciences Society 2006: 240). Control and care needed adaptation to local conditions and cultural factors. Education was imperative to overcome the stigma of the disease since the Chinese considered it hereditary and a 'family disgrace'. 'Weak lungs' were thought to be the causative factor, thereby delaying modern medical treatment (as opposed to using TCM) until haemoptysis occurred. Indiscriminate spitting (an increase usually noted after an influx of mainland refugees necessitating 'anti-spitting patrols') and overcrowded dwellings spread the disease (Wu 1948: 37). In April–June of 1957, the outbreak of influenza type A/Asian/57 (originating in China) affected 300,000 people (about 10% of the population) and no doubt complicated the problem by increasing coughing and driving people indoors (Director of Medical and Health Services 1957–1958: 15).

Economic development and welfare assistance helped to improve nutritional standards but overcrowding and substandard housing needed to be addressed. The government's planned resettlement of squatter areas (rehousing 439,000 people by 1961), followed by the dispersal of the population in 'New Towns' developments in Kowloon and the New Territories in the 1970s under the Housing Authority, began to make inroads into this long-standing problem (Director of Medical and Health Services 1961–1962: 1; Miners 1998: 70). Density of population would not decline so the solution was to create high-rise residential structures for low-income families. Two factors helped to accelerate the process: the riots of 1966–1967 influenced by the radical politics of China's ongoing cultural revolution was a warning that livelihood issues and living conditions in Hong Kong must be rapidly improved; and the 'touch base' policy, that is, accepting refugees from China if they made it across the border, needed to be revised to repatriate them back to the mainland. Complicating the problem was a move by the PRC to issue exit visas to the disaffected allowing them to leave. These 'legal' emigrants numbered over 55,500 in 1973, with 32,000 legal and 28,000 illegal emigrants crossing the border in 1974. Secret talks were held between British and Chinese representatives to stop the flow (*Far Eastern Economic Review* 11 June 1976). The Deputy Director of Medical and Health Services warned that health resources were strained to the limit and outbreaks of infectious diseases, many of them eliminated or controlled in Hong Kong, might reappear or escalate (*The Standard* 14 January 1979).

Vaccine-preventable diseases

Smallpox, that deadly scourge of the past, was finally brought under control with the last cases reported in 1952 (Director Medical and Health Services 1971–1972: 18). An annual diphtheria vaccination campaign began in 1959, with the last reported cases in 1982. Poliomyelitis campaigns began in 1963 around the lunar New Year (January to March) in order to reach the floating population who ceased fishing during that period. The last reported case was in 1985. Measles vaccination campaigns began in 1967, a disease with high mortality due to complications of bronchopneumonia and resistance by the local population to vaccinating their children because of traditional medical beliefs that contracting it was 'necessary for future health' (Topley 1977: 263). Vaccination campaigns were brought 'close to home' to overcome local prejudices and to reach children in squatter areas and fishing boats, though biennial outbreaks continued. Children who received the P.T.A.P. vaccinations were given a figurine symbolizing 'Health' as an incentive, which flopped, and was replaced with sweets to great success (Director of Medical and Health Services 1960–1961: 19).

Overcoming local reluctance to accept the benefits of vaccinations was boosted by the outbreak of cholera El Tor in 1961, spreading from Guangdong province (although this was denied by the PRC). The government successfully inoculated over 1.8 million people (75% of the population) with the help of vaccine donated by foreign countries (Director of Medical and Health Services 1961–1962: 75–110). Disposable syringes were first used in 1966 in mass immunization drives and may have had an impact on reductions in viral hepatitis infections (notification was not compulsory at this time) that began to decline from 386 cases in 1966 to 191 in 1968. Hepatitis B was of acute interest due to the progression to liver cancer (the second highest cancer reported in Hong Kong). However, the true extent of viral hepatitis infections (types A, B, C, D and E) in the community (and in China, where types A, B and E were understood to be endemic) would be revealed by the 1970s and would constitute the third most common notifiable disease after tuberculosis and food poisoning, and the incidence would match that of Guangdong province by the 1990s (Chau et al. 1997: 261–265; Huang et al. 2002: 832–836; Lai 1997: 79). Beginning in 1975, donor blood supplies were screened for hepatitis B virus (HBV) and in 1988 the HBV vaccination programme was introduced for all newborn infants.

Blood donations were another area where education had to overcome traditional prejudice. The Hong Kong branch of the British Red Cross Society began to solicit blood from volunteers beginning in 1952 but only 5% of the blood collected came from Chinese donors because of 'Confucian concepts of filial piety' that precluded any harm to one's body that was bestowed by one's parents. By 1962, the proportion was 10%; by 1982, 90% of the blood was donated by Chinese under the age of 30, showing a change in societal attitudes. Securing a safe and adequate blood supply was imperative since there were reports surfacing in the 1960s of private blood sales (Hong Kong Museum Medical Sciences Society 2006: 273–274).

Health policy development

The basic remit and underlying philosophy that would guide the development of the medical and health services was 'to provide, directly or indirectly, low-cost or free medical and personal health services to that large section of the community which is unable to seek medical attention from other sources' (Director of Medical and Health Services 1963–1964: 2). The government's white paper, *The Development of Medical Services in Hong Kong* (1964), was updated in 1974 to expand quantitatively and qualitatively the provision of public hospitals (90% of all hospital beds are in the public sector) and clinical services to meet the needs of the community (Medical Development Advisory Committee 1974). The Medical and Health Department would be reorganized as the Hospital Services Department and the Department of Health in 1989 to reflect these changes. In 1993 and again in 1999, consultative documents were published addressing changing disease patterns tied to social, economic and demographic trends. Preventive medicine was emphasized due to longer life expectancies and changing lifestyles; smoking was targeted in particular as it was linked to lung cancer, the highest cause of death, and escalating health-care costs. However, Hong Kong has favoured an 'incremental' and 'cost rationalistic' rather than 'cost reduction' approach in the health sector (Gould 1995: 105–115) – an artefact of its historical development.

Another aspect of government health policy in Hong Kong's historical development was the ambiguous status of TCM. In the 1950s, evidence was accumulating as to the extent of malpractice and quackery in the treatment of eye diseases by unqualified persons, including Chinese herbalists who were unregistered. The Hong Kong Opthalmological Society found that 80% of blindness in Hong Kong was preventable and came out forcefully to support the Medical Registration (Amendment) Ordinance (1958) to prohibit the treatment of eye diseases by unregistered practitioners. Chinese herbalist associations, the directors of the Chinese Chamber of Commerce, civic organizations and the Chinese press protested the proposed bill on the basis that: (1) Chinese medicine had a long history; (2) TCM doctors, although never required to register before, had their own professional associations with regulations and paid their business license fees; (3) the bill would restrict their freedom to treat eye diseases of patients 'who had confidence in them'; (4) 'herbalists should not be included in the classification of quacks'; and (5) that eye clinics and doctors were insufficient and the poor would be deprived of a source of treatment leading to more cases of blindness. The bill passed after the director of Medical Services assured the TCM associations that the ordinance would not affect 'genuine classical Chinese herbalists' but only those practicing 'under the cloak of Chinese herbalist methods' (Hong Kong Opthalmological Society 1958: 194–201). After the signing of the Joint Declaration in 1984, a working group was set up to review the status of TCM and to formulate policies to develop Chinese and Western medicine (TCM development is enshrined in the Chinese constitution) which was included in the Basic Law (1990). Although aspects of TCM were studied in the medical school of the University of Hong Kong from the 1970s and the medical school of the Chinese University of Hong Kong (established in 1981) from the 1980s, it was after the establishment of the Chinese Medical Council in 1997 that schools of Chinese medicine were established at both universities as well as the Hong Kong Baptist University leading to full-time degree courses. Legislation was gazetted in 2002 to register TCM practitioners in line with mainland policy (Ho 2002: 257–285).

China and public health convergence

If the emplacement of medical infrastructure, sanitation, creation of pure water supplies, preventive health measures, hospitals and public health institutions in Hong Kong and the treaty port enclaves or concessions acted as a catalyst in traditional Chinese society – by practical example – they also served as conduits for the transfer of medical theories and practice in the establishment of private (and missionary) and public medical schools. One measure of the success of these institutions was that, by the turn of the twentieth century, Chinese students were being trained not just in major medical schools in Japan, Europe and America, linking China to an international medical circuit extending throughout the world, but increasingly in China's major cities. These promising developments must be read against a background of politically disruptive times as well as the seriousness of continued major outbreaks of epidemic or pandemic diseases in China. Although the Qing government began to institute reforms in education, local self-government, the establishment of urban health departments and sanitary control organized under the police, a system borrowed from Japanese and German models, after the debacle of the anti-foreign Boxer rebellion in 1900, change came too late to save the traditional dynastic system. The establishment of the Republic in 1912 and the eventual unification of China under the Guomindang (the Nationalist party) from 1927 to 1937 saw medical practice (both traditional and modern), education and hygiene, urban and rural hospitals and clinics, epidemic disease control and the gathering of vital statistics reorganized under the newly founded National Ministry of Health.

Pneumonic plague and public health in China

The dramatic shift in the trajectory of modern public health in China can best be illustrated by the response to the outbreak of pneumonic plague in Manchuria in 1910–1911, with 60,000 deaths, compared to the bubonic plague epidemics at the turn of the century. The first large-scale epidemic prevention service in China, the Manchurian Plague Prevention Service, was created in 1912, and was the model for the National Quarantine Service organized in 1930 by Cambridge-educated Dr Wu Lien-teh, a medical modernizer who was internationally famous for his work on plague prevention (Flohr 1996: 361–380). The new government convened an international plague prevention conference, the recommendations of which were partly adopted, short of establishing a central health department and an effective national medical education system, though sanitary and public health efforts at the municipal level proceeded apace. In Guangzhou, the temporary revolutionary capital from 1917 to 1926, the Ministry of Health had to develop de novo the regulatory and health machinery that was non-existent under the Manchu (Qing) regime. The need for infectious diseases control was urgent particularly for a port city that was regularly devastated by bubonic plague and other contagious diseases. An infectious diseases hospital was established and port health inspections were enforced. Similar to colonial Hong Kong, registration of births and deaths was made mandatory, although this was difficult to implement though presumably resistance by the population was not due to 'anti-foreignism'. Interference with vested economic interests seemed to be the cause when undertakers went on strike because coffins could not be sold without evidence of a death certificate signed by a registered medical practitioner. For several days burials ceased and Guangzhou was described as 'a city of the dead'. Undertakers only reopened their shops after the government imported coffins and sold them at cost. New regulations enforced over the collection of night soil and its removal from the city were ignored by the monopoly that controlled the trade, leading to the arrests of some workers and resulting in a strike, thereby stopping this essential service in a city without proper sewerage. When the police arrested the leaders, the 'night men' resumed work. Health inspectors, besides their duties in port health, market inspections and anti-plague control measures such as disinfection of dwellings, rat collection and laboratory examination of the specimens and segregation of lepers, were posted at the city gates with instructions to cut the queues of male pedestrians entering the city for reasons of hygiene (lice infestations) and patriotic symbolism since the hairstyle had been forced on the population by the Manchu dynasty as a symbol of subjugation (Li 1958: 164).

Rockefeller Foundation and the China Medical Commission

International cooperation was welcomed. In 1914, the Rockefeller Foundation, a charitable corporation dedicated to promoting 'the well-being of mankind throughout the world', set up the China Medical Commission to study all aspects of medicine and health for a country believed to have the highest death rate in the world. The Commission, facilitated by both the United States and Chinese governments, visited 11 of the 18 provinces of China and inspected 88 hospitals (including Hong Kong), 59 Protestant missionary establishments, four run by Catholic missionary establishments, and 35 run by Chinese central or local governments including those supported by private individuals, foreign settlements and concessions or Chinese societies (China Medical Commission of the Rockefeller Foundation 1914: vi, 53–54). The Commission's report, which would guide the priorities for funding of activities, recommended the advancement of medical education and capacity-building at the local level in hospitals, particularly those attached to medical schools, but acknowledged that large-scale public health assistance was not feasible.

In the Commission's opinion, south China, an area 'most subject to epidemics of tropical diseases', would best be served by establishing a medical college in Guangzhou rather than relying on the University of Hong Kong's medical school for several reasons: the University of Hong Kong was too expensive, taught in English and required 'unessential' subjects like English literature for admission. Furthermore, its graduates seemed 'to go into British government employ or into private practice in one of the British colonies, and it is alleged that they become more or less alienated from their people' (China Medical Commission of the Rockefeller Foundation 1914: 52). The Commission recommended that Beijing, the traditional capital (this would change in 1927 when Nanjing became the capital), would be the best site for the location of 'a strong and influential medical school' (China Medical Commission 1914: 43–44). Thus, the Union Medical College, founded by six missionary societies, was transformed into the Peking Union Medical College (PUMC) and formally dedicated in 1921 as the key medical educational centre in China, modelled after the innovative curriculum of the Johns Hopkins University Medical School. Its public health curriculum and urban health-care system, designed by Dr John B. Grant and his Chinese colleagues and students, would be 'internationally emulated' (Bullock 1980: 6).

In effect the Commission – with the establishment of the China Medical Board – used its organizational, educational and fiscal resources to draw together the various foreign and Chinese non-governmental public health providers who had assumed responsibility for the management, control and notification of diseases in their hospitals and clinics. Communication was critical as there were 254 missionary hospitals of various denominations in China by 1937. Communication was also sustained through the Medical Missionary Association founded in 1886. Its journal, *The China Medical Missionary Journal*, changed its name to the *China Medical Journal* in 1907, no doubt reflecting changed perspectives and the increase in Chinese modern medical practitioners amongst their ranks. The Medical Missionary Association changed its name to the China Medical Association at a meeting in Hong Kong in 1925, held jointly with the British Medical Association. In China, plans for a National Medical Association with its own journal were drawn up by Dr Wu Lien-teh and established in 1914. The two merged in 1932 and became the China Medical Association, with a branch in Hong Kong.

The nationalist decade, 1927–1937

With the successful conclusion of the Northern Expedition and the unification of the country under the nationalist government, political, economic and social reconstruction of the nation was linked to the modernization of medicine, and public health was the vehicle for achieving national strength and wealth. The Ministry of Health was reorganized in 1931 and placed under the Ministry of the Interior. In 1936, it once again became an independent administration directly under the Executive Yuan of the central government. Its functions were divided into two agencies: the National Health Administration, responsible for regulatory and supervisory functions (such as regulations governing doctors, dentists and nurses), legislation and policy; and the Central Field Health Station, the technical and coordinative arm of what now constituted the National Health Service.

After technical advice from the League of Nations, a three-year plan was implemented and the Central Field Station functioned as a 'centre of disease control' with branch laboratories and stations (35 stations in 8 provinces by 1934) to train postgraduates and public health officials, collect epidemiological data, vital statistics, epidemic control, sanitation, school hygiene, industrial health and safety and child and maternal welfare. A Central Hospital was established in Nanjing for research and teaching, while a Central Hygienic Laboratory in Shanghai was to manufacture 40 kinds of sera, vaccine and antitoxin drugs for use against communicable diseases. A Central Medical School to train public health professionals was opened in Jiangxi province in 1937, but the Japanese invasion in the coastal cities and provinces necessitated its relocation, along with other medical schools and institutions, with their personnel to the interior. (Yip 1995: 50–58; 109).

In 1929, the government passed restrictive regulations to control traditional medicine practitioners who had appropriated some aspects of modern medical practice, the use of some medical instruments and equipment as well as the growing trend to package herbal medicines to mimic modern pharmaceuticals. This was not the first effort by the government to abolish traditional medical practice, whose adherents in various cults and sects had organized themselves into societies and established schools (36 of them by 1915) supported by drug guilds and private benefactors. It was also in response to competition from the modern medical sector which was no longer an exclusively foreign import and which could be resisted on cultural or nationalistic grounds. It was both a 'scientific' and 'Chinese' profession (Bretelle-Establet 2002: 190–193 Crozier 1968: 70–104). Another dimension of the issue was economic, since livelihoods were threatened, as well as a substantial and profitable trade in herbal medicines. In 1914, the minister of education refused to register a traditional medical society stating that 'I have decided to prohibit the native practice and do away with crude herbs' (Wong and Wu 1936: 159). A Medical Salvation Society was organized to protest but the authorities made clear that the advancement of public health and preventive medicine required conformity to international scientific standards in medical education and practice. One exception was the Guangdong Medical College, a provincial government supported school that provided a mix of modern (scientific) and traditional medical education following the example of Hong Kong's Tung Wah hospitals.

In response to the restrictive legislation of 1929, the Shanghai Native Medical Society 'raised a hue and cry' by telegraph and in newspapers calling for a mass rally in the city, and over 2,000 practitioners closed their clinics in protest. The rally was fittingly held in the General Chamber of Commerce and attended by 131 organizations from 13 provinces. They organized the Institute of National Medicine, and lobbied the government successfully to pass regulations for Chinese medicine (which meant the institute could qualify practitioners and the government would license them) in 1935. They also demanded a vice-directorship in the National Health Administration, which was not granted. Ultimately the majority of traditional medical doctors would remain outside of the regulatory scheme and the public health sector during the Republican period (Wong and Wu 1936: 160–168; Yip 1958: 60–62).

Public health therefore became synonymous with the state (King 1943: 690–691). It was understood that to reduce an excessive mortality rate of 4 million people a year from infectious and parasitic diseases, and to increase the health infrastructure to treat on a daily basis 60 million people at no or little cost, state or socialized medicine would be necessary (Lim and Chen 1937: 781–796). State capacity however was limited by a lack of resources, foreign-controlled areas and interests protected by treaty rights, internal threats to its authority, by regional warlords, the newly founded Communist Party in 1921, and externally by the rising power of Japan, all of which shaped its fiscal priorities. Public health expenditures trailed that of the military, economic and infrastructural spending and accounted for only 0.7% of the total budget in 1936, amounting to 'roughly 2.4 cents per Chinese citizen' (Yip 1995: 63). Although firmly anti-imperialist, the Nationalist government countenanced foreign assistance when deemed appropriate, or cooperated when deemed prudent, while assiduously working to overturn the 'unequal treaties'. In Shanghai, a city divided into three jurisdictions – the International Settlements with its independent Municipal Council created in 1854; the French Concession with its Conseil Municipal; and the Chinese-administered area, which became the Municipality of Greater Shanghai in 1927 – public health authorities cooperated across jurisdictions regarding disease surveillance and other preventive measures affecting the entire city of over 3.5 million people. Technical assistance was welcomed from the Health Section of the League of Nations (China was a member) and information on communicable diseases was shared with its Far Eastern Bureau in Singapore (Shanghai Municipal Council 1934: 4–5, 17).

Urban vs. rural health

Urban centres were the focus of initial public health measures but in a country of over 450 million people, curative and preventive measures needed to move out to the rural areas where 80% of the population lived. Adopting new concepts on community health service that were gaining currency in the West, as well as building on the success of the Peking First Health Station founded in 1925 by PUMC's Dr John B. Grant, Dr J. Hung Liu, who headed the National Ministry of Health (renamed the National Health Administration in 1931) from 1929–1938, helped design and implement rural health stations supported by a mix of private and public initiatives that would serve as disease surveillance points, demonstrate modern public health measures and train medical students as well as paramedical personnel – the forerunners of the post-1949 'barefoot doctors' (Yip 1995: 71–99).

If there was any doubt as to the need for such services, the rural health stations began to reveal the appalling health conditions in the countryside. Although nationwide standardized statistics would not become a reality during the Nationalist decade, statistics were available at the local level from municipal health departments and public and private hospitals. In the Gaoqiao district health station near Shanghai, research showed that infant mortality up to the first year of age was 199.4 per 1000 live births, mostly due to tetanus neonatorum probably caused by unhygienic practices of traditional midwives who for superstitious reasons often contaminated knives by plunging them into the earth before severing the umbilical cord. In the same district this rate was cut to 40.3 per 1,000 live births using modern trained midwives (Chang *et al*. 1936: 581–582; Shu 1963: 4). Maternal and child health-care services developed jointly under the Central Field Health Station and local urban and rural health bureaus and stations began to attract greater attendance at maternity clinics and hospitals in the larger cities. In 1936, 25% of all deliveries were attended to by the service in Nanjing (Liu 1936: 1420). Birth control was supported by the National Health Administration in 1934 in maternity health centres but appealed only to the better-off and well-educated classes (Bullock 1980: 178–180).

Helminthic and parasitic diseases were rampant because of the universal use of night soil as fertilizer which prompted important scientific surveys in the Yangzi river delta and in north China by Ernest Carroll Faust and his colleagues at PUMC showing an 80% infective incidence of all cases and many harbouring more than one parasite (Faust 1924: 411–437). Schistosomiasis, or 'snail fever' was endemic in Yunnan, Jiangsu, Zhejiang, Anhui, Jiangxi, Hubei and Guangdong provinces, affecting approximately 10 million people. Kala-azar (*leishmania donovani*), a deadly parasitic disease vectored by the sand fly, was found to be endemic in specific areas of China with high infectivity. Surveys revealed that over 200,000 people were infected in one endemic area in northern Jiangsu (Liu 1936: 1409).

Plague, malaria and smallpox epidemics as well as the incidence of typhoid, diphtheria, dysentery and other gastro-intestinal infections continued although preventative measures made inroads into their prevalence and important research was undertaken to understand the best means of control. Cholera epidemics with 46 invasions of varying intensity from 1820 to 1932 spread through most of China and transmissions increased as the lines of communication improved. In 1932, 100,000 cases were reported with 34,000 deaths. Refugees in the years 1932 and 1937 spread the epidemic to Hong Kong, most likely by asymptomatic vibrio carriers, although this was not well understood at the time (Director of Medical and Health Services 1961–1962: 17–18). Improved sanitation, the provision of potable water, food safety and the advent of anti-cholera inoculations and intravenous saline treatment helped to control and reduce morbidity of the disease (MacPherson 1998: 487–519). Although these contagions were theoretically controllable by environmental hygiene, or vaccinations, popularizing individual sanitary knowledge and personal hygiene was essential in preventive work and encouraged eclecticism. In Shanghai as early as 1908, 'fuglemen' with bells to attract an audience were hired to recite the cholera prevention notices in the local dialect and continued to be used successfully for other sanitary and vaccination campaigns. 'Fly Brigades' were organized to control the insects and used colourful and graphically illustrated flyers and posters as well as lantern slide shows, the latter particularly effective in anti-venereal diseases campaigns in following decades (Shanghai Municipal Council 1934: 70–73; Stanley 1908: 331–333).

Leprosy, a lesser priority of government, was estimated to affect 1 million people, or 2.5 per 1,000 population with available care for only one-third of their numbers. Some care was provided by missionary hospitals or those established by private benefactors like the Tai Lam Leper Hospital near Guangzhou in 1928 (Leung 1928: 40–43). The Government in 1935 opened a National Leprosarium in Shanghai for the training of physicians and nurses, and with the potential to house up to 500 patients. Scarce funding dictated that the majority of cases would have to be handled as outpatients in clinics, depending on early detection for successful treatment (Liu 1936: 1409).

The greatest cause of death in China, as it was in Hong Kong in the twentieth century, was tuberculosis. This was particularly difficult to eradicate in growing, crowded cities where there was a change of working environments due to manufacturing and industrialization. According to Dr Wu Lien-teh, tuberculosis killed a reported 1.2 million people each year during the 1930s, and more than 10 million people were thought to have an active form of the disease. Eighty per cent of the urban population, 15 years or older, were infected, with the highest numbers in the cities gradually diminishing in the countryside (Zhang and Elvin 1998: 523–533). Unless poverty and malnutrition were addressed and housing conditions improved, there was little that public health officials could do to contain the disease until the advent of chemotherapy and BCG vaccinations in the 1950s.

Wartime public health

The war with Japan created unprecedented challenges, particularly in epidemic control, for the National Health Administration for coping with military medical emergencies and the condition of the civilian refugee population fleeing the Japanese-controlled areas. There was evidence that grain and rags contaminated with plague bacilli and fleas were scattered from Japanese planes causing outbreaks of bubonic plague in Zhejiang and Hunan provinces (Barenblatt 2004: 21–36; King 1943: 705–706). The National Red Cross Society of China and other civil relief agencies worked with the Administration and the Military Medical Administration to coordinate emergency hospitals, train staff and provide services for the wounded. Epidemic control was organized with the help of the League of Nations which trained paramedics, nurses and students to serve in travelling antiepidemic corps. The National Epidemic Prevention Bureau and its laboratories were relocated to the interior and began emergency preparation of sera and vaccines, supplemented by 10 million doses of cholera vaccine provided by the League and other foreign health services, and a National Anti-epidemic Corps was formed in 1938 (King 1945: 831–832; Yen 1938: 46). The United States Public Health Service was commissioned to send medical and sanitary officers and entomologists to supervise malaria control and the health of 250,000 labourers employed in constructing a railroad in Yunnan linking free China to the Burma Road (*Science* 1941: 228–229). The war and the presence of numerous epidemics finally impressed diffident provincial and municipal governments to fund and expand public health work. Medical schools that had relocated to the interior readjusted their curriculum to meet wartime requirements. After 1941 and the capture of Hong Kong, some of the University of Hong Kong's medical students continued their training in China and had their degrees recognized by the University after the war (Yen 1938: 45–48).

Even with substantial economic and medical relief from the international community through the United Nations Relief and Rehabilitation Administration (J. Heng Liu was a medical coordinator), the American Bureau for Medical Aid to China, and substantial plans for the medical reconstruction of the country, after eight long years of war, corruption, inflation and the resumption of civil war with the Communists, the Nationalist government was defeated and withdrew to Taiwan. The defeat brought an ignominious end to the era of medical 'progressivism' and the international cooperative spirit in public health on the mainland (Bullock 1980: 203–204). Many medical professionals fled to Taiwan or to Hong Kong where the government waived Hong Kong's medical qualification regulation because of the need for doctors to cope with the mass influx of refugees (Hong Kong Director of Medical and Health Services 1949–1950: 2). Most medical personnel however stayed on the mainland to carry on the hard-won legacy (unacknowledged by the communist regime) and use that experience to build the 'new China'.

The PRC and the politics of public health, 1949–1978

After the establishment of the PRC in 1949, medicine and public health were subsumed under a soviet-style, state socialist planning system. Mao Zedong declared that the Chinese people had 'stood up', rejecting capitalism and adhering to a policy of 'self-reliance' in the face of a hostile international environment during the 'War to Resist U.S. Aggression and Aid Korea' (1950–1953). The majority of United Nations members refused to recognize the PRC as the legitimate government of China, and the Security Council seat was held until 1971 by the Nationalist government of the Republic of China in exile on Taiwan. In Mao's view, 'elite' medicine and health institutions like the PUMC that developed under the previous regime benefited the cities at the expense of the countryside and medical practitioners trained under 'imperialist' influence needed to be 're-educated' to the proper socialist goals of society. Foreign-directed or -funded medical schools and missionary hospitals and institutions, now equated with 'imperialist aggression', were nationalized and foreigners expelled. Curriculums were shortened and revised according to Russian scientific thought like Lysenkoism (characterized as 'Marxian theory as applied to genetics'), which had disastrous consequences for the development of biomedicine and genetic research (Schneider 2003: 117). Compulsory courses on Marxism-Leninism were introduced as well as political indoctrination and mass meetings. Hospitals were reorganized on the soviet model of specialized institutions. The mass production of medical personnel was the educational target: 40,000 graduates of first-level medical and pharmacological schools and 153,000 graduates of the second-level public health schools with two or three years training by the end of the first decade (Chen 1961: 155). But the struggle between 'red' and 'expert' – meaning the ascendancy of ideological 'correctness' over technical expertise – particularly in the Anti-Rightist campaign of 1957 when quotas of individuals accused as 'Rightists' had to be filled, some medical personnel were executed for suspected espionage, imprisoned or sent for 'rehabilitation', but others were protected because of the need for modern medical doctors, especially for 'ensuring the health (*baojian*)' of the communist leadership (Minden 1994: 134).

Public health was subordinated to politics and the Communist Party (CCP). Ideological struggles over the ensuing years meant that health policy and administration shifted from bureaucratic to centrally coordinated systems, all of which demoted the role of medically trained personal in the decision-making process. Thus command and control techniques were used to achieve public health objectives and social change, such as the elimination of prostitution and drug addiction. Mass 'patriotic' political and health campaigns launched by the CCP to 'eradicate' specific diseases such as venereal diseases (the entire population of Shanghai was tested in 1954), plague, cholera, smallpox or parasitic infections such as schistosomiasis (in anti-snail campaigns), *kala-azar*, or the 'four pests' (rats, flies, mosquitoes and grain-eating sparrows) and the training and deployment of paramedical personnel – the 'barefoot doctors' – to deliver basic health care in the countryside, were heralded as the great successes of the socialist system (Horn 1969: 86). Of the reported 10 million cases of schistosomiasis, 4 million were reportedly cured. Over 10.5 million people were given BCG vaccinations and tuberculosis rates, at least in Beijing, fell from 230 per 100,000 in 1949 to 46 per 100,000 in 1958. Although there are no reliable national statistics before the 1953 census, a spectacular decline in mortality was reported with a crude death rate of 17 per 1,000 reduced to 11 per 1,000 in 1957, coupled with a sharp population increase (Salaff 1973: 552–563).

The Great Leap Forward

Under the Great Leap Forward campaign of 1958–1959, a programme of forced industrialization (to surpass the West) and collectivization of the countryside into communes, a three-tiered hierarchical system of medical and health services was organized. The lowest level of primary care was provided in the townships and rural areas and increasingly sophisticated services provided at the higher administrative levels. The Sino-Soviet split ended Russian technical assistance and aid in 1959. Modern trained medical practitioners were directed to study TCM which was accepted by medical insurance schemes (covering workers, soldiers, government employees and students). Since population mobility was strictly controlled through the workplace (*danwei*) and household (*hukou*) registration systems in the urban areas or in the agricultural communes, individual medical expenses were heavily subsidized by state-owned enterprises and institutions reflecting economies of scale and facilitating epidemic and infectious diseases control. However the radical reorganization of the society and economy produced one of the largest recorded famines in world history with an estimated excess of 30 million deaths and a breakdown in public health measures. Retreat from the disastrous collectivist policies, and reinstating private agricultural plots as incentives, helped to restore the food supply after 1962 (Smil 1999: 1619). An estimated 140,000 refugees – 'the great exodus' – fled to Hong Kong (*Far Eastern Economic Review* 13 May 1972).

The Great Proletarian Cultural Revolution

The Great Proletarian Cultural Revolution (GPCR) launched by Mao Zedong in 1966 'officially' ended in 1969, but in fact lasted until his death in 1976. From hindsight it represented the 'ten lost years' in all sectors of the society and economy. Essentially it was a power struggle within the CCP. The campaign or 'revolution' was then extended to the general population to root out counter-revolutionaries, 'capitalist-roaders' and to put politics in command under a coalition of workers/peasants/soldiers and to radically remake society. Schools were closed and millions of students or 'Red Guards' circulated around the country fomenting revolution, resulting in an estimated 400,000 deaths. Medical education ceased in 1966, but medical schools reopened in 1970 to 'serve the people' (workers/ peasants/soldiers). The curriculum was ideologically oriented and stressed practical training instead of basic science and in the spirit of egalitarianism, entrance examinations and diplomas were eliminated (Reynolds and Tierney 2004: 2141). TCM and its practitioners, previously embraced as a national cultural symbol and as a cheaper alternative to scientific medicine, were attacked in the anti- 'four olds' (old ideas, culture, customs and habits) campaign as a vestige of the feudal past. Modern trained doctors suffered a similar fate if they had any foreign or Guomindang links or if their 'class background' was suspect (people were required to carry identification cards that listed their class background). Amidst open class warfare in the cities, public health departments and hospitals were taken over and directed by non-medical personnel, making it difficult to maintain services until the army restored order. Cholera El Tor emerged in 1961 and 'huge' epidemics of meningococcal meningitis, subgroup III in the 1960s and subgroup V in the 1970s occurred (Achtman 1994: 16).

During the GPCR, state statistics and epidemiological data ceased to be kept and had to be reconstructed in 1978. In 1975, the 'four modernizations' (agriculture, industry, science and technology) were announced, a campaign to reverse the radical and destructive policies of the preceding decade no doubt helped by the policy shift ending international isolation with the normalization of relations with the United States and admission to the United Nations as the legitimate government of China. National entrance exams were reinstated in 1977, and previous graduates of the medical schools were required to take remedial coursework as were the barefoot doctors – about 5 million of them – to upgrade standards (Reynolds and Tierney 2006: 2141). TCM, 'the great treasure house' as Mao called it, was integrated with modern medicine putting it on a scientific basis (Taylor 2005: 152). To accelerate economic development the population needed to be reduced and stabilized since population increase showed a rise from 562 million in 1950 to 820 million in 1970 with 30 million babies born from 1962 to 1972. An increase in life expectancy, though problematical to ascertain with varying parameters, was one obvious contributor, as was fertility. A national birth control campaign was launched in 1972, with limited results, but draconian birth control methods and the 'one-child policy' were enforced from 1980 due to the rise in rural births to increase the labour supply after the liberalization of the economy in 1978 (Scharping 2002: 29–80). In 1995, a new law on maternal and infant health to prevent the birth of children with 'hereditary defects' was passed to international outcry as a throwback to the eugenics laws of Nazi Germany (Reichman *et al.* 1996: 425–426; *The Times* 5 June 1995).

Reform and transition

No lengthy review of the multiplicity of economic, political or social policies pursued since 1949 is necessary here to indicate the failure to achieve acceptable levels of modernization. The reforms of 1978–1979 were ample testimony to that fact. 'Opening up to the outside world' meant that key policy changes to the socialist system would be benchmarked against international standards. Economic liberalization, the dismantling of underperforming state-owned enterprises, collective farms and their welfare provisions, the switch to market principles (albeit with 'socialist' characteristics) and fiscal decentralization stimulated unprecedented economic growth. State medicine and public health services that had developed basically in isolation from world influences were financially and managerially devolved to provincial and local governments (with the exception of the military and other strategic state enterprises like the railways, which maintained their own medical schools and hospitals) and made responsible for 'cost recovery' or fee-for-service with the aim of reducing inefficiencies through price and service innovations. The commitment to and acceleration of reforms in all sectors of the economy and society were critical to the opening of negotiations over the future of Hong Kong resulting in the Sino-British Joint Declaration of 1984 returning Hong Kong to Chinese sovereignty in 1997.

The attenuation of the state's monopoly in health services reflected these trends. Private medical practice was legalized in 1985 and privately owned and financed hospitals established in line with the policy commitment to diversity and 'multiple forms' of health services outlined in the seventh five-year plan (1986–1991). But the profit-oriented approach to public health had a profound impact on preventive health measures – fees charged for basic immunizations and drugs – and curative services such as public hospitals and health-care personnel were dependent on charges to fund salaries and ongoing costs, to the detriment of the urban and rural poor not covered by the various insurance schemes that covered party members, soldiers, labourers and students (Hillier and Shen 1996: 260–262).

Speaking of these changed directions and China's re-engagement with the international scientific, medical and public health communities, Liming Lee of the Chinese Center for Disease Control and Prevention (CDC), established in Beijing in 2002, noted that 'in the past 20 years of reform and opening, public health enterprise in China has achieved world spotlight success'. Lee cited the dramatic increase in average life expectancy from 35 years (this number varies considerably) in 1949 to 71.4 years in 2000 as evidence of this remarkable change (the change in average life expectancy in the period since the reforms in 1978 is an increase from 68 years to 72 years in 2006) (Lee 2004: 328). However, in a population estimated to be 1.3 billion people in 2006, the so-called eradicated diseases have re-emerged, diseases said to have been controlled are on the rise and the rapid spread of new diseases such as HIV/AIDS, H5N1 or SARS and the lack of 'transparency' in addressing the extent and control of these diseases has exposed weaknesses in epidemiology and the inadequacies of a public health system that was underfinanced and essentially unaccountable.

Hong Kong and China: convergence or integration?

The convergent evolution of public health in Hong Kong and China since the nineteenth century diverged in important ways with the establishment of the PRC in 1949, reflecting the historical differences in the political, economic, social and legal systems which prevailed. Hong Kong people from 1841 to 1997 enjoyed a high degree of personal freedom protected by the rule of law, limited representative government and compliance to international covenants on human rights, and the colony was involved with international organizations such as the World Health Organization since its founding in 1948. Hong Kong's Department of Health exchanged information, sought expert advice, and in turn advised the WHO, regularly reporting to its Epidemiological Intelligence Station in Singapore on quarantinable infectious diseases. Its Virus Laboratory functioned as a WHO National Influenza Centre when the 'Hong Kong' flu (H3N1) emerged in 1968 affecting 500,000 people in the territory before it became pandemic. The flu was named for its place of identification but it originated in China where access was problematical, as the PRC was in the throes of the GPCR (Director of Medical and Health Services 1967–1968: 9).

Hong Kong has maintained a continuous engagement (and the freedom to do so) with a growing international circuit of public health associations, preventive health programmes and strategies and professionals, importing expertise to combat cholera, tuberculosis, malaria and other infectious diseases, many of them conditioned by the geopolitical situations we have reviewed. The form and functioning of its public health establishment distinguished it from the mainland despite its human and ecological interdependence with south China.

From the signing of the Sino-British Joint Declaration in 1984 to the handover and beyond, Beijing has stressed the need for 'convergence' and a smooth transition to Chinese sovereignty. As An-Chia Wu surmised, this rationale for the 'one country, two systems' formula was reminiscent of Brzezinski and Huntington's cold war 'convergence theory' of the 1960s (with reference to the USA and USSR) (Brzezinski and Huntington 1964: 10–13; Wu 1987: 155–177). Jan Tinbergen, who developed the theory in 1961, argued that capitalist and socialist polities and their inherent ideological contradictions would under reciprocal influence change and 'converge' under the forces of industrialization, urbanization and economic growth which would give rise to a common culture (Tinbergen 1961: 333–341). Although the theory has been roundly criticized by comparative economists for its lack of theoretical and empirical precision, what is important here, as Wu implied, is the perceived (and desired) direction of long-term change: for Marxists, capitalism, defeated by its own imperfections, will become socialist; for proponents of capitalism, the irrational (idealistic) socialist system will revert to a rational market economy (Andreff 1992: 58–59). For Hong Kong, the transitional period was summed up in the slogan, '*wushi nian bu bian*' ('no change for 50 years') before the two systems become one. In other words, before China's 'socialist system and polices shall be practiced in Hong Kong' (The Basic Law of the Hong Kong Special Administrative Region of the People's Republic of China, Article 5).

Convergence theory has also been extended to the public health sector suggesting that social, political and economic organization and scientific technologies in developed countries are productive of similar outcomes in policies and health strategies (Field 1989: 1–3). Critics have argued that the theory does not recognize the extent to which national public health systems are embedded in their histories and cultures which determine social norms, values and interactions (Saltman 1997: 449).

Since the opening up of China 'to the outside world', the liberalization of the economy has meant a remarkable expansion of national economic growth. Not surprisingly, the first site chosen for creating a market-oriented economy, or 'socialism with Chinese characteristics', was Shenzhen on the Hong Kong /PRC border in 1979. This 'window of technology, management, knowledge and foreign policy' according to the late premier Deng Xiaoping, grew from an agricultural backwater of approximately 300,000 people to a county-level urbanized area of over 10 million people primarily due to its economic and technological cooperation with Hong Kong. Economic integration has proceeded apace with the Closer Economic Partnership Agreement (CEPA) signed in 2003, improving cross-border connectivity along with the Hong Kong Economic and Trade Office in Guangdong assisting Hong Kong businesses to navigate the Guangdong market. This also reflects the fact that over 70,000 Hong Kong-financed or -owned factories operate in the province and 60% of inbound investment in Guangdong comes from Hong Kong (*South China Morning Post* 26 June 2006). Cross-border traffic has increased exponentially and over 218,000 residential properties have been purchased, built or rented by Hong Kong residents, with 88% located in Guangdong. As of 2005, 91,800 Hong Kong people were living across the border and an equal amount would like to do so in the next 10 years, according to a recent survey by the Hong Kong Government Census and Statistics Department (Census and Statistics Department 2005; *The Standard* 7 July 2006). The province also supplies most of Hong Kong's water and up to 70% of Hong Kong's food and Shenzhen is the largest export base of live chickens in China. Although briefly discussed here, the notion of 'convergence' at least economically, from both mainland and Hong Kong perspectives, would seem to be following a 'through train' in this transitional period.

However, questions of public health practices and policies have not fared so well under the 'one country, two systems' formula, partly explained by the historical differences in development. Questions of public health provisions are interdependent with the 'right to health' particularly, rights 'to seek, receive and impart information and ideas through any media and regardless of frontiers' (Universal Declaration of Human Rights (UDHR) 1948: Article 19), of which China is a now a signatory. Repeatedly China has warned foreign states or international organizations against intervening in its domestic affairs, including the rights of its citizens, using human rights as a pretext (*Liaowang* [Outlook] 26 March 1990: 7–8).

How does this affect Hong Kong, since it enacted a Bill of Rights Ordinance in 1991 which implements the International Covenant on Civil and Political Rights (ICCPR) that both China and Britain in the Joint Declaration agreed would remain in force (Wacks 1992: 225)? As Nobel Laureate John Polanyi opined in *Science* in 1997, 'As scientists we share the belief that freedom of thought and expression are vital to achieving new insights. "One country, two systems" is a slogan we can embrace if it becomes an invitation to openness and tolerance' (Polanyi 1997: 881). Has this been achieved and how has it impacted on the health of Hong Kong, China and the world?

Emerging and re-emerging infectious diseases

HIV/AIDS

Jonathan Mann and his co-authors have argued in the inaugural issue of *Health and Human Rights: An International Journal* that 'health and human rights are complementary approaches for defining and advancing human well-being' and that '[t]he interdependence of health and human rights has substantial conceptual and practical implications' (Mann *et al.* 1994: 6–23).The authors present a tripartite framework for examining this relationship that includes understanding the 'optimal balance between public health goals and human rights norms'; 'that promotion and protection of health are inextricably linked to promotion and protection of human rights'; and 'that violations of rights have important health effects'. Perhaps no emerging infectious disease provides a better case study than HIV/AIDS first notified in Hong Kong in 1984 (HIV) and in China the following year (Lee *et al.* 1996: 70–76).

The profile of patients in both places is similar except the transmission route in Hong Kong is primarily due to sexual contact where China reports injecting drug users (IDU), though 'foreigners and prostitutes' were initially blamed for the epidemic. Hong Kong has had a voluntary reporting system for HIV/AIDS since 1985 to assist in epidemiological investigations. The government moved quickly to screen the blood supply, and set up the AIDS Advisory Council in 1990, composed of public and private representatives to devise prevention strategies in consultation with the WHO. It also decriminalized homosexuality to encourage testing. China reacted to the epidemic by requiring 'AIDS-free' health certificates in 1986 from foreigners residing or intending to reside in China, and then extended the requirement to frequent visitors from Hong Kong, creating a storm of controversy particularly when random testing was done at the border in 1993 in contravention of WHO guidelines (*The Standard* 22 February 1993). The tests were criticized by health officials in Hong Kong for 'unreliability, poor safety standards and infringement of human rights' and were suspended after cross-border talks, helped no doubt by local tour companies cancelling trips to China because of the testing requirements (*South China Morning Post* 24 February 1993). Ironically, it was Hong Kong health experts who wrote China's first three-year plan for AIDS control and at the 43rd annual meeting of WHO's Western Pacific Regional Committee they were singled out for praise for their 'ability to transfer its technology and energy to China' (*South China Morning Post* 12 September 1992).

China's denial of the extent of HIV/AIDS infections hampered efforts to control and prevent the disease, as evidenced by under-reporting, and treating AIDS-related information as 'state secrets' including the knowledge of the scope of national blood sales and contamination of blood supplies first exposed by Dr Gao Yaojie and others in Henan province (Cohen 2004: 1431; *The New York Times* 6 February 2007). As stated by AIDS activist and director of the Beijing AIZHI Education Institute, Dr Wan Yanhai (who was held under arrest for over a month in 2002 for allegedly leaking state secrets on the extent of the AIDS problem in China), 'State Secrets Law contains no provisions relating to health information. In 1999, the Ministry of Health issued a note to all provincial health departments stating very clearly that AIDS-related information is not a state secret' (United States Congressional-Executive Commission on China 2003: 6, 25). However, as Zunyou Wu from Beijing's Center for Disease Control admitted recently, 'In the face of infectious disease epidemics the primary responsibility of public health is to contain and control the epidemic in order to protect the uninfected. In the areas of HIV/AIDS, we have not always remembered that principle' (Wu *et al.* 2006: 1475–1476).

At the end of 2005, due to international pressure and aided by cooperation and access to the Global AIDS Fund, China's accounting had significantly improved, revealing that there is an estimated 650,000 HIV sufferers with an estimated 60,000–80,000 new cases reported. China had consistently denied having an HIV problem until one month after the Global AIDS Fund was announced in 2002. As Kevin R. Frost, vice president of the Clinical Research and Prevention Program, American AIDS Foundation in New York, recalled, 'the number of people officially said to be infected in China went from 30,000 to 1 million in a single day' (United States Congressional-Executive Commission on China 2003: 26).

The number of HIV sufferers in Hong Kong remains low (the cumulative figure from 1984 to 2005 is 2,825) but the increase in HIV infections in Guangdong (one of the highest in China) and Shenzhen has raised alarms in Hong Kong because of the 'extensive mobility across the border and high-risk behaviours' according to Homer Tso, chairman of the HKAIDS Advisory Council, 'especially if men travel to the mainland for sex'. Because of the extension of the border-crossing hours, relaxation of entry regulations and the prospect of increased earnings, the number of mainland visitors engaged in prostitution arrested in Hong Kong rose from 2,977 in 2000 to 10,903 in 2005, many of them admitting to unsafe sex. Shenzhen reported a year-on-year increase of 136% in 2004 mostly due to IDUs but also an increase in sexual and mother-to-child transmissions. Guangdong experts estimate the actual numbers of HIV carriers to be 40,000 in 2006 (*The Lancet* 30 December 2002; *South China Morning Post* 2 November 2004).

'Spiralling' outbreaks of HIV amongst IDUs in a substantial population of 900,000 estimated drug users may lead to an upsurge in cross-border infections. The costs have to be counted. Losses to the mainland economy due to AIDS may reach USD 40 billion over the next five years according to the biennial report of UNAIDS. Dr Peter Piot of UNAIDS argued that 'AIDS was no longer a humanitarian crisis...but could undo decades of economic progress and threaten global security' (*Newsweek* 5 June 2006: 39; *The Standard* 8 June 2006).

H5N1 'bird flu'

In April 1997, just months before the handover, several chicken farms in Yuen Long and the Cheung Sha Wan wholesale market experienced mass deaths of poultry. Reports surfaced that Guangdong chicken farms, where most of Hong Kong's chickens are sourced, experienced similar events between February and April. In May the first case of avian influenza A (H5N1) occurred in Hong Kong acquired directly from chickens without an intermediate host. By December, 18 individuals were confirmed to have the infection, six of whom died. A massive cull of more than 1.5 million chickens commenced on 29 December and all poultry imports from the mainland were halted. No new cases were reported until 2003, when this emerging highly virulent influenza strain rapidly disseminated through Asia and the world, possibly through chicken imports and migratory birds. The Chinese Ministry of Health confirmed the presence of the virus only in 2004 in samples taken from a Guangxi duck farm (*WHO Epidemic and Pandemic Alert Response* (EPR) 27 January 2004). China did not verify its first human case until November 2005, though in February of 2003, two cases were confirmed in Hong Kong of family members who had travelled to Fujian province and contracted the infection there (*WHO EPR* 27 February 2003).

Suspicions in Hong Kong that the H5N1 virus originated in China surfaced early in 1998, but Dr Lavanchy of the WHO fact-finding mission in China denied that there was any evidence to support that speculation and Guangdong health authorities expressed skepticism over Hong Kong's testing methods for the virus (*The Standard* 19 and 24 January 1998). Despite the expanding threat of increased virulence to humans from the virus, a laboratory run by universities in Hong Kong and China suspended their surveillance studies due to stringent new regulations issued by Beijing after the team published an article in *Nature* confirming the presence of H5N1 in China and that wild birds in Qinghai were infected by poultry (Chen *et al.* 2005: 191–192; *New Scientist* 11 July 2006). Even more disconcerting was the revelation that a 24-year-old man had died in November 2003 of H5N1 and not SARS as previously thought, months before China admitted the virus was circulating in its poultry and two years before the first reported human case (*New Scientist* 1 July 2006).

International collaborative efforts organized in partnership with the WHO to investigate H5N1 have been hampered by China's resistance to sharing samples, viewed by many scientists as a competitive approach to discover a vaccine first. Furthermore, the existence of a new subtype (Fujian) of H5N1, identified by researchers at the University of Hong Kong and the United States, was denied by Beijing amid ongoing criticism from the WHO of the failure of China to share recent samples of the virus. One day after

Dr Margaret Chan Fung Fu-chun (Hong Kong's former director of Health Services) was voted in as the head of the WHO, China released 20 samples from 2004 and 2005 to the WHO laboratory in the United States (*South China Morning Post* 11 November 2006). Whatever the state of surveillance competency in China, the Hong Kong experience with bird flu and its human and economic consequences, as well as cross-border relations, would be further strained with the advent of SARS (Enserink 2005: 1409).

SARS

SARS (severe acute respiratory syndrome), an emerging highly transmissible coronavirus, was globalized through Hong Kong in February 2003 (SARS Expert Committee 2003). The story of its spread from Hong Kong and its control through the cooperation of many governments, health organizations, medical personnel and scientists has been ably examined by the recent WHO publication, *SARS: How a global epidemic was stopped* (2006). For Hong Kong people, of whom 1,755 were infected and with 300 deaths (worldwide there were 8,000 infected with 900 deaths), the social, economic and political impacts, as well as the shattering of confidence in the health-care system, left many scars (SARS Expert Committee 2003: 12–23). The lack of transparency and the denial of critical information from the mainland where the disease originated were severely damaging to China's credibility internationally. If timely intelligence of the initial spread of 'atypical pneumonia' cases in Guangdong had been communicated to Hong Kong health authorities in the months preceding the arrival of the index case, instead of vague newspaper reports and cell phone calls from relatives and friends in the province, much expertise and palliative care may have attenuated the epidemic. The director of Health Services, Dr Margaret Chan, testified to the Select Committee that she was informed by Guangdong officials that information concerning infectious diseases was classified as 'state secrets'. The Secretary of Health, Welfare and Food, Dr Yeoh Eng-kiong, resigned and Dr Margaret Chan, was criticized for her 'inadequate performance' (Legislative Council Select Committee 2004: 34). The economic costs on local consumption and export services related to tourism and travel for Hong Kong were considerable in the short term, although the impact on manufacturing and exports across the border was negligible (Siu and Wong 2004: 62–83).

Environment

China and Hong Kong share a common ecosystem and one rationale made by Britain during the negotiations for the return of Hong Kong to China was its utter dependence on food and water from the mainland. Furthermore, the reservoirs for H5N1 and SARS are zoonotic in origin and environmental degradation could have enhanced the emergence of these diseases. The Chinese State Environmental Protection Administration (SEPA) in its new report issued on 4 June 2006, admitted that 60% of China could be described as 'environmentally fragile'. Problems cited ranged from energy consumption, desertification, coastal and marine ecosystem degeneration, pesticide and fertilizer overuse, as well as increasingly scarce water supplies, all related to human population impacts. Significantly, there is no comprehensive environmental protection law to give force to a maze of regulatory regimes and policies, and no systematic attempt to promote public discussion and awareness of environmental problems. According to Zhou Shengxian, the minister of SEPA, mass protests over pollution increased in 2005 by over 29%, and 50% of the 51,000 disputes reported related to the lack of potable water, a basic public health parameter. In Guangdong, less than 2% of waste water in cities and towns is treated and almost half of the rivers managed by the province are polluted. China's Gross Domestic Product (GDP) growth is projected to be well over 7.5% over the next five years but half of this growth rate could be 'wiped off the books' if the annually recurring pollution costs were taken into account (*South China Morning Post* 23 June 2006; *People's Daily* 22 May 2006). Hong Kong has had its own accountings. Rising levels of air pollution directly related to the manufacturing and industrial boom across the border since the 1990s (much of it financed and owned by Hong Kong people) are costing Hong Kong over 1,600 lives and at least HKD 2 billion – HKD 1.5 billion for health-care costs and HKD 504 million in lost productivity a year, according to a recent study. The city's concentration of air pollutants exceeded WHO standards by 200% (Hedley *et al.* 2006: 1–4; *South China Morning Post* 9 June 2006). Only cross-border enforcement of emissions regulations will alleviate the problem.

Food safety

China has over 200 laws and regulations on standard food safety but 'a lack of unified supervision and control', according to Professor Luo Yunbo, dean of the China Agricultural University's College of Food Science, has led to major problems in the industry. Rapid development and the proliferation of food industries 'struggling to adjust to a capitalist system' are to blame for weak enforcement of standards, said Dr Gerald Moy of the WHO Food Safety Programme. Another technical officer with the WHO was of the opinion that 'the growing awareness of the food safety problems in China is partly because the perception that food in the past was safe. This is not the case' (*The Straits Times* 1 September 2005).

Hong Kong has had long experience with tainted food supplies imported from the mainland. Vegetables contaminated with banned pesticides imported from Shenzhen began surfacing in the 1980s, sending hundreds to hospital, 500 in 1988 (*South China Morning Post* 13 June and 28 October 1988). Oysters contaminated with cadmium, and shellfish with hepatitis A virus (*South China Morning Post* 11 December 1983), and traditional Chinese medicine with high levels of arsenic, lead and mercury (a considerable problem since 75% of the 99,000 tonnes of Chinese medicine exported from Guangdong was consumed in Hong Kong in 2006) prompted the Hong Kong government to set up more stringent border checks and in cooperation with the Guangdong local authorities a system of inspection and registration of farms exporting food to Hong Kong

(*South China Morning Post* 31 January 2006). However food scares including fish and eels containing malachite green panicked Hong Kong consumers and there was a 40% drop in live fish sales as well as a 25% drop in pork sales because of pig-borne disease (from *Streptococcus suis*) in 2005. It was found that 18 accredited fish farms (eight in Shenzhen) on the list provided by the State General Administration for Quality Supervision, Inspection and Quarantine did not exist (*South China Morning Post* 22 September 2005). Guangdong provincial party secretary, Zhang Dejiang, acknowledged to Hong Kong legislators and the Chief Executive Donald Tsang that China's most prosperous province and the pioneer in the open economic reform was facing severe environmental crises related to rapid economic growth. Guangdong and Hong Kong authorities agreed to open a direct daily channel of communications and to a package of proposals to combat food scares and air pollution in September of 2005 (*The Standard* 29 September 2005).

Despite such promising initiatives to strengthen cross-border cooperation and coordination, the chronicle of food hygiene goes on. Problems continue with imported fish from Guangdong contaminated with either banned chemicals or antibiotics (*South China Morning Post* 10 November 2005, 13 June, 8 July and 20 December 2006). In November 2006, fresh water garoupa containing malachite green prompted a temporary ban on fresh water fish imports from China, which was extended to saltwater fish two weeks later after samples were found to contain the antibiotic nitrofuran. Hong Kong's testing standards were criticized by the Guangdong Inspection and Quarantine Bureau as 'vague' and the state-owned company that controls the trade in fresh water fish in Guangdong refused to resume sales to Hong Kong. Fish farmers claimed that 10,000 workers in the industry were 'gravely affected' with losses of HKD 150 million (*South China Morning Post* 27 November and 8 December 2006). Eggs were found tainted by the industrial dye, Sudan Red, and tests on fruits and vegetables imported from Guangdong revealed that 25% were contaminated with banned pesticides, with 50% of the strawberries having an excessive lead content (*South China Morning Post* 21 December 2006).

The Chinese Ministry of Agriculture released the findings of nationwide food safety checks claiming that 90% of food products in the mainland were safe and 'scare-free'. Hong Kong's head of the Expert Committee on Food Safety, Kwan Hoi-shan, praised the mainland for becoming more transparent on health issues, but the deputy chairman of the Legislative Council panel on food safety and environmental hygiene cautioned that 'it might be a warning sign. Could there be food contaminated with large doses of banned drugs that we are yet to know about?' (*South China Morning Post* 28 November 2006). This has been revealed after Zheng Xiaoyu, director-general of the State Food and Drug Administration from 1998 to 2005 and a 'model worker' with a reputation for enforcing stringent standards in the manufacture of pharmaceuticals (a sector plagued by fake or tainted drugs, including infant formula), went on trial and was summarily executed for taking bribes to approve drugs (*The Standard* 1 January 2007; *South China*

Morning Post 16, 21, 23 August 2007).[1] In Southeast Asia, twelve brands of antimalarial drugs in circulation produced by Guilin Pharma in China were tested and identified as fakes. China has been credited as the 'source of most of the world's fake drugs' (*International Herald Tribune* 21 February 2007; Newton *et al.* 2006: 752–755).

Health-care funding

Hong Kong, long touted as the 'free enterprise capital' of the world, ironically, has the most socialist of health-care systems, funding 97% of the public health bill of HKD 30 billion a year through one of the lowest tax regimes. Public or government subvented hospitals and clinics provide excellent service at minimal or free cost to Hong Kong people who opt to patronize them. Hong Kong's funding for health care amounts to 5.7% of the GDP, low by developed world standards, though the health indices compare favourably with them. In 2000, life expectancies at birth for men (78 years) and women (83.9 years) were the highest life expectancies for men and the second highest for women in a ranking of the 191 WHO Member States (Law and Yip 2003: 43–47). In 2006, life expectancy has continued to rise for a population of 6,900,000 people to 78.8 years for men and 84.4 years for women and the age structure has changed dramatically with only 16% of the population under 15 years and 11% over 65 years, focusing public health planning on the needs of an aging population. Critical to this demographic trend is the decline in fertility to 1.2 per 1,000 people, a natural decline since there are no population control measures as in China, prompting some government officials to call for incentives to increase the birth rate. On the other hand, Hong Kong's reputation for high-quality and low-cost maternal and infant health care in the public sector and the 2001 Court of Final Appeal judgment allowing mainland babies born in Hong Kong to have right of abode has attracted a rising number of mainland women to give birth in the SAR – 13,398 in 2005–2006, or one-third of all children born. This has prompted local controversy due to the overburdening of maternity services, the lack of antenatal care of expectant mainland women prior to their arrival, many of whom default on their payments (*South China Morning Post* 13 December 2006). With rising costs and deficits, the government has pursued a decade of health-care reform and financing, creating the Hospital Authority to rationalize the system. Proposals currently under review include those aimed at encouraging private health insurance schemes for those that can afford them.

Since 1949, China's socialist health-care system was lauded by many as a successful example of a poor country with limited resources creating an equitable distribution of services where its health status and disease control experience might have important lessons for developed nations (Sidel and Sidel 1973). Others, however, understood that China's health-care system was embedded in its economic and political system and therefore not exportable (Blendon 1979: 1453–1458). Under a centrally planned system health care was delivered through a highly stratified fixed residency (*hukou*) and workplace (*danwei*) registration system where agricultural collectives and state-owned enterprises at various levels enrolled their workers in low-cost insurance schemes. With the reforms of 1978 and the divestiture of underperforming state-owned enterprises, including hospitals, state subsidies were cut and costs rose significantly (Liu and Mills 2002: 1691–1693).

The annual report on the state of the nation's health 'Green Book on Health' is a sobering account of the past decade of reforms on a system that had prided itself on controlling diseases like schistosomiasis which are now resurgent due to a decrease in funding for preventative programmes (*Asian Economic News* 7 November 2005). Tuberculosis was claimed to have been brought under control, but the Vice Minister of Health, Wang Longde, admitted that only 600,000 people out of 4.5 million TB sufferers (the second largest number in the world) received treatment with 130,000 deaths recorded (*South China Morning Post* 26 March and 25 May 2006). The report cited the lack of government financial support, inadequate official supervision and improper government intervention in the health-care system, as well as collusion between public hospitals and government health authorities in fee structuring, as the most critical issues. China's reported expenditure on health care dropped from 2.53% of total government expenditure in 1986–1990 to 1.66% in 2000–2005 (*South China Morning Post* 7 December 2006). In the 2006 budget, out of more than CNY 3 trillion, only CNY 120 billion was earmarked for health care. Furthermore, 80% of health-care funding goes to urban as opposed to rural areas. The WHO ranked China the fourth worst in the world in equitable distribution of medical resources, and the *China Legal News* labelled it an 'extortionate industry' (Akin *et al.* 2005: 87–89; *China Legal News* 20 February 2006; *South China Morning Post* 20 February and 25 May 2006). The government announced it will allocate CNY 1 billion to seven central and western regions to lower costs and improve health-care delivery to redress the imbalances in 2007 (*South China Morning Post* 7 December 2006).

Smoking and tobacco control

Dr Wang Ruotao, from China's CDC, warned that compounding problems in controlling the legacy of communicable diseases is the rapid rise in cancer, heart diseases, diabetes and high blood pressure – diseases associated with changing lifestyles and an aging population – creating a 'double burden' on the health system and absorbing 'a huge percentage of the health budget' (*South China Morning Post* 14 October 2006). One example is the preventable epidemic in smoking. Over 350 million people smoke, with an estimated 1 million premature deaths and 460 million are affected by second-hand smoke, accounting for another 45,000 premature deaths from smoking-related diseases. China's tobacco industry is the largest in the world and with increased disposable income China's people consume 25–30% of the world's cigarettes. Increasing the tax on tobacco, a control policy used in many countries for decades, and banning smoking in public venues, has faced resistance paradoxically because of the potential loss to government revenue since the domestic tobacco companies are state-owned enterprises (Hu 2006: 6; Liu *et al.* 1998: 1421).

Hong Kong passed legislation in the 1960s to control tobacco by increasing taxation, banning smoking on public transport and public institutions like schools and hospitals, and annual anti-smoking campaigns targeting youths, since a study confirmed that 25% of all deaths of people aged 35–69 in 1998 were attributable to tobacco (Lam *et al.* 2001: 361–362). After years of debate, The Smoking (Public Health) Amendment was gazetted in April 2005 and passed into law on 19 October 2006. On 1 January 2007, smoking was banned in all public venues, including public spaces, with a few exceptions such as mahjong parlours and bars that do not serve food; these places will come under the ban by June 2009. In 2003, with the introduction of the individual visit scheme, over 12 million mainland tourists, many of whom smoke, visited in 2004 with no sign of abatement. Enforcing the new legislation and collecting the fines may prove difficult (*Asian Economic News* 31 January 2005). These challenges to the public health of China as outlined above will have a continuing impact on the future of Hong Kong in this transitional period.

Conclusion

It is almost a decade since the retrocession of Hong Kong to Chinese sovereignty and the operation of the 'one country, two systems' formula. Responses to newly emerging diseases such as SARS and H5N1, unprecedented as they were, have highlighted the weaknesses of a system unable to cope with the openness that modernization demands. The pattern of official response, regardless of China's professed commitment to 'open up to the outside world', has a long history as far as Hong Kong is concerned, and the minimizing or denial of epidemics and suppression of health-related information will continue to challenge Hong Kong's integration with the mainland. Speaking in Hong Kong, the director of CARE USA's health unit, Sanjay Sinho, said: 'preventing avian flu in Hong Kong means preventing avian flu in the world' (*South China Morning Post* 23 June 2006). But does Hong Kong wish to function as the first line of defence in the spread of diseases?

One promising development is the selection of Guangdong province (the epicentre of emerging influenza strains) as the venue for the WHO Collaborating Center for Surveillance, Research and Training on Emerging Infectious Diseases on 13 June 2006. WHO country director in Beijing, Henk Bekedam, indicated that Guangdong's Center for Disease Control 'has long been a tried-and-tested warrior in the fight against infectious diseases well known during the SARS epic'. Be that as it may, when a Shenzhen man contracted bird flu, Guangdong officials notified the Hong Kong Centre for Health Protection immediately since Hong Kong has been free of any new cases since 2003. However, Shenzhen health bureau authorities denied there was a suspected case, although security was stepped up at the Donghu hospital and reporters were barred entry and allegedly punched by security guards (*South China Morning Post* 14 June 2006). Over two hundred attacks on Guangdong hospitals and staff were recorded in the first half of 2006. Lian Zhenhui, former director of the Shenzhen Luohu district health bureau, was imprisoned for thirteen years for accepting CNY 1.7 million in bribes from 1995–2006 (*South China Morning Post* 10 September 2006). Cai Hangang, the former head of the Immunization Planning Institute's vaccination section under Guangdong's CDC and his boss Luo Yaoxing, both frontline workers during the SARS epidemic, were charged with accepting CNY 11.6 million in bribes from pharmaceutical companies from June 2002 to February 2006 (*South China Morning Post* 13 December 2006). One month later, defective immunoglobulin tainted with hepatitis C (sold nationwide) produced by Guangdong's Bioyee Pharmaceutical firm was identified, though Guangdong's propaganda department banned the media from investigating the scandal (*South China Morning Post* 25 January 2007).

Beijing has drafted a specific (besides the Law on the Protection of State Secrets) law forbidding journalists to report on disease epidemics and other 'emergencies' before the government releases the information (*The Standard* 5 July 2006; *South China Morning Post* 26 June 2006). Under PRC law, 'freedom of the press' is guaranteed but is controlled in the interests and security of the State, particularly by a strict and burdensome licensing system and censorship by the Communist Party Central Propaganda Department, the General Administration of Press and Publications and the National Administration of State Secrets. The Law on the Protection of State Secrets, previously rather vague on what matters might be considered a state secret if it gave rise to consequences that might 'hinder health work', will now has teeth. The fear that the restrictions to press freedom will apply to Hong Kong (as part of the one country) despite its guarantee of freedom of speech and the press under the Basic Law (the two systems) has raised a storm of protest.[2] As one legal expert has said, 'can China be held internationally responsible for failing to perform international obligations?' (Mushkat 1997: 34).

Margaret Chan's election to head the WHO, supported by China's government, promises a new era in cooperation with the mainland and the world. However, there were mixed feelings expressed publicly in Hong Kong questioning whether she would be able to function independently from her base of support. An editorial in a local paper stressed the need for China in matters of health to 'bridge the credibility gap' (*South China Morning Post* 11 November 2006). The day after her election and China's release of 20 bird flu samples to the WHO, she was quoted as saying 'I won't wear my nationality on my sleeve. I'll leave it behind' (*South China Morning Post* 11 November 2006).

If Hong Kong's future political, social and economic development, which is inextricably linked to the public's health as promised under the Basic Law, is convergent to progress on the mainland, what are the implications for Taiwan? According to the late Premier Deng Xiaoping, the 'one country, two systems' formula was originally devised with Taiwan in mind in order to settle the last issue of national sovereignty, unresolved since 1949. Although China signed a memorandum of agreement with the WHO accepting the principle that preventive measures against epidemics have no national boundaries, Taiwan has consistently been barred even from observer status in the WHO under the 'one China policy' by member nations of the UN (*Taipei Times* 15 March 2006; Wachman 2000: 183–203). As Robert Zoellick, a former US deputy secretary of state, stated: 'It is time to take our policy beyond opening doors to China's membership into the international system: we need to urge China to become a responsible stakeholder in that system' (*South China Morning Post* 21 June 2006). Hong Kong and the world's health will depend on it.

Notes

1 Although Hong Kong has faced escalating food and drug safety problems from mainland products for the past 25 years, it was only after international outcry over melamine-contaminated products imported from China and used in the manufacture of pet, chicken, pig and fish food in the United States and Canada, cough syrup contaminated with diethylene glocal (with 100 deaths reported in Panama) as well as toothpaste (in Panama and the United States), toys manufactured in China with excessive lead content (the Hong Kong owner of the factory in Guangdong hanged himself ostensibly over more than USD 30 million of debt when the US company recalled the products), 'excessive' levels of formaldehyde found in Chinese manufactured clothing and blankets in New Zealand and Australia, and so on, that China has agreed (faced with global trade sanctions and product recalls) to close cooperation with the United States, the European Union and other countries over product safety and to invest CNY 8.8 billion by 2010 to improve food and drug safety, whilst continuing to protest that the majority of its products are safe (*The Standard* 2, 4, 6, 9 and 27 August 2007; *South China Morning Post* 16, 21, 23 August 2007).
2 The protest to the draft 'emergency response law', along with the poor record of local governments to respond to emergencies has had some impact. At the third reading of the draft law during the meeting of the National People's Congress in August 2007, it was reported that the controversial clause allowing local governments to impose stiff fines and penalties on media agencies who report on 'disasters' without official sanction, has been dropped (*The South China Morning Post* 25 August 2007).

References

Achtman, M. (1994) 'Clonal Spread of Serogroup A Meningococci: A Paradigm for the Analysis of Microevolution in Bacteria', *Molecular Microbiology*, 11(1): 15–22.
Akin, J., Dow, W. H., Lance, P. M. and Loh, P. A (2005) 'Changes in Access to Health Care in China, 1989–1997', *Health Policy and Planning*, 20(2): 80–89.
Andreff, W. (1992) 'Convergence or Congruence between Eastern and Western Economic Systems', in Dallago, B., Brezinski, H., and Andreff, W. (eds) *Convergence and System Change*, Aldershot: Dartmouth Publishing Company, 47–86.
Atkinson, J. M. (1896) 'Medical Report on the Prevalence of Bubonic Plague in the Colony of Hong Kong During the Years 1895 and 1896', *Hong Kong Legislative Council Sessional Papers*, Hong Kong: Government Printers.
Barenblatt, D. (2004) *A Plague upon Humanity: The Secret Genocide of Axis Japan's Germ Warfare Operation*, New York: HarperCollins.
Blendon, R. J. (1979) 'Can China's Health Care be Transplanted without China's Economic Policies?', *The New England Journal of Medicine*, 300(26): 1453–1458.
Bretelle-Establet, F. (2002) *La Santé en Chine du Sud (1898–1928)*, Paris: CNRS Editions.
Brzezinski, Z. and Huntington, S. P. (1964) *Political Power: USA/USSR*, New York: Viking Press.

Bullock, M. B. (1980) *An American Transplant: The Rockefeller Foundation and Peking Union Medical College*, Berkeley: University of California Press.
Census and Statistics Department (2005) *Hong Kong Residents Working in the Mainland of China*, Hong Kong: Government Census and Statistics Department.
Chadwick, O. (1882) 'Report on the Sanitary Condition of Hong Kong: With Appendices and Plans', Eastern No. 38, London: Colonial Office.
Chadwick, O. and Simpson, W. J. (1902) 'Report on the Question of the Housing of the Population of Hong Kong', *Hong Kong Legislative Council Sessional Papers*, Hong Kong: Government Printers.
Chang, T. S., Lai, D. G., and Chu, H. J. (1936) 'A Note on Infant Mortality Rate in Kao-Chiao Shanghai', *Chinese Medical Journal*, 50: 581–582.
Chau, T. N., Lai, J. Y., Yuen, H. (1997) 'Acute Viral Hepatitis in Hong Kong: A Study of Recent Incidences', *Hong Kong Medical Journal*, 3(3): 261–266.
Chen, H., Smith, G. J. D., Zheng, S. Y., Qin, K., Wong, J., Li, K. S., Webster, R. G., Peiris, J., and Guan, Y. (2005) 'H5N1 Virus Outbreak in Migratory Water-fowl', *Nature*, 436(July 14): 191–192.
Chen, W. Y. (1961) 'Medicine and Public Health', *China Quarterly*, 6: 153–169.
China Medical Commission of the Rockefeller Foundation (1914) *Medicine in China*, New York: The University of Chicago Press.
Ching, R. (1951) 'A Review with Comments of the Medical Records of the Tung Wah East Hospital Eye Service', *The Bulletin of the Hong Kong Chinese Medical Association*, 3(1): 11–17.
Choa, G. (1981) *The Life and Times of Sir Kai Ho Kai: A Prominent Figure in Nineteenth Century Hong Kong*, Hong Kong: Chinese University Press.
Cohen, J. (2004) 'An Unsafe Practice Turned Blood Donors into Victims', *Science*, 304 (5676): 1438.
Colonial Office (1894) Original Correspondence, CO 129/263: 187–193; 548–564.
Colonial Surgeon (1879) Annual Report, *Administrative Reports*, Hong Kong.
Crozier, R. C. (1968) *Traditional Medicine in Modern China*, Cambridge: Harvard University Press.
Director of Medical and Health Services (1949–50) *Annual Departmental Report*, Hong Kong: Government Printers.
—— (1950) *Annual Departmental Report*, Hong Kong: Government Printers.
—— (1957–1958) *Annual Departmental Report*, Hong Kong: Government Printers.
—— (1960–1961) *Annual Departmental Report*, Hong Kong: Government Printers.
—— (1961–1962) *Annual Departmental Report*, Hong Kong: Government Printers.
—— (1962–1963) *Annual Departmental Report*, Hong Kong: Government Printers.
—— (1963–1964) *Annual Departmental Report*, Hong Kong: Government Printers.
—— (1966–1967) *Annual Departmental Report*, Hong Kong: Government Printers.
—— (1967–1968) *Annual Departmental Report*, Hong Kong: Government Printers.
—— (1968–1969) *Annual Departmental Report*, Hong Kong: Government Printers.
—— (1970–1971) *Annual Departmental Report*, Hong Kong: Government Printers.
Director of Medical Services (1939) *Annual Medical Report*, Hong Kong: Government Printers.
Endicott, G. B. (1964) *A History of Hong Kong*, Hong Kong: Oxford University Press.
Enserink, M. (2005) 'Talk on Underground Bird Flu Rattles Experts', *Science*, 310 (5753): 1409.
Faust, E. C. (1924) 'Observations on North China Intestinal Parasites of Man', *Journal of Tropical Medicine*, 4(4): 411–437.

Field, M. G. (1989) (ed.) *Success and Crisis in National Health Systems: A Comparative Approach*, London: Routledge.

Flohr, C. (1996) 'The Plague Fighter: Wu Lien-teh and the Beginning of the Chinese Public Health System', *Annals of Science*, 53(4): 361–380.

Gould, D. B. (1995) 'Implementation of Health Policy in Hong Kong', *Asian Journal of Public Administration*, 17(1): 105–115.

Hedley, A., McGhee, S., Wong, C., Barron, B., Chau, P., Chau, J., Thach, T., Wong, T. and Loh, C. (2006) *Air Pollution: Costs and Paths to a Solution*, Hong Kong: Civic Exchange.

Hennessy, J. P. (1881) 'Address of Governor, Sir John Pope Hennessy, K. C. M. G. on the Census Returns and the Progress of Hong Kong', *Administrative Reports*, Hong Kong: Government Printers.

Hillier, S. and Shen, J. (1996) 'Health Care Systems in Transition: People's Republic of China. Part 1: An Overview of China's Health Care System', *Journal of Public Health Medicine*, 18(3): 258–265.

Ho, P. L. H. (2002) 'Agenda-Setting for the Regulation of Traditional Chinese Medicine in Hong Kong', *Asian Journal of Public Administration*, 24(2): 257–285.

Hong Kong Museum of Medical Sciences Society (2006) *Plague, SARS and the Story of Medicine in Hong Kong*, Hong Kong: Hong Kong University Press.

Hong Kong Opthalmological Society (1958) 'Medical Registration (Amendment) Ordinance, 1958', *The Bulletin of the Hong Kong Chinese Medical Association*, 10(1): 193–201.

Hooper, A. S. (1990) 'The Sanitary Board', in Wright, A. and Cartwright, H. A. (eds) *Twentieth Century Impressions of Hong Kong*, Singapore: Graham Brash, 157–187.

Horn, J. (1969) *Away with All Pests: An English Surgeon in People's China*, London: Hamlyn.

Housing Commission (1938) *Report of the Housing Commission 1935*, Hong Kong: Government Printers.

Hu, T. W. (2006) 'Balancing Interests: The Economics of Tobacco Control in China', *China Brief: A Journal of Analysis and Information*, 6(19):6–9.

Huang, P., Ye, G., Zhong, J. and Sha, Q. (2002) 'Assessment of Current Epidemiological Status of Viral Hepatitis in Guangdong Province, China', *The Southeast Asian Journal of Tropical Medicine and Public Health*, 33(4): 832–836.

Humphries, M. (1996) *Ruttonjee Sanatorium: Life and Times*, Hong Kong: Wing Yiu Company.

Keith, O. (1922) 'Commission Government in Canton', *Far Eastern Review*, 18(2): 101–103.

Kerr, J. G. (1888) 'The Sanitary Condition of Canton', *The China Medical Missionary Journal*, 2(3): 134–138.

King, P. Z. (1943) 'Public Health', *The Chinese Year Book*, Shanghai: The Commercial Press.

—— (1945) 'Public Health', *The Chinese Year Book*, Shanghai: The Commercial Press.

Lai, J. Y. (1997) 'Hepatitis A and E in Hong Kong', *Hong Kong Medical Journal*, 3(1): 79–82.

Lam, T. H., Ho, S. Y., Hedley, A. J., Mak, K. H. and Peto, R. (2001) 'Mortality and Smoking in Hong Kong: Case-Control Study of All Adult Deaths in 1998', *British Medical Journal*, 323(7301): 361–362.

Law, C. K. and Yip, P. S. F. (2003) 'Health Life Expectancy in Hong Kong Special Administrative Region of China', *Bulletin of the World Health Organization*, 81(1): 43–47.

Lee, L. M. (2004) 'The Current State of Public Health in China', *Annual Review of Public Health*, 25: 327–329.

Lee, S. S., Lo, Y. C. and Wong, K. H. (1996) 'The First One Hundred AIDS Cases in Hong Kong', *China Medical Journal*, 109(1): 70–76.
Legislative Council Select Committee (2004) *Report to Inquire into the Handling of the Severe Acute Respiratory Syndrome Outbreak by the Government and the Hospital Authority*, Hong Kong: Hong Kong Government.
Lethbridge, H. J. (1971) 'A Chinese Association in Hong Kong: The Tung Wah', *Contributions to Asian Studies*, 1: 144–158.
Leung, G. K. (1928) 'Tai-Lam, A Paradise for Lepers', *The China Journal*, 8: 40–43.
Li, S. F. (1958) 'Reminiscences of 50 Years of Medical Work in Hong Kong and China', *The Bulletin of the Hong Kong Chinese Medical Association*, 10(1): 161–173.
Lim, R. K. S. and Chen, C. C. (1937) 'State Medicine', *Chinese Medical Journal*, 51: 781–796.
Liu, B. Q., Peto, R., Chen, Z. M., Boreham J., Wu, Y. P. and Li, J. P. (1998) 'Emerging Tobacco Hazards in China: 1. Retrospective Proportional Mortality Study of One Million Deaths', *British Medical Journal*, 317: 1411–1422.
Liu, J. H. (1936) 'Public Health', *The Chinese Year Book*, 1: 1392–1427.
Liu, X. Z. and Mills, A. (2002) 'Financing Reforms of Public Health Services in China: Lessons for Other Nations', *Social Science & Medicine*, 54: 1691–1698.
MacPherson, K. L. (1987) *A Wilderness of Marshes: The Origins of Public Health in Shanghai, 1843–1893*, London: Oxford University Press.
—— (1997) 'Conspiracy of Silence: A History of Sexually Transmitted Diseases and HIV/AIDS in Hong Kong', in Lewis, M., Bamber, S. and Waugh, M. (eds) *Sex, Disease and Society: A Comparative History of Sexually Transmitted Diseases and HIV/AIDS in Asia and the Pacific*, Westport: Greenwood Press, 85–112.
—— (1998) 'Cholera in China: An Aspect of the Internationalization of Infectious Disease', in Elvin, M. and Liu, T. J. (eds) *Sediments of Time: Environment and Society in Chinese History*, Cambridge: Cambridge University Press, 487–519.
—— (2001) 'Health and Empire: Britain's National Campaign to Combat Venereal Diseases in Shanghai, Hong Kong and Singapore', in Davidson, R. and Hall, L. A. (eds), *Sex, Sin and Suffering: Venereal Disease and European Society since 1870*, London: Routledge, 173–190.
Mann, J. M., Gostin, L., Gruskin, S., Brennan, T., Lazzarini, Z. and Fineberg, H. V. (1994) 'Health and Human Rights', *Health and Human Rights: An International Journal*, 1(1): 6–23.
Medical and Sanitary Reports (1914) *Administrative Reports*, Hong Kong.
—— (1915) *Administrative Reports*, Hong Kong
—— (1917) *Administrative Reports*, Hong Kong.
—— (1918) *Administrative Reports*, Hong Kong.
—— (1924) *Administrative Reports*, Hong Kong.
Medical Committee Report (1895) *Hong Kong Legislative Council Sessional Papers*, Hong Kong.
Medical Development Advisory Committee (1974) *The Further Development of Medical and Health Services in Hong Kong*, Hong Kong: Medical and Health Department.
Minden, K. (1994) *Bamboo Stone: The Evolution of a Chinese Medical Elite*, Toronto: University of Toronto Press.
Miners, N. (1987) *Hong Kong under Imperial Rule, 1912–1941*, Hong Kong: Oxford University Press.
—— (1998) *The Government and Politics of Hong Kong*, Hong Kong: Oxford University Press.

Mushkat, R. (1997) *One Country, Two International Legal Personalities*, Hong Kong: Hong Kong University Press.
Newton, P., McGready, R., Fernandez, F., Green, M. D., Sunjio, M., Bruneton, C., Phanouvong, S., Millet, P., Whitty, C., Talisuna, A., Proux, S., Christophel, E., Malenga, G., Singhasivanon, P., Bojang, K., Kaur, H., Palmer, K., Day, N., Greenwood, B., Nosten, F. and White, N. (2006) 'Manslaughter by Fake Artesunate in Asia – Will Africa be Next?', *Public Library of Science, Medicine* (PLoS Med), 3(6): e197. DOI: 10.1371/journal.pmed.0030197.
Phillips, D. R. (1988) *The Epidemiological Transition in Hong Kong*, Hong Kong: Centre of Asian Studies.
Platt, J., Jones, M. and Platt, A. (1998) *The Whitewash Brigade: The Hong Kong Plague of 1894*, London: Dix Noonan Webb Ltd.
Polanyi, J. (1997) 'Science and "One Country, Two Systems" ', *Science*, 277(5328): 881.
Registrar General (1892) Report for the Year 1891, *Hong Kong Legislative Council Sessional Papers*, Hong Kong: Government Printers.
—— (1894) Report for the Year 1894, *Hong Kong Legislative Council Sessional Papers*, Hong Kong: Government Printers.
Reichman, J. M., Brezis, M. and Steinberg, A. (1996) 'China's Eugenics Law on Maternal and Infant Health Care', *Annals of Internal Medicine*, 125(5): 425–426.
Reynolds, T. A. and Tierney, L. M. (2004) 'Medical Education in Modern China', *Journal of the American Medical Association*, 291(17): 2141
Rogaski, R. (2000) 'Hygienic Modernity in Tianjin', in Esherick, J. (ed.) *Remaking the Chinese City: Modernity and National Identity, 1900–1950*, Honolulu: University of Hawaii Press, pp. 30–46.
Salaff, J. (1973) 'Mortality Decline in the People's Republic of China and the United States', *Population Studies*, 27(3): 551–576.
Saltman, R. B. (1997) 'Convergence Versus Social Embeddedness: Debating The Future Direction Of Health Care Systems', *European Journal of Public Health*, 7(4): 449–453.
SARS Expert Committee (2003) *SARS in Hong Kong: From Experience to Action*, Hong Kong.
Scharping, T. (2002) *Birth Control in China 1949–2000: Population Policy and Demographic Development*, London: Routledge.
Schneider, L. (2003) *Biology and Revolution in Twentieth Century China*, Lanham: Rowman & Littlefield.
Science (1941) 5 September, 94(2436): 228–229.
Selwyn-Clarke, P. S. (1939) *Report of the Technical Committee for the Reorganization and Improvement of Existing Official Hospital and Clinical Facilities of the Colony of Hong Kong*, Hong Kong: Noronha & Co.
—— (1946) *Report on Medical and Health Conditions in Hong Kong for the Period 1st January, 1942–31st August, 1945*, London: His Majesty's Stationary Office.
—— (1975) *Footprints: The Memoirs of Sir Selwyn Selwyn-Clarke*, Hong Kong: Sino-American Publishing Co.
Shanghai Municipal Council (1934) *Health Department Annual Report for the Year 1934*, Shanghai: Kelly & Walsh.
Shu, H. Y. E. (1963) *The Developmental History of Medicine in China*, Seattle: Wah Young Co.
Sidel, V. W. and Sidel, R. (1973) *Serve the People: Observations on Medicine in the People's Republic of China*, Boston: Beacon Press.
Simpson, W. J. (1902) 'Preliminary Memorandum on Plague Prevention in Hong Kong', *Hong Kong Legislative Council Sessional Papers*, Hong Kong: Government Printers.

Siu, A. and Wong Y. C. (2004) 'Economic Impacts of SARS: The Case of Hong Kong', *Asian Economic Papers*, 3(1): 62–83.

Smil, V. (1999) 'China's Great Famine: 40 Years Later', *British Medical Journal*, 319: 1619–1621.

Soloman, T. (1997) 'Hong Kong 1894: The Role of James A. Lowson in the Controversial Discovery of the Plague Bacillus', *The Lancet*, 350(9070): 59–62.

Stanley, A. (1908) 'Extracts from the Health Officer's Report', *The China Medical Journal*, 22: 331–333.

Sun, K. (1919) 'Dushi guihua lun' (Essay on urban planning), *Jianshe*, 1(5): 1–17.

Sun, X. T. (1957) *Zhongguo jindai gongye shi ziliao* (Historical Materials on the Industrial Development of Modern China), Beijing: Kexue chubanshe.

Taylor, K. (2005) *Chinese Medicine in Early Communist China, 1945–63*, London, Routledge.

Tinbergen, J. (1961) 'Do Communist and Free Economies Show a Converging Pattern?', *Soviet Studies*, 12(4): 333–346.

Topley, M. (1977) 'Chinese Traditional Etiology and Methods of Cure in Hong Kong', in C. Leslie (ed.) *Asian Medical Systems*, Berkeley: University of California Press, 243–265.

Tseng, F. I. (1949) 'Retiring President's Report 1948/49', *The Bulletin of the Hong Kong Chinese Medical Association*, 2(1): 8–9.

United Nations (1948) *Universal Declaration of Human Rights*, adopted and proclaimed 10 December by UN General Assembly Resolution 217A(III).

United States Congressional-Executive Commission on China (20 October 2003) 'China's Mounting HIV/AIDS Crisis: How Should the United States Respond?' Washington DC.

Wachman, A. M. (2000) 'Taiwan: Parent, Province, or Blackballed State', *Journal of Asian and African Studies*, 35(1): 183–203.

Wacks, R. (1992) (ed.) *Human Rights in Hong Kong*, Hong Kong: Oxford University Press.

Whitehead, T. H. (1896) Report on the Tung Wa Hospital, *Hong Kong Legislative Council Sessional Papers*, Hong Kong: Government Printers.

Wong, K. C. and Wu, L. T. (1936, 2nd edn) *History of Chinese Medicine*, Tientsin: Tientsin Press.

WHO (2006) *SARS: How a Global Epidemic was Stopped*, Geneva: WHO Press, 155–180.

Wu, A. C. (1987) 'Can the Hong Kong Settlement Serve as a Model for Taiwan', in Chiu, H. D., Jao, Y. C. and Wu, Y. L. (eds) *The Future of Hong Kong*, Westport: Greenwood Press, 155–180.

Wu, T. P. (1948) 'Fighting Tuberculosis in Hong Kong', *The Bulletin of the Hong Kong Chinese Medical Association*, 1(1): 32–39.

Wu, Z. Y., Sun, X. H., Sullivan, S. G. and Detels, R. (2006) 'HIV Testing in China', *Science*, 312(5779): 1475–1476.

Yen, F. C. (1938) 'The National Health Administration during War-time', *The People's Tribune*, 23(3–4):45–47.

Yersin, A. (1894) 'La Peste Bubonique à Hong Kong', *Archives de Médecine Navale*, 62: 662–667.

Yip, K. C. (1995) *Health and National Reconstruction in Nationalist China*, Ann Arbor: Association for Asian Studies.

Zhang, Y. X. and Elvin, M. (1998) 'Tuberculosis and Environment in Modern China', in Elvin, M. and Liu, T. J. (eds) *Sediments of Time: Environment and Society in Chinese History*, Cambridge: Cambridge University Press, 520–544.

2 History of public health in modern Japan

The road to becoming the healthiest nation in the world

Masahira Anesaki

Introduction

The objectives of this chapter are to review the history of public health in modern Japan in a socio-historical context and to discuss how Japan became the healthiest nation in the world. Since the concept and the practice of public health has expanded historically (Brockington 1979: 1–8; Hanlon and Pickett 1984: 3–7; Winslow 1923: 1), this chapter covers the history not only of preventive and environmental health but also of medical care delivery; and the history of the population's health status as well as modern health promotion.

Japan's history is divided into the pre-modern and modern eras by the Meiji Restoration in 1868. The focus of the chapter is on the period since 1868, itself divided into two periods by Japan's surrender in 1945. The period before World War II has three stages: the beginning of modern Japan; industrialization and militarization; and time of war. The period from 1945 may be divided into recovery; rapid economic development; and slow economic growth.

The beginning of Modern Japan (1868–1900)

In 1853, the feudal government of the Shogun was forced by the American Commodore Perry and his fleet (the 'Black Ships') to end its two-hundred-year policy of isolation. In 1854, a treaty was signed whereby Japan opened two ports to the Americans for trade and allowed an American consul to be resident in Japan. Similar peace and friendship treaties were signed with Britain, Russia and the Netherlands, one after another. In 1858, trade treaties (later called 'Unequal Treaties' due to extra-territorial rights for foreigners) were signed with Russia, Britain, France, the Netherlands and the United States.

In 1868, administrative power was regained by a modern monarchy from the Shogunate in what is now called the 'Meiji Restoration'. The capital of the country was transferred from Kyoto to Yedo, which was renamed Tokyo. The emperor issued 'The Charter of Oath': 'Knowledge shall be sought for all over the world and thus shall be strengthened the foundation of the imperial polity'.

The foundation of the public health system

In 1872, the Department of Medical Affairs was set up in the Ministry of Education. A year later the department became a bureau, and in 1875 the bureau was moved to the Home Office and renamed the Bureau of Hygiene. In 1871–1873, a mission visited the United States and various European countries, attempting to revise the Unequal Treaties, though having no success. In the mission was Sensai Nagayo, who later became the second chief medical officer of the Ministry of Education. Having studied public health systems in the United States and Europe, he finalized the draft of the Medical Law, called 'Isei' in Japanese. The Law was the first comprehensive health statute in Japan. Enacted in 1874, it consisted of 76 articles, which covered public health administration, medical education, hospitals, licensing of health professionals, medical practitioners, midwives and acupuncturists and regulation of pharmaceutical matters.

The threat of acute infectious diseases

Towards the end of the feudal era, epidemics of old and new infectious diseases broke out. The principal causes were civil wars, the opening of ports to foreigners and poor quarantine inspection under the 1858 Unequal Treaties.

Smallpox was an old, fatal epidemic disease in Japan, originally brought by ships from the Korean Peninsula. While staying in Japan in 1848–1850, Otto Mohnicke, medical officer of the Dutch Trading House, introduced cowpox vaccination. The Shogunate established an anti-smallpox vaccination centre in Yedo, which later became the University of Tokyo Medical School. As early as 1870, the new government began to issue laws and regulations relating to smallpox prevention. However, large smallpox epidemics appeared four times: 1883–1885 (32,000 deaths); 1892–1894 (24,000 deaths); 1896–1897 (16,000 deaths); and 1904 (4,000 deaths).

Cholera came from India in 1822 for the first time. After Japan opened her ports, a second epidemic broke out in 1858. In three years more than 100,000 people died in Yedo alone. In 1877 the arrival of a cholera epidemic forced the Meiji government to issue Cholera Prevention Guidelines. In 1879, when the number of deaths was more than 100,000, the government issued Provisional Regulations for Cholera Prevention and Quarantine Inspection Regulations for the Prevention of Cholera Infection. The government also established the Central Sanitary Council and a Local Sanitary Council in each prefecture. Even after the establishment of Regulations, 500,000 people died in 1881–1882, 150,000 in 1885–1886, 40,000 in 1890 and 50,000 in 1895.

In 1880, Regulations for the Prevention of Infectious Diseases were issued. The regulations applied not only to cholera but also to typhoid, dysentery, diphtheria, typhus, smallpox and other diseases listed by local authorities, although the death rates for typhoid, dysentery and typhus were lower than those for smallpox and cholera. The regulations provided for mandatory reporting of cases by physicians, disinfection methods and compulsory admission of patients to isolation hospitals.

As well as the government efforts to control acute infectious diseases by legislation and administrative reform, a voluntary organization called the Great Japanese Sanitary Association was founded in 1883 to promote awareness of sanitation among the general populace. In 1893, local public health administration became the responsibility of the police.

Victory in the Sino-Japanese War of 1894–1895 enhanced Japan's international standing. The Unequal Treaties were revised in 1894, and new treaties negotiated in 1899. In 1897, the Infectious Diseases Prevention Act was enacted. In 1899, the Seaport Quarantine Act was enacted. A Seaport Quarantine Station and an Institute for Research on Infectious Diseases were established. Quarantine inspection was now carried out under Japanese jurisdiction. This system proved a success with those returning from China after the Sino-Japanese War. By 1900, Japan had managed to ride out the storms of the first period of the acute infectious diseases era.

German medicine as a model

In 1868, the Shogunate government had allowed Western medicine to be introduced. The new Meiji government supported it, renouncing Chinese medicine. The government decided to follow Germany as a model and to build 'a rich country with a strong army'. It thus aimed to emulate the German medical system. In 1870, the forerunner of the Medical School at Tokyo University invited two instructors from the German army school to visit. In 1871, they established a new medical education system at Tokyo University from where Western medicine spread all over Japan. From 1876, a licence to practice medicine was granted only to those trained in Western medical science. The excluded practitioners of Chinese medicine were still in a majority, but their struggle for inclusion in the new system failed against a background of officially endorsed westernization of the country.

From public to private dominance of hospitals

Before the Meiji Restoration there was only one hospital which had been built by the Shogunate, on the advice of Dutch naval surgeon Pompe van Meerdervoort, to assist in the modernization of medicine. After 1868, both central and local governments began to build public hospitals attached to medical schools. But due to the heavy cost of medical schools and the centralization policy of the central government, in 1887, an ordinance banned support for medical schools from prefectural taxes and forced many prefectural hospitals to be closed. Private practitioners then began to convert their clinics into hospitals. By 1898, there were 136 government hospitals and 518 private ones. Except for military hospitals and leading national university hospitals, the private sector dominated health-care delivery from the end of the nineteenth century (see Table 2.1).

Table 2.1 Number of hospitals by owners in the Meiji period

Year	Total	Government			Private
		Sub-total	National	Local	
1874	52	23	—	—	29
1875	63	41	—	—	22
1876	97	65	—	—	32
1877	159	124	12	112	35
1878	235	175	29	146	60
1879	309	219	42	177	90
1880	363	241	28	213	122
1881	510	355	29	306	175
1882	626	330	—	—	296
1883	—	—	—	—	—
1888*	556	225	—	—	339
1889	573	222	—	—	351
1890	577	214	—	—	363
1891	579	197	—	—	382
1892	576	198	—	—	378
1893	579	198	2	106	382
1894	597	189	2	187	408
1895	589	174	2	172	415
1896	592	166	2	164	426
1897	624	159	3	156	465
1898	654	136	3	133	518

Source: Japan Ministry of Health and Welfare (1955): 818.

Note
* Figures from 1883 to 1887 are unavailable.

Industrialization and militarization (1900–1930)

The government promoted industrialization in order to compete with the advanced Western powers. Towards the end of the nineteenth century, Japan experienced an industrial revolution in light industries like textiles which was followed by the development of heavy industry. In the meantime, it established a colonial empire in Asia. After the Sino-Japanese War, Japan colonized Taiwan, and after the Russo-Japanese War, in 1910, it colonized Korea. It should be noted that Japan's rapid industrialization and militarization were achieved through the exploitation of industrial workers and peasants and colonial peoples.

Control of chronic diseases

After the establishment of the acute communicable disease control programme, chronic diseases attracted government concern. These included venereal diseases, leprosy, mental disorders, tuberculosis, silicosis, beriberi, trachoma and some particularly unpleasant parasitic diseases endemic to the country. In 1900 the

Table 2.2 Number of hospitals in the Meiji period

Year	Total number	Hospitals	Branch hospitals	Insane asylums	VD hospitals	Beriberi hospitals	Leper houses	Others
1875	63	59	—	—	3	—	—	1
1876	97	89	—	—	7	—	—	1
1877	159	146	—	—	12	—	—	1
1878	135	124	63	1	40	—	4	3
1879	309	165	71	3	61	—	6	3
1880	363	234	55	3	57	3	6	5
1881	510	281	73	5	135	4	5	7
1882	626	402	64	6	130	5	5	14

Source: Japan Ministry of Health and Welfare (1955): 821.

government set up a system of medical examination of prostitutes for venereal diseases and passed the Law for Care and Custody of Mentally Disordered Persons. In 1904 the Cattle Tuberculosis Prevention Act was introduced.

Venereal diseases

Venereal disease (VD) first appeared in Japan in 1515 and it spread quickly across the country. In the early 1880s, medical examination of conscripts revealed that about two-thirds of examinees suffered from VD. Table 2.2 illustrates the number of VD hospitals at the beginning of the modern era.

Officially permitted red-light districts were common in most cities during the latter half of the feudal era. The prostitutes were usually girls from poor backgrounds who had been sold to brothels as a means of raising money for the family. The system continued until 1957 when the Anti-Prostitution Law came into force; it lasted so long because of a long history of licensed quarters for brothels, strong opposition to the abolition movement from the owners of brothels and the relative indifference of a male-dominated political world.

A system of inspection of prostitutes was introduced after a request in 1860 from the Russian Admiral, Evfimii Vasilievich Putiatin, whose crew were allowed ashore while their damaged vessel was undergoing repairs. The inspections were organized by Pompe van Meerdervoort and his students. Similar checks were organized in Yokohama in 1867 to protect British soldiers after a request by the British minister, Harry Smith Parkes. In the same year the system was expanded to cover the whole country. Records of the day show that in 1878, 65.1% of employed prostitutes were infected with VD; by 1883, 75.8% were infected and by 1888, this figure had reached 92%. Under the Prostitution Control Law of 1900, inspection became compulsory and an officially sanctioned prostitution system continued. Further legislation, the Venereal Disease Prevention Law, was passed in 1927. This law targeted not only prostitutes but other vulnerable groups of people like geisha girls. It provided for the establishment of VD clinics by the local governments, central government subsidies for the establishment of clinics and the punishment of prostitutes who knowingly passed on infections.

Leprosy

People with leprosy had traditionally faced vicious discrimination. Rejected by their families and the community, they were condemned to a life as wandering beggars or vagabond pilgrims. Some remote temples and shrines organized loosely-knit communities for sufferers. Foreigners were particularly appalled by the conditions of the patients; their complaints to the authorities caused the Japanese government some considerable embarrassment. Several private 'leprosaria' had been set up in the mid-nineteenth century, and from the 1890s Christian missionary groups ran another group of facilities. Neither the leprosaria nor the university dermatology departments were capable of doing much for sufferers. The government finally took radical action in 1907, introducing the Lepers Control Regulation. This established five public, regional leprosaria and empowered local authorities to detain homeless patients. Administration of the Leprosy (Hansen's disease) Control Act rested with the police who had similar powers for the control of acute infectious diseases. Since Hansen's disease was not curable, those detained were essentially condemned to a life sentence in the leprosaria, which offered little therapy for residents. In 1931, the 1907 Regulation was revised and the Leprosy Prevention Law provided for free, in-patient care for all leprosy patients at government-run facilities.

Mentally ill people

Japan has historically paid little attention to the welfare and rights of mentally ill people. In feudal times they were sent to a prison or a remote island. In 1878, the Tokyo Metropolitan Police Board issued an order that whoever intended to keep a mentally disordered person in a private house had to seek permission from the police and to furnish a medical certificate signed by a doctor. The Criminal Law of 1880 was the first to state that crimes committed by a mentally disturbed person should not be punished. In 1900, the Mentally Disordered Persons Supervision and Protection Law was enacted. This law made it the liability of the family, or the mayor of the town or village where there was no family, to supervise a psychotic person. It prohibited confinement without sufficient reason. These laws were progressive but the reality was different. In 1918 a Tokyo University professor of psychiatry carried out a comprehensive survey of mentally-ill patients detained in private houses and revealed the misery of many. There were 18 government mental hospitals with about 1,000 beds and 37 private hospitals with about 4,000 beds. But an estimated 130,000 to 140,000 mentally disordered persons were denied the benefit of modern medicine. They had been forsaken by both the state and the community. In 1918 the Mental Hospital Law was enacted to promote the establishment of public and private mental hospitals through provision of subsidies and to give care and protection to patients through hospitalization. Even so, progress in the establishment of mental hospitals was slow. Many mentally disordered persons are still put under restraint in a private house without medical attention.

Tuberculosis

From the beginning of the nineteenth century, epidemics of tuberculosis broke out. The majority of patients were working girls. When found ill, a girl was sent back home. It was not long before tuberculosis spread in her family and then around the community.

A hygienist, Dr Osamu Ishihara, did an excellent epidemiological survey on 'female factory workers and tuberculosis', which was published in 1913. He described in detail the horrendous living and working conditions of factory workers and presented his theory on the spread of tuberculosis from the girls to the rest of the community. Dr Ishihara compared mortality rates for females in the same age groups in the community and in factories. He blamed industrialists for the deaths of 5,000 female workers annually. His work promoted the introduction of the Factory Act in 1916. This Act prescribed an 11-hour working day for women and children, and a minimum working age of 13 years.

In 1913, the Tuberculosis Prevention Association was organized as a private organization to campaign for tuberculosis prevention. The next year a law providing for subsidization of new sanatoria was enacted. However, the only treatment available at the time was fresh air, rest and a nutritious diet. Different therapies were tried with little success, and not until after World War II was the disease brought under control.

Silicosis, endemic parasitic diseases, beriberi and trachoma

Around 1900, legislative and other measures were taken to combat silicosis, endemic parasitic diseases, beriberi and trachoma. In 1890, the Water Supply Act and the Mining Industries Act were passed. Partly to deal with trachoma among school children, in 1897, the Regulations for School Cleanliness and for Periodical Physical Examinations were issued. In 1900, further public health legislation was enacted: the Nuisances Removal Act; the Sewerage Act; and the Regulations of Food and Drink Act. In the same year, the Department of School Health was founded at the Ministry of Education. Soon after came the Mining Industry Act in 1905 and the aforementioned Factory Act in 1911.

Socialization of the medical care payment system

Payment for medical services was not regulated so doctors charged their patients any level of fees they wished and high fees became a concern. In 1911, the emperor issued an imperial proclamation on charitable medical care. Money donated by the emperor and public donations allowed the government to set up an imperial charitable foundation. By 1936 this foundation ran 15 hospitals, 3 sanatoria, 1 maternity hospital, 1 nursery, 10 visiting medical units, 12 mobile nurses units and 61 clinics in various parts of the country.

Also in 1911, a dedicated physician, ex-businessman and parliamentarian set up a chain of discount clinics. The clinics had such strong support, especially among the working class, that clinic development became a national movement. The clinics promoted the organization of medical cooperatives and the introduction of social health insurance. Towards the end of the nineteenth century mutual aid associations (predecessors of health insurance societies) had become well organized among employees of mines, textile companies and government agencies such as railways, printing offices, mints, postal and telecommunications offices.

Japan's first social health insurance law was passed in 1922 and came into force in 1927, almost 50 years after the world's first health insurance law was passed by the German Reichstag. It provided for medical treatment and cash benefits for up to 180 days, but included only 2 million out of an estimated 4.7 million workers.

Independence of Japanese medicine in education and research

In 1887, the last two German professors in the Tokyo University Medical School retired, and all chairs came to be occupied by Japanese. From 1890, following the establishment of the Japan Medical Society, specialist societies were organized. By 1912, there were 14 such societies, covering hygiene, anatomy, otorhinolaryngology, paediatrics, ophthalmology, surgery, gastrology, dermatology, psychiatry and neurology, dentistry, obstetrics and gynaecology, internal medicine, pathology and urology. Moreover, Japanese medical researchers were now making significant medical discoveries.

The road to World War II (1930–1945)

In this period, economic crises affected working and living conditions. The incidence of tuberculosis was high and growing. The infant mortality rate was also high. Many areas lacked doctors, clinics or hospitals. Even if a doctor was available, the number of the insured was so limited that most people could not afford to use his services.

The early 1930s saw two notable attempts to remedy these deficiencies. One was the movement for cooperative medical care facilities, and the other was the communist movement for medical care facilities for poor workers. The cooperative movement, in association with other groups like the agricultural cooperative association, was taken over during the war by the Japan Medical Corporation, the official body in charge of wartime medical services. The authorities closed down the facilities of the second group.

In the 1930s, extremists in the military took Japan down the path of militarism. Japan started the 'Fifteen-year War' with China and became involved in World War II. The Japanese government had established medical schools in its colonial territories, Taiwan, Korea and Manchuria (northeast China), from the beginning of the twentieth century. In Taiwan and Korea, medical faculties were established at imperial universities in addition to a couple of junior medical colleges in each territory. Those imperial university medical faculties catered for Japanese and local elite students. The majority of patients seen at affiliated hospitals were Japanese. These medical institutions and the rest of the public health infrastructure were for the benefit of the colonial elite rather than the local people. In Manchuria the notorious bacteriological warfare research department, Unit 731, under the command of Lieutenant General Shiro Ishii, did medical experiments on Chinese and other prisoners and the Manchuria Medical School became associated with this unit.

The military forces were so worried about the poor health of conscripts they demanded the establishment of an independent Ministry of Health and Welfare intended to produce 'healthy and strong soldiers'. In 1938, the Ministry was established, and community public health centres started to offer preventive services and health education. Also in 1938, the National Health Insurance Act was passed and this covered self-employed people such as farmers and fishermen and their families.

On 8 December 1941, the Pacific War began. The National Medical Service Act of 1942 regulated all matters relating to the medical and health professions, establishing the Japan Medical Corporation to control a network of medical facilities across the country. But the war ended before the establishment of a national, pyramidal, medical care delivery system. Nevertheless, the war years saw some expansion of the health insurance system and by 1945 approximately one-third of the population was covered by some insurance. On the other hand, the war severely limited the availability of health care because bombing destroyed many facilities and interrupted production of drugs and medical supplies; it also forced male physicians into the military forces.

Post-war rehabilitation (1945–1961)

Ten million out of a population of 73 million had been called up as soldiers, of whom 2 million died on the battlefield; between 300,000 and 1,000,000 civilians were killed in air raids and other wartime emergencies; and 3.1 million houses were burnt down. Transport and communications were almost totally paralyzed. Immediately after the war, the health of the people was at a low ebb. Food shortages sapped people's resistance to disease and shortened life expectancy markedly. Insanitary conditions aggravated by the repatriation of 7 million people caused epidemics of acute infectious diseases not known since the period when Japan opened its ports under the Unequal Treaties. Tuberculosis, venereal disease and parasites like roundworm were major problems.

Epidemics of acute infectious diseases

Lice and typhus

Under the insanitary conditions in the years just before and after the war, there were plagues of fleas, lice, flies and mosquitoes. Only 100 cases of typhus were reported in 1943, but the number of typhus cases increased to 3,941 in 1944, 2,461 in 1945 and 32,366, (of whom those who died numbered 3,351) in 1946. The pathogens were brought into the country from continental Asia.

Smallpox

Smallpox had been virtually forgotten following the Regulations for the Prevention of Smallpox of 1876. It was reported again soon after Japan began to fight the Fifteen-Year War with China and became serious in 1941 when Japan began to fight the Pacific War and sent soldiers to different parts of Asia. Some brought back the infection from smallpox-contaminated areas. Cases increased: 385 in 1942, 546 in 1943, 311 in 1944, 1,614 in 1945 and 17, 945 (of which 3,029 were fatal) in 1946. The last was the highest number since 1908.

The suppression of epidemics

The General Headquarters (GHQ) of the Allied Powers brought hundreds of thousands of pounds of Dichloro-Diphenyl-Trichloroethane (DDT) into Japan to spray from planes and at the street corners to exterminate lice-spreading typhus. This massive spraying campaign quickly brought the epidemic under control.

The Ministry of Health and Welfare dispatched health officials to various parts of the country to give advice and provide preventive inoculations against typhoid fever, paratyphoid and typhus, and to ensure DDT spraying was carried out. As a result, the number of the cases of infectious disease decreased remarkably even in 1947. From 1948, the Preventive Vaccination Law provided for periodic, compulsory inoculations against infectious diseases such as smallpox, typhoid, paratyphoid, diphtheria, whooping cough and tuberculosis. The law also provided for temporary inoculations against other six diseases: typhus, cholera, plague, scarlet fever, influenza and Weil's disease. Infectious diseases appeared in the chaotic situation after the war and then quickly vanished, with the last three cases of typhus being reported in 1951. However, the side effects of DDT and the compulsory inoculations became problems later. In the early 1970s, the use of DDT was prohibited and a law of compensation for inoculation victims was enacted.

Other problems: tuberculosis, VD, parasites and poliomyelitis

Tuberculosis

Tuberculosis was called Japan's national disease for it was pre-eminent among the causes of death. In 1947, the death rate was as high as 187.2 per 100,000 population.

The Ministry of Health and Welfare promulgated in 1948 the Preventive Vaccination Law which required people under the age of 30 years to have a tuberculin test once a year and, where necessary, to be inoculated with the BCG vaccine. The new Tuberculosis Control Law, enacted in 1951, provided for routine examinations, registration of patients, preventive measures, medical treatment and public financial support for tuberculosis patients.

In 1952, the domestic production of streptomycin and para-aminosalicyclic acid (PAS) began, and isoniazid joined them. The combined chemotherapy worked so miraculously that the number of deaths decreased almost by half to 60,000 in 1950–1958. In 1951 tuberculosis was replaced by cerebrovascular diseases as the greatest killer. Japan can be proud of these effective control measures.

Venereal disease

Traditionally, venereal diseases were considered to be primarily diseases of prostitutes and control involved their periodic examination. As the GHQ of the Allied Powers regarded this as worthless from a medical standpoint, they abrogated all laws that authorized licensed prostitution in 1946. From 1948 the Venereal Disease Prevention Law provided for premarital education and examination for VD, required physicians to report cases treated and patients to seek treatment, and authorized government subsidization of medical fees as well as establishment of VD clinics. The advent of penicillin improved dramatically the effectiveness of treatment (Sams 1962: 472–480).

Parasites

In 1947, national statistics revealed that roundworms were found in 60% of the population. This high prevalence was attributable mainly to the use of human excrement as manure, and the habit of eating raw fish and fresh vegetables and a shortage of good quality vermicides.

Post-war recovery and promotion of welfare and health

The new constitution, called the Constitution of Pacifism and Democracy, came into force in May 1947. Article 25 states: 'All people shall have the right to maintain the minimum standards of wholesome and cultural living. In all spheres of life the state shall use its endeavors for the promotion and extension of social welfare and security and of public health'. It was a revolution that the new constitution guaranteed the right to life and established state responsibility to promote welfare, social security and public health. This article became the foundation of social and health policy.

Some intellectuals saw the British welfare state as a model for Japan. During the early period of the occupation, government committees drew up idealistic blueprints for a social security system based upon social insurance.

After a period of hyperinflation around 1950, Japan's economy stabilized. Consumption expenditure reached 80% of the pre-war level in 1950 and exceeded it in 1953. The Korean War broke out in 1950 but the pacifist constitution prohibited Japan from participating directly. The country reaped large economic benefits from the war. The Japanese Peace Treaty came into force on 28 April 1952, the occupation ceased, and Japan became an independent nation again.

Universal health insurance was achieved, finally, in 1961. The number of health facilities steadily increased so that the number of hospitals by 1947 exceeded the total in 1941. In 1948 the Medical Service Act, the Medical Practitioners Act, the Dental Practitioners Act, the Nurses Act and the Dental Hygienists Act were passed. The aim was to improve the quality of health services and the effectiveness of the health professions. Legislation concerning other health professions soon followed.

Rapid economic development and new health problems (1961–1973)

Health protection measures

Rapid industrialization disrupted the natural environment and people's health. From 1953 to the early 1960s, in a fishing village called Minamata, a strange disease causing spastic paralysis was prevalent. The cause of Minamata disease was identified as sea food contaminated with organic methyl mercury discharged from a chemical factory. In 1964, cases of the same disease were found along a river the water of which was contaminated by another large factory. The disease was called 'Ouch ouch' disease. Air pollution produced by petrochemical complexes caused many cases of asthma.

From the mid-1950s, subacute myelo-opticoneuropathy (SMON), caused by clinoquinol, an antidiarrhoeal, appeared. Pregnant women, who took thalidomide pills, gave birth to babies with deformed limbs. Public concern about health hazards heightened. In 1967, the Public Nuisance Basic Act was passed, and in 1968 the Air Pollution Prevention Act. The 1970 Diet session was called the 'public nuisance session', at which six new laws and eight amendments passed including the Water Pollution Prevention Act, the Ocean Pollution Prevention Act and the Control of Poisons and Powerful Drugs Act.

Expansion of health-care delivery

In order to address the oversupply of physicians after the war, the government restricted the training of new physicians for some time. However, because a sharp increase was predicted in the demand for medical care after the introduction of universal health insurance, the government planned to increase the intake of medical students and even allowed the establishment of new medical schools from 1970. The 'one medical school at one prefecture' policy was instituted in 1973. The government's target was to reach 150 physicians per 100,000 population by 1985. This goal was achieved two years earlier. Private sector dominance in the field of health care was restored in the period of high economic growth and strengthened after heavy political pressure from the Japanese Medical Association which represented the interests of private practitioners and physician-owned, private hospitals. Moreover, private hospitals have since 1950 enjoyed tax exemption. In 1960, the new Medical Finance Corporation began to provide hospitals with long-term, low-interest loans, and the government limited the increase in public hospital beds. Thus private hospitals came to enjoy a favorable position.

Changes in mortality and morbidity

The death rate was 14.6 per 1,000 population in 1947. It continued to fall sharply and in 1963 it was down to 7.0.

From the mid-1930s to 1950, tuberculosis was the premier cause of death while pneumonia and bronchitis ranked second. Thanks to anti-tuberculosis drugs and antibiotics and other measures, deaths due to these diseases continued to fall steadily. In 1951, tuberculosis fell to second place, being replaced by cerebrovascular diseases. In 1960, cerebrovascular diseases, cancer and heart diseases, lifestyle-related or degenerative diseases, became the first, second and third causes of death. Tuberculosis fell to seventh place. In 1960, death by accidents was in fifth place for the first time, reflecting rapid industrialization. An increase in suicide deaths in the 1960s is noteworthy. A large shift in the main causes of death from infectious diseases to lifestyle-related diseases occurred at the end of the 1950s.

A turning point (1973 to the beginning of the twenty-first century)

From expansion to containment in health-care finance

The year 1973 was a turning point for the social security system. The government instituted free medical care for the aged, reduced the percentage of co-payment required of dependants from 50% to 30%, and introduced a ceiling on the total amount of co-payment. Japan also introduced a new universal pension scheme. Tragically, all of these benefits originating in Japan's era of high economic growth came to a halt in October of the same year, when the Fourth Arab-Israeli War began. The Organization of Oil Exporting Countries (OPEC) used oil supplies as a diplomatic weapon and restricted the exports to the countries supporting Israel. Most Western countries as well as Japan were affected, and oil prices increased by 30% to 70%. Japan's high economic growth, which relied almost wholly on imported oil as its energy source, slowed. Eventually, the government had to introduce cost-containment measures in all areas including the health services.

Primary health care and health promotion

In 1978 at Alma-Ata in Soviet Russia, at an international conference on primary health care, the Alma-Ata Declaration was agreed upon as was the principle of 'Health for All by the Year 2000'. The gist of the declaration was the promotion of community health care. In response to the declaration, the Japanese government encouraged autonomous health promotion projects by local communities and introduced model cases. The government also formulated a National Health Promotion Plan which involved comprehensive, lifetime, health promotion measures. This was the first ten-year plan; the second plan started in 1988. From 2000, under the new revised plan, Healthy Japan 21, the government mapped out measures to promote mental and physical health including prevention of lifestyle-related diseases.

Japan had a higher smoking rate (more than 40% among men) than Western nations. The state monopoly tobacco industry from 1898 to 1997 contributed to this high smoking rate. A new problem is an increase in smoking among minors. The government has regarded anti-tobacco measures as one of the important themes in public health. Healthy Japan 21 has four goals concerning smoking: diffusion of sufficient knowledge about the effects of smoking on health; elimination of smoking by minors; thorough separation of smokers from non-smokers in common areas; and the promotion of a support program for smokers hoping to stop smoking.

Japan has begun to produce leaders in international health administration. In 1979, Dr Hiroshi Nakajima became the Director of World Health Organization (WHO) Western Pacific Region. In 1988, he was elected director-general of the WHO, retaining this position until 1998. In 1979, the WHO declared the eradication of smallpox from the earth, a task which had been performed by a WHO team led by Dr Isao Arita. From 1999, Dr Shigehiro Omi was the director of the WHO Western Pacific Region.

In 1982 the Health Service System for the Elderly Act was passed. This law introduced a co-payment for medical care of elderly patients and a cost-sharing arrangement with other insurers. It also provided for preventive measures like health checkups and health education for people over 40 years of age.

To address the rapid ageing of the population (and sharp increase in the number of senile elderly), measures to promote home and community care were introduced under the Gold Plan in the 1990s. The latest version of the plan, Gold Plan 21, was to be revised in 2005. The Gold Plan comprises ideological principles and specific numerical targets for home and community care for the elderly. The principles are the creation of a vital image of the elderly, the securing of the dignity of the elderly and the establishment of long-term care services. The numerical targets cover the numbers of home helpers, home-visit nursing care stations, day-care centres, short-stay centres, welfare facilities, health-care facilities, group homes, care houses and living-support houses.

The number of elderly people in need of long-term care was estimated to increase so rapidly as to be 5.3 million in 2005 (it was only 2.8 million in 2000). Long-term care provided by local government was so limited that a heavy burden was carried by family members. Moreover, the caretakers themselves were ageing.

In accordance with the Gold Plan and to support the cost of long-term care, in 2000, the Long-Term Care Insurance Act for elderly people was passed. Under this act municipalities are insurers and those people 40 years old and over are the insured. Benefits paid out under the system are 50% funded by public money (25% from the central government and 25% from prefectural governments) and 50% by premiums and co-payments. Those who need domiciliary or institutional long-term care services and are 65 years of age and over apply for care to the municipal governments and those certified as requiring long-term care are classified into six groups according to the level of care they require.

The number of people receiving care almost doubled from April 2000 to December 2003. This scheme is reviewed every five years. In 2005, revisions were being made concerning prevention of deterioration; enhancement of domiciliary services; care for the elderly with dementia; and a response to increased costs from the increasing number of users (Ministry of Health, Labour and Welfare 2004: 175–178).

Measures against infectious diseases

At least in economically advanced countries, people have been free from serious bacterial diseases since the advent of vaccines, antibiotics and DDT. However, more recently, serious viral diseases such as HIV/AIDS, SARS, West Nile fever, avian influenza, Ebola hemorrhagic fever and an infectious protein as in Creutzfeldt-Jacob's disease have appeared as new threats. Japanese haemophiliacs have caught HIV/AIDS through contaminated blood products. HIV carriers and AIDS patients are increasing in number, in particular, among young people and homosexual males.

Japan has succeeded in preventing a SARS, avian flu or Ebola haemorrhagic fever outbreak. There has been one Creutzfeldt-Jacob's disease patient who had spent 24 days in Britain in 1990 where he had eaten beef; he died in December 2004. The new Infectious Disease Law of 1999, which was revised in 2003, provides for stricter quarantine inspection, prevention and disinfecting measures, food safety measures (including the restriction of beef imports to prevent Bovine spongiform encephalopathy (BSE)-infected cattle meat from being imported), the detection of avian influenza-infected birds, and more efficient international cooperation and communication. It is claimed that Japanese hygienic habits like regular hand-washing and gargles may also contribute to the high level of prevention of infections.

Conclusion

Key health indices like average life expectancy and infant mortality suggest that Japan has become the healthiest country in the world (see Figures 2.1; 2.2 and 2.3). The following factors are considered to have contributed to this outcome: (1) the long period of peace after World War II; (2) the public health policies of the occupation forces, measures against acute infectious diseases, DDT spraying and vaccinations to protect the occupying troops also benefited the Japanese; (3) antibiotics that could be produced and distributed by Japanese firms; (4) a universal health insurance system that made health care easily accessible; (5) an excess of physicians

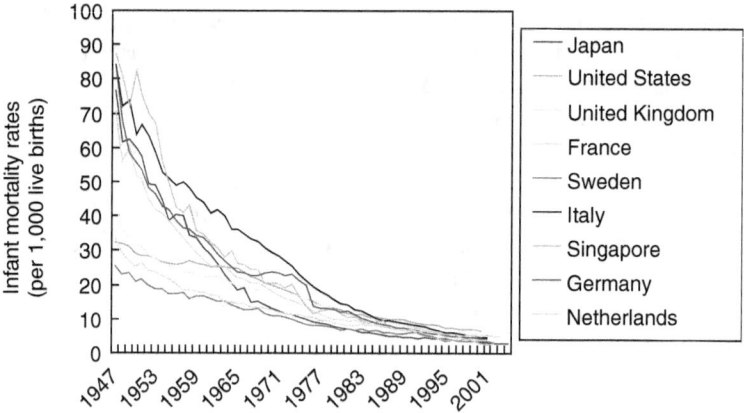

Figure 2.1 Infant mortality rates in selected countries (1947–2004).

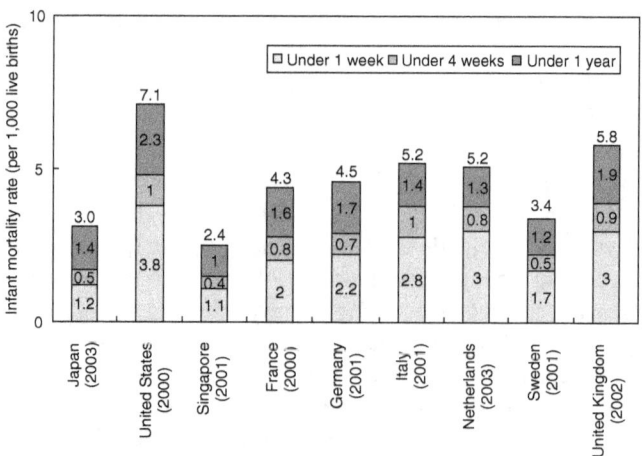

Figure 2.2 Infant mortality rates by age in selected countries.

History of public health in modern Japan 71

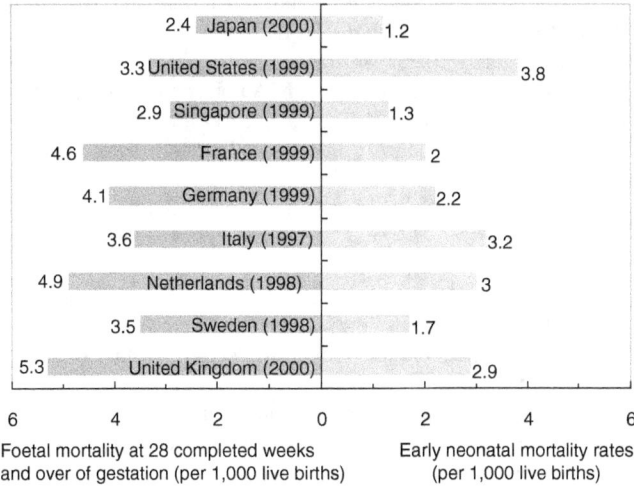

Figure 2.3 Perinatal mortality rates in selected countries.
Sources: Ministry of Health, Labour and Welfare (2004: 23, 25 and 33).

produced in war time that facilitated access to health care; (6) Japan's economic growth that raised the standard of living; (7) development of maternal and child health, school health, occupational health and health care for the elderly; and (8) underlying these factors, a compulsory education system dating from the beginning of the modern era.

As the healthiest country, Japan may reasonably be expected to collaborate with other countries to promote global health; not only through large aid projects but also provision of personal health services and infrastructure such as safe water supplies.

Notes

The general history is based upon Storry (1960). Information on public health matters is drawn from Anesaki and Munakata (2001), Kawakami (2002), Ohtani (1971), Powell and Anesaki (1990) and Tatara (1991).

With thanks to Doctors Kiyohiko Katahira, Yukiko Katsumata, Takeshi Kawakami, Milton J. Lewis, Ayumi Mishiro, Ryu Niki, Saburo Nishi, Fujio Ohtani, Eikichi Urata and Mitsuhiro Ushio for their advice on this chapter.

References

Anesaki, Masahira and Munakata, Tsunetsugu (2001) 'Health, Illness, and Health Policy in Japan', in William C. Cockerham (ed.) *The Blackwell Companion to Medical Sociology*, Oxford: Blackwell Publishers, 441–455.

Brockington, C. Fraser (1979) 'The History of Public Health', in W. Hobson (ed.) *The Theory and Practice of Public Health* (5th edn), Oxford: Oxford University Press, 1–8.

Hanlon, John J. and Pickett, George E. (1984) *Public Health: Administration and Practice*, (8th edn), St. Louis: Times Mirror/Mosby.

Hashimoto, Masami (1981) 'National Health Administration in Japan', in Masami Hashimoto, Nobuhiro Maruchi, Yuji Kawaguchi, Akira Matsuda and Kazuo Nishioka (eds) *Sekai no Koshueisei* (Public Health in the World), Tokyo, Japanese Society of Public Health: 769–809.

Imukyoku (Bureau of Medical Affairs), Kouseishou (Japan Ministry of Health and Welfare) (1976) *Isei 100 nenshi (One Hundred Year History of the Medical System in Japan)*, Tokyo: Gyosei.

Japan Ministry of Health and Welfare (1955) *Isei 80 nenshi* (History of Medical Care for Eighty Years), Tokyo: Government Printing Office.

Kawakami, Takeshi (2002) *Sengo Nihon Byoninshi* (Post-war History of Patients in Japan), Tokyo: Nosangyosonbunnkakyokai.

Maruchi, N. and Matsuda, M. (1991) 'Provision and Financing of Health Care Services in Japan', in Walter W. Holland, Roger Detels and George Knox (eds) *Oxford Textbook of Public Health*, Oxford: Oxford University Press, 333–346.

Ministry of Health, Labour and Welfare (2003) *Annual Report on Health, Labour and Welfare 2002–2003*, Tokyo: Japan International Corporation of Welfare Services.

—— (2004) *Annual Report on Health, Labour and Welfare 2003–2004*, Tokyo: Japan International Corporation of Welfare Services.

—— (2005) *Annual Report on Health, Labour and Welfare 2004–2005*, Tokyo: Japan International Corporation of Welfare Services.

Ohtani, Fujio (1971) *One Hundred Years of Health Progress in Japan*, Tokyo: International Medical Foundation of Japan.

Onodera, Nobuo (1991) 'Public Health Services in Japan', in Walter W. Holland, Roger Detels and George Knox (eds) *Oxford Textbook of Public Health*, Oxford: Oxford University Press, 253–260.

Powell, Margaret and Anesaki, Masahira (1990) *Health Care in Japan*, London: Routledge.

Regional Office for Europe, World Health Organization (1978) *Glossary of Health Care Terminology*, Regional Office for Europe, World Health Organization: Copenhagen.

Sams, Crawford F. (1962) *Medic*, Hoover Institute on War, Revolution and Peace, Stanford University, unpublished memoir.

Storry, Richard (1960) *A History of Modern Japan*, Middlesex: Penguin Books.

Tatara, Kozo (1991) 'The Origins and Development of Public Health in Japan', in Walter W. Holland, Roger Detels and George Knox (eds), *Oxford Textbook of Public Health*, Oxford: Oxford University Press, 35–48.

University of California, Berkeley, Public Health Library. *What is Public Health?* Online. Available <http//www.lib.berkeley.edu/PUBL/whatisph.html> (accessed 8 December 2004).

Winslow, C.-E. A. (1920) 'The Untilled Fields of Public Health', *Science*, 51(1306): 23–33.

—— (1923) *The Evolution and Significance of the Modern Public Health Campaign*, New Haven: Yale University Press.

3 A history of public health in Korea

In-sok Yeo

Introduction

This chapter will focus on the introduction and development of a modern public health system in Korea over the past one hundred years, a period dramatic in its impact on Korean society and its health.

The 'opening' of the country in 1876, Japanese colonization and occupation (1910–1945), liberation from Japan (1945), the subsequent division into South Korea and North Korea, the Korean war (1950–1953), a military coup in 1961, and more recently, rapid economic development, have all influenced the history of public health and determined its characteristics. Although the history of medicine and health in pre-modern Korea will be touched upon, this disproportion is in a sense inevitable, given that public health is a relatively modern concept, and it was the modern state that began to realize its importance in maintaining social stability. Furthermore, the focus will be on South Korea as North Korea is beyond the purview of this essay. This general survey will highlight the interaction of medicine and society and state/society relationships in the foundation of public health in Korea.

Public health in the pre-modern period

In the pre-modern period, health was viewed more as a problem of the individual than as a problem of society. *Yang-saeng* (養生, nurturing life), based on Chinese medical theory and practice, was the key term that represented the traditional concept of maintaining or 'preserving' the health of an individual including diet, clothing and housing. The word originated from Taoist thought with the ultimate goal of prolonging life, but it was also widely used in Confucian culture since preserving one's body was a tenet of filial piety, one of the main Confucian virtues. Along with *yang-saeng*, *wi-saeng* (衛生, guarding life) was another term that bore almost the same connotation as *yang-saeng*. It was used later as the translation for 'hygiene' in China, Japan and Korea, which referred to health of a population as a whole (Park 2003: 35).

In pre-modern Korea, as elsewhere in Asia, the main problem of public health was the outbreak of epidemics. Records of epidemics in official dynastic histories date back for almost two thousand years. *Chosen Wangjo*

Shilok (朝鮮王朝實錄, 'The authentic chronicle of the Chosen dynasty, CE 1392–1910') records numerous epidemics but it is difficult to make a retrospective identification of the diseases (except for smallpox) due to the differences between traditional and modern thinking and terminology.

Thus, evil spirits that roamed between heaven and earth were believed to be responsible for the outbreaks of epidemics. Ritual offerings of rice, broth, liquor and meat were made to appease these spirits. The central government sent officials to carry out these rituals in areas where the epidemics had occurred (Shin 1997: 29). Medical treatment was not clearly distinguished from non-medical treatment. Traditional medical texts such as *Byuk Yeok Shin Bang* (辟疫新方, 'New prescriptions for warding off epidemics') did attribute the outbreaks of epidemics to unseasonable climate and meteorological activities and recommended treatment using fumigation by certain aromatics. However, fumigation was probably believed to ward off evil spirits and medical texts also recommended wearing protective talismans. Epidemic control measures such as isolating infected persons in a remote place or burning the belongings of the victims were helpful, though hardly effective as when cholera epidemics broke out in the early nineteenth century with high mortality (Shin 1997: 26). The understanding of the causes of epidemics and their control remained unchanged until the introduction of Western medicine and modern knowledge of hygiene and etiology of diseases.

The introduction of Western medicine and emergence of a public health system

Western medicine was introduced to Korea in two stages. The first stage covers the period from the seventeenth to the early nineteenth century when translations of Western medical texts were imported from China. The second stage is the period from the late nineteenth century when Western medical practices and treatment were introduced by medical missionaries. In the first period, Korean scholars such as Yi Ik (李瀷, 1681–1763) and Yi Kyu-kyung (李圭景, 1788–?) reproduced in their writings what they had learned from these books. The knowledge that they acquired, however, was not that of contemporary Western medicine. In other words, it was not the anatomy of Vesalius or physiology of Harvey (Lee 1954: 213), but the medieval version of Galenic medicine. Furthermore, no special mention of public health or hygiene is to be found. The writings of Choe Han-ki (崔漢綺, 1803–1877), however, mark a new period in understanding Western medicine. He wrote a medical work entitled *Shin Ki Chon Hum* (身機踐驗) that was based on the five medical books of Benjamin Hobson (1816–1873), a British medical missionary in China. Hobson's medical books, published in the 1850s, were very popular not only in China, but also in Korea and Japan. His books dealt with anatomy and areas of clinical medicine such as paediatrics, gynaecology and internal medicine (全體新論, 西醫略論, 內科新說, 婦嬰新說, 博物新編). In addition, hygiene in the modern sense takes up a considerable portion of Hobson's books. We can presume that Choe Han-ki learned the modern concept of hygiene from these works, but it was not generally known outside of a small circle of scholars (Yeo 1993: 78).

The formation of a modern public health system in Korea began to take shape when Korea, a 'closed country', opened up to the outside world in 1876. Learning from the earlier experiences of the 'opening' of China and Japan to foreign trade and residence, Korea was compelled to strengthen the nation in the face of imperialism. A strong nation needed a large and healthy population. To that end, the Korean government sent educational missions consisting of government officials and young intellectuals to the West and Japan to study their political, economic and health systems. Their reports stressed the importance of social and personal hygiene and the building up of a public health system, particularly the necessity of providing a pure water supply and a sewerage system as keys to making the nation wealthy and strong (Park Y. J. 2002: 13). Their reports, however, were not immediately reflected in government policy for several reasons but mainly because neither the high government officials nor the reporters themselves were sufficiently aware of the scientific foundations of these systems. Although they were impressed by the social effect of a sanitary system, its adoption was retarded by this lack of basic understanding of Western medicine. An institute was necessary in which Western medicine could be taught to people who could then reproduce it (Shin 1997: 50).

Dr Horace N. Allen, the first medical missionary in Korea, with the support of the Korean government, opened the first modern hospital in1885; a medical school attached to the hospital was opened in the following year. The opening of the hospital, Je Joong Won (濟衆院, House of Caring People), was a symbolic event in the sense that it marked the official introduction of Western medical practice to Korea (Park H. W. 2002: 69). Moreover, the hospital was a success. According to the first annual report, more than 10,000 patients were treated (Allen and Heron 1886: 21). Within a decade, 7 hospitals and 12 dispensaries were founded by Western missionaries. Although these hospitals were far from satisfying all the medical demands of the time, their existence played an important role in medicalizing Korean society. In addition, magazines and newspapers such as the *Independent Daily* and *Whansung Daily*, which were published in the 1890s, abound in articles promoting social and personal hygiene and the necessity of establishing Western sanitary facilities such as running water and sewerage (*Independent Daily* 27 June 1896).

The Korean government launched a smallpox vaccination campaign on a national scale in the 1890s as part of efforts to establish a public health system. But the project met with strong resistance and the public hostility is partly explained by the antipathy towards Western civilization that persisted after the opening of Korea. The antipathy was amplified by the traditional practitioners of variolization and the shamans who made a fortune by performing rituals of 'seeing off' evil spirits which were believed to be responsible for smallpox.

Another symbolic event that provoked resistance was a consequence of the 'Order for Cutting the Top Knot' issued under the influence of the Japanese who had gained much power in Korea after they had defeated China in 1895. Traditionally, when Korean males married they made a top knot with their hair as a symbol of becoming an adult. Furthermore, according to Confucian teachings, one's body, hair and skin are inherited from one's parents and therefore to preserve them is one of the important duties in filial piety. Given these traditional and cultural contexts, it was only natural that the order for cutting top-knots met with strong resistance. The government's order was carried out in the name of hygiene but Koreans regarded it as a severe challenge to their traditional values and a negation of their customs. Some conservative Confucian literati strongly resisted the order saying 'You can cut off my head, but not my top knot!' The act was regarded 'as one of the first and important parts of a scheme to blot out Korea's national identity, and merge her into one with Japan' (Underwood 1908: 170).

There were several modalities to the emergence of a modern health-care system. Western health care and medicine, initially of little importance, became dominant, and indigenous medicine and health care began to be marginalized. When Korea was opened to the outside world, the Korean government thought it was able to select some Western health-care methods without changing the existing social order. However, because of the shifting external political situation surrounding Korea and the turmoil of internal uprisings aimed at destroying the existing dynasty, more fundamental changes were needed.

The institution of political and social reforms during 1894–1895 was the product of these movements. As a result of the reform movements, the government health-care system, previously based on a Confucian ideology which regarded governmental health care as a product of a ruler's grace toward his beloved subjects, was modernized in order to manage the population in terms of both quality and quantity. The change in ideas resulted in a change in the response to epidemics. Confronted by the outbreak of cholera epidemics in 1895, the Sanitary Board was formed, consisting of Korean officials and Western and Japanese doctors. Dr O. R. Avison, a Canadian missionary who was in charge of the Che Chung Won, was appointed as the head of the Sanitary Board and with his missionary colleagues and government support he attempted to check the spread of the disease and provide care for its victims. The cholera epidemics led to the establishment of several isolation hospitals and quarantine stations and compelled the Korean government to realize the importance and effectiveness of modern medical measures against such dreadful epidemics and to accelerate the reform of the system of public health in general. Yet, reform of the public health system could not be carried out without reform of the whole society.

Thus, most of the modern health-care system was established during the Kwangmu Reform Period (1896–1904) under orders issued by Emperor Kojong and his successors. The system consisted of health-care organizations, public health, medical care and surveillance of private practitioners (of both modern and traditional medicine). In appearance, the health-care system that emerged during this period seems quite similar to the present system, but it reflected the contemporary acceptance of paternalistic authority rooted in the authority of the emperor, unlike the present system which is based on individual rights. Despite these promising efforts, the growing influence of Japan and the annexation of Korea meant that the health-care system became a tool of colonial power.

Public health under Japanese occupation

After opening the country in 1876, Korea established diplomatic relations with other countries. Due to Korea's geographical accessibility, many Japanese, including diplomats, officials, soldiers and civilians, came to Korea and the Japanese soon opened clinics for their compatriots. At first, military doctors took charge of the clinics and although there were some civilian Japanese doctors in Korea, they served the Japanese, not Koreans. Nevertheless, there were substantial connections between Japanese and Korean medicine. Several Koreans went to Japan to study Western medicine, and the Government Medical School, founded by the Korean government in 1899, hired a Japanese doctor as an instructor. However, there is hardly any evidence to indicate that Japan tried to transplant Japanese medicine [based on German medicine] before 1905 when Korea was compelled to agree to the Protectorate Treaty which ultimately led to its annexation. In contrast, Western missionary doctors were more active in spreading Western medicine since medicine was regarded as a powerful tool in Christian evangelical work.

In 1905, Japan took steps to establish a colonial health-care system in Korea. The Residency-General merged three medical institutes, Kwang Je Won, the Government Medical School and the Red Cross Hospital, previously run by the Korean government. The new institute was called the Taihan Hospital and it was a centre for controlling the national health system, medical education and sanitary administration.

The general policy of the health-care system

In 1910, Japan formally annexed Korea and the health policy was fundamentally revised. Japan assumed control of medical institutions and built high-quality, Western-style hospitals for the care of Japanese residents. They eliminated Korean traditional medicine in the public sector by expelling all the traditional practitioners working in hospitals and the military. The Japanese also strengthened the control of infectious diseases by civil and military policing. In the name of hygiene, police powers and surveillance were applied in the daily life of Koreans.

With the beginning of the Japanese occupation, some fundamental changes occurred in the public health system. Before the occupation, the Sanitary Bureau of the Home Department was in charge of health affairs, and the Police Department played only a minor role. But during the occupation, all public health affairs were managed by the Police Department, which meant that the Japanese applied their own medical policing system in colonized Korea. According to Rosen, medical police is a concept relating to theories, policies and practices originating in 'the absolute, mercantilist German state during the seventeenth and eighteenth centuries for action in the sphere of health and welfare, so as to secure for the monarch and the state increased power and wealth' (Rosen 1974: 141).

In Korea, however, Japan's autocratic approach was reinforced by militarism which was used to exert even stronger control over the colonized people. Japan occupied Korea from 1910 to 1945 and the basic Japanese policy for colonial public health system remained the same with only minor variations in response to changes in the domestic and international situation. We can divide the Japanese occupation of Korea into three periods.

The changes of policy in three periods

The first period was from 1910 to 1919 during which a nationwide movement for the restoration of independence, called the March First Movement, flourished. Japanese control was very harsh and the colonial system was maintained by military police under an army general who was appointed as the governor-general. This militarism manifested itself in the field of public health. All public health and health-care affairs including quarantine measures were managed by the civil and military police. In addition, army or naval doctors were appointed as the directors of most of the provincial hospitals established in each province after the annexation.

The second period (1919–1941) saw Japanese expansionism in East Asia resulting in war against China and European colonial possessions in the region. Having faced strong resistance from the Korean people, Japan changed its policy. The governor-general advocated so-called enlightened administration, which meant more 'civilized' government. For the public health system this meant the replacement of military with civil police and the decentralization of authority.

The third period began in 1941 and ended with the Japanese defeat in 1945. The entire public health and health-care system was used by the Japanese to recruit human resources to serve the war effort (Yeo 2002: 151). Many young Korean men were sent to the battlefields against their will and numerous young women were sent to give 'comfort' to Japanese soldiers. Most of the surviving 'comfort women' are still suffering from the terrible memories of what happened during the war. In order to recruit from a healthier and stronger population, Japan stressed physical improvement and promoted so-called Physical Training for National Defence. Throughout the occupation period, the health of Koreans had never been an end in itself, but had always been a 'tool' to advance the good of Imperial Japan, and this approach intensified during this last period (Shin 1986: 319).

Japan advertised its public health-care system as a contribution to the modernization of Korea and as a means of legitimizing its rule. Japan established more than 40 provincial hospitals between 1909 and the 1940s. At first, they were called 'provincial charity hospitals' established to treat poor Koreans. However, these hospitals were in reality built mainly for the Japanese inhabitants. Another important aspect to note is that they were built along the important railroad lines and some of the hospitals were even called 'Railroad Hospitals'. Given the fact that railroads were very important infrastructure for exploiting the natural resources of the colonized country, it is not difficult to imagine that the hospitals were founded to take care of the personnel who were economically developing the provinces (Shin 1986: 117).

Control of infectious diseases

Control of infectious diseases is crucial for the maintenance of social stability. Accordingly, every government has a fundamental interest in controlling them, and the Japanese Government-General in Korea was no exception. But the basic policy of the Japanese was to identify and isolate patients rather than promote prevention and treatment despite issuing regulations to that end in 1915. While the Japanese built several isolation hospitals, the facilities of the hospitals were usually poor, they were overcrowded and they offered inadequate diets. Furthermore, the Japanese civil or military police were often abusive in finding infected people and forcing them into the hospitals. These practices made Koreans hostile to the isolation hospitals. In addition, many preferred to be treated by traditional herbal therapy rather than the Western therapy practiced by Japanese doctors, and they resisted admission to the isolation hospitals. Conflict frequently occurred between patients' families who were trying to hide them and the police (Park 1998: 39).

The Korean people's antipathy towards public isolation hospitals gave rise to a movement to establish private hospitals. A committee was formed and a campaign to raise funds was launched. The movement failed to raise sufficient funds for a separate hospital and what was raised was used to establish a contagious diseases ward in the Severance Hospital (the first Western missionary hospital in Korea). Nevertheless, the movement illustrates the level of resistance to Japanese policy for the prevention of epidemic diseases (Park 1998: 44).

Western medical missionaries also played an important role in controlling infectious diseases during the occupation period. In particular, they made considerable contributions to the control of tuberculosis (TB) and leprosy. TB was, perhaps, the most critical infectious disease in the early twentieth century before effective chemotherapy was discovered. The exact prevalence rate of TB during the occupation period is not known, but it was presumed to be around 15% of the Korean population which was about 20 million. The Japanese Government-General had issued regulations for preventing TB in 1918, but was far from active in controlling the disease. However, medical missionaries were. In 1920, the first TB ward was built in the Severance Hospital and the first anti-tuberculosis society was organized in the same hospital (*The Severance Bulletin* 1929: 64). A Canadian medical missionary, S. H. Martin, and his Korean colleagues, Dr Lee Yong-suel and Dr Paul D. Choy, were the founding members of the society (*The Severance Bulletin* 1929: 61). In 1927, another Canadian medical missionary, Florence Jessie Murray, opened a TB ward in Hamheung, a northern city.

The first sanatorium in Korea was established by Dr Sherwood Hall in 1928 (Hall 1978: 390). It was built in Hyejoo, Hwanghye province. The opening was much opposed not only by the people living nearby but also by the governor of the province. The fear was that when the sanatorium was opened, TB patients would flock to the city, thus spreading the disease. Dr Hall, however, succeeded in obtaining permission to open the sanatorium after convincing the governor otherwise. He introduced pioneering treatment modalities, and after several years, the sanatorium became famous with many patients coming to be treated. From 20 beds, it expanded to 50 beds in 1934 and there were 297 inpatients in 1936–1937 (Lee 2003: 810). Dr Hall also introduced the practice of selling Christmas seals (postage-like seals) to raise funds.

The Japanese authorities were prodded into action by the activities of the Western missionaries. The Chosen (Chosen is an old name for Korea) Society for Preventing Tuberculosis was organized in 1936 and branches were established in each province. Its activities were focused mainly on prevention. More substantial activities were initiated during the early 1940s and several sanatoria were opened. BCG vaccinations began in 1943 and 300,000 persons were to be given free vaccinations. Since Western missionaries were forced to leave after Japan began the War, the anti-tuberculosis activities were mostly carried out by the Japanese during the early 1940s (Kim 1998: 275).

Another infectious disease that was important during the occupation period was leprosy. Again it was medical missionaries who launched health care of lepers. There are no reliable statistics of the numbers for the second decade of the twentieth century, but it is presumed to be over 20,000. Most of the lepers were scattered over the southern part of Korea. They led very hard lives, were often deserted by family and friends, and were thus forced to become beggars or criminals because of the social stigma associated with the disease. Most were homeless and the situation became worse when Koreans began to understand that leprosy is contagious (Wilson 1914: 65). The first leper asylum was opened in 1910 by Dr C. H. Erwin in Pusan, a southern harbour city, with the help of the British Leprosy Mission. Two years later, Dr R. M. Wilson, a medical missionary of the Southern Presbyterian Mission, opened another asylum in Kwangju. In 1914, Dr A. G. Fletcher of the Northern Presbyterian Mission opened the third asylum in Taegu. In 1913, Mr Bailey and his wife, who founded the International Leper Mission, visited Korea and were so deeply impressed by the work in Korea that they raised substantial funds for construction of better and larger buildings. Hearing the news of the opening of these asylums, many lepers sought refuge there. However, only a small number could be housed. In 1917, each asylum could accommodate about one to two hundred lepers. The asylums were hospitals, working places and communities at the same time. The lepers who were healthy enough learned carpentry, masonry and brick-making, and raised cattle, pigs, rabbits, poultry and cows. They supplied their own daily necessities. Religious activities were also an important part of the life of asylums. These humanitarian ways of treating lepers in missionary leprosaria were in marked contrast to the conditions in those run by the Japanese authorities.

In 1916, the authorities opened a leper asylum on a beautiful island called Small Deer Island (So Rok Do) situated in the Southern Sea. The island became the symbol of the leprosarium in Korea. The number of inmates increased from 99 at its opening to 6,000 in 1939. Since isolation was adopted as the first means of controlling the disease, the colonial authorities planned to accommodate as many as lepers in the asylum as possible. The inmates complained about the imposition of Japanese ways of life: they had to wear Japanese clothes and to live in Japanese-style houses.

The authorities issued regulations for preventing leprosy in 1935 under which any leper could be compulsorily interned. In fact, many vagrant lepers were sent to the island. The lepers were at the complete mercy of the staff. The director was given the right to imprison an inmate for up to 60 days. While in the early years the lepers received comparatively humane treatment, the asylum soon became more like a concentration camp or Gulag. In addition, a jail was established on the island to which leper-criminals were transferred. The colonial authorities advertised the asylum as a paradise but the reality was very different. Thus, the patients were forced to construct buildings and pave roads, leading to many attempts to escape. Even married couples had to live separately and could only live together on the condition the man underwent sterilization. Toward the end of the occupation, life on the island became harsher than ever and there were riots and the director was assassinated by one of the inmates (National So Rok Do Hospital 1996: 84). The asylum on Small Deer Island was symbolic of the whole approach to public health in colonized Korea.

Public health in the late 1940s and 1950s

Korea was liberated after Japan's surrender in 1945. American forces established the Military Government which soon created a Health Ministry; it took over public health from the police department. But the Military Government was reluctant to make long-term policy for public health because their primary concern was protecting American forces stationed in Korea. As a result, the control of chronic infectious diseases such as TB had a low priority. The system of public health under the Japanese can be defined as 'public' in the sense that the colonial government took charge of public health. By contrast, the Military Government entrusted a large part of public health to the private sector following the American model. The budget for provincial public hospitals under the Japanese amounted to 34% of the whole budget for health care. But in 1947 it decreased to 7%. The Military Government promoted the expansion of the private sector, and this policy determined the basic characteristics of the health-care system of today (Shin 2000: 213). Korean doctors were also sent to the United States to study public health and they played an important role in establishing a public health system after the American model.

A Korean government was founded in 1948. However, the Korean war which broke out soon after helped transplant features of American medicine and the health-care system due to extensive American involvement in the war. Of course, the war itself generated many public health problems as well as controversy over the use of biological weapons (Endicott and Hagerman 1998). A new infectious disease, Korean hemorrhagic fever, appeared during the war, and poor nutrition and poor hygiene aggravated the population's health. TB, leprosy and parasitic infections were still major problems during and after the war: for example, egg detection rates for *Ascaris lumbricoides*, one of the major parasites in Korea, were 82.4% in 1949 and 81.9% in 1957.

Public health problems in the 1960s and 1970s

After the war, parasitic infections ranked first in terms of prevalence. Although an extensive survey was carried out during the period of Japanese rule (Seo 1992: 47; Yeo 2004: 246), no substantial preventive measures were implemented. Furthermore, these infections did not draw as much attention as TB and leprosy simply because they were not as deadly or as socially burdensome. After the Korean war, parasitic infections began to be regarded as one of the most important problems of public health in Korea. It was estimated that more than 90% of the population were infected with parasites of various kinds in the late 1950s because of poor hygiene and the traditional way of fertilizing vegetables with human excrement. Parasitologists drew public attention to the problem and underlined the urgency of eradicating human parasites. The Korea Association of Parasite Eradication (KAPE) was founded in 1964 with a national campaign launched as the 'Ten year movement for zero percent national parasite infection rate'. KAPE provided health education and mass anti-helminthic treatments and supported research on parasites. At the beginning its control activities encountered many difficulties mostly due to lack of financial resources. But from the beginning of the 1970s the Korean government provided support. This, indeed, was the typical way public health issues were addressed in the 1960s, 1970s and even into the 1980s. Usually the Korean government was not directly involved; rather, it was doctors and civilian specialists in public health or medicine who organized an association for handling the problem in question. Lacking resources, they received technical and financial support from overseas. As the Korean economy developed, the governmental contribution became larger, as was true with the schemes for control of TB and leprosy.

After the government provided more support, mass examinations and treatment for parasitic infections were carried out on all primary, middle and high school students beginning in 1969. The first national survey of intestinal helminthic infections amongst rural people was made in 1971. The rate of infections decreased remarkably in the 1980s. One of the most common intestinal parasites in Korea, *Ascaris lumbricoides*, showed a nationwide egg positive rate fall from 41% in 1976 to 2.1% in 1986. The causes were multifactorial: mass chemotherapy, environmental sanitation, public health education, improvement in socio-economic status, better anti-helminths, increased use of chemical fertilizers and acceleration in national industrialization (Seo 1992: 63). Korea's success in controlling parasitic infections in a relatively short period was internationally recognized and Korean parasitologists continue to share their experiences with other developing countries, providing technical and financial help through the Korea International Cooperation Agency (KOICA).

Another important issue in public health during the 1960s and 1970s was family planning. The population increased from 25 million in 1960 to over 29 million in 1966. Like other developing countries, a large and rapidly growing population was regarded as a burden on the growth of the national economy. Specialists in public health such as Yang Jae-mo drew the attention of the government to the urgency of the population problem. As a result, a model project for family planning was launched in a rural county near Seoul in 1962 and an urban project commenced in 1964. On the basis of the success of these two model projects, family planning became a nationwide policy. Its success was so dramatic that a large number of family planning leaders of other countries came to Korea from 1965 to be trained, only five years after the beginning of family planning in this country. Since family planning was carried out under the auspices of the government and the Catholic community was small in Korea, the campaign met with little resistance.

The results were spectacular. The birth rate fell dramatically to 1.17 in 2002 from 4.5 in 1970. The unusual success can be attributed to effective co-operation between the government and its civil partners. The government provided the necessary drive along with the organization. Each unit of administration had its corresponding unit for family planning.

The Korean government took the lead in family planning because it regarded it as an urgent economic problem rather than as a problem of public health. The government understood that a 'population explosion' would severely retard economic development. This explains why family planning was included in the Five-Year Plan for Economic Development, which commenced in 1962. Satisfaction with the success soon faded because the abrupt decrease in the birth rate is now menacing the economy's growth. The Korean government is now encouraging young couples to have more children but so far this has proved ineffective.

Public health in the age of globalization

As globalization advances so too do the problems of public health. HIV/AIDS, for instance, has spread to every part of the world since it was identified for the first time more than twenty years ago. In Korea, since the first HIV/AIDS patient was notified in 1985, the number of infected has reached 3,829 (2005). The number is relatively small compared to neighbouring Asian countries, but the increasing rate of newly infected individuals is quite high. In 2005, 680 new cases were reported. Most of the patients were infected through sexual intercourse, both homosexual (49.8%) and heterosexual (50.2%). Since most of the infections are attributed to sexual behaviour, the Korea Centre for Disease Control and Prevention is carrying out public education programmes in order to prevent further transmission. Although no victim of severe acute respiratory syndrome (SARS) or 'mad cow disease' was reported in Korea, the threat of these infections impacted greatly on the whole society.

The life expectancy of Koreans has increased markedly in recent years (Table 3.1), but the problem of 'traditional' infectious diseases still remains to be

Table 3.1 Life expectancy of Koreans (in years)

	1983	1993	2002	2003
Female	71.47	76.80	80.44	80.82
Male	63.21	68.76	73.38	73.87

Source: Korean Statistical Information System (2006).

solved. For example, the TB case notification rate per 100,000 persons was 56.2 in 2004, which is one of the highest rates among Organisation for Economic Cooperation and Development (OECD) countries. The high notification rate may be attributed to the increase of the homeless after the national financial crisis of 1998.

Chronic diseases originating from lifestyle are another important problem. Diseases such as hypertension, diabetes and obesity are believed to be caused mostly by overnutrition and lack of exercise. Those in their fifties and sixties who were poorly nourished during their childhood (because of World War II and the Korean war) are especially susceptible to these diseases because of their richer diet in the era of rapid economic growth. It is estimated that there are 4 million diabetes patients and each year 500,000 new patients are diagnosed. The mortality rate due to diabetes is 34.7 per 100,000 persons, the highest among OECD countries, which signifies that diabetes is poorly controlled. The high rate of smoking is another issue for public health since as of 2004 nearly 60% of adult males smoke. Radical legislation that attempts to prohibit sales of tobacco is being prepared, and Korea's ratification of The Framework Convention on Tobacco Control (WHO) in 2005, which bans all promotional policies or advertisements for tobacco use as well as insisting on mandatory health warnings, will start the difficult process of control and smoking cessation (*China Daily* 2005; Park 2004: 759–80).

The low coverage rate (50%) of national health insurance is also a problem. The present 'leftist' government, paradoxically, is trying to solve this problem by introducing private insurance which many fear will severely damage social solidarity.

Another important issue is the dual system of medical care (Son 1998: 278). The origin of the system dates back to the time when Western medicine was introduced in Korea and it was officially established when the Japanese authorities decided to issue different licences to Western-trained doctors and herbal doctors (Yeo 1999: 307). Since then the competition between the two systems has intensified and herbal doctors have tried to establish a system equivalent to that of their rivals. They have built their own 'hospitals' and are trying to award 'specialist licences' after the model of Western medicine. Ironically, all these efforts have tended to blur the distinction between traditional medicine and Western medicine in terms of the way service is provided. Today a patient who visits a private clinic can hardly tell which medicine is practiced since it will be equipped with modern medical equipment and herbal doctors will be attired in white gowns.

The present dual system poses health-care challenges. Frequent disputes between Western-trained and herbal doctors are burdensome for policymakers. For example, policymakers who allowed herbal doctors to use modern diagnostic apparatus such as Computerized Tomography Scanners were strongly criticized by Western-trained doctors. An important task for improving public health will be the integration of traditional medical practices, which many people rely on, into the national health-care system.

Conclusion

This chapter has attempted to delineate the impact of historical changes in the political, social and economic regimes on the development of public health in Korea. In the pre-modern period, the control of epidemics as a nascent public health measure was conceived of in terms of Confucian ideology centred on the emperor's benevolence toward his subjects. The introduction of modern medicine and concepts of public health was a product of Korea's opening to Western and Japanese influences at the end of the nineteenth century where survival of the country demanded a host of state-directed reforms and private initiatives to improve the nation's health. During the Japanese occupation, public health policies were instituted to facilitate Japanese control. After the Korean war (which divided the country), South Korea's economy and public health system were 'liberalized' and basically modelled on those of America. Family planning in the 1960s and 1970s, a response to rapid population growth, proved so successful in reducing the growth rate that recently reversal of the decline has become part of the national agenda because it threatens economic progress. As with other countries in Asia, rising living standards and changes to lifestyles have transformed the epidemiological profile so that chronic diseases are becoming more prominent as advances in infectious disease control have made significant inroads into the burden of long-standing afflictions such as leprosy and TB.

Korea, like its Asian neighbours, in this era of globalization will have to grapple with the consequences of new or newly emerging diseases and address the problem of the close relationship between public health problems at the national and international levels. If the past is any guide, we must not forget how the changing political, social and economic contexts have shaped public health, and how future challenges will continue to reflect these changes in Korean society, the nation and the world.

References

Allen, H. N. and Heron, J. W. (1886) *First Annual Report of the Korean Governmental Hospital*, Seoul: R. Meiklejohn.

Anonymous (1929) 'The Foundation of Severance Anti-Tuberculosis Society', *The Severance Bulletin*, 11: 61–62. (Korean)

China Daily, 26 April 2005.

Endicott, S. and Hagerman, E. (1998) *The United States and Biological Warfare*, Bloomington: Indiana University Press.

Hall, S. (1978) *With Stethoscope in Asia: Korea*, McLean: MCL Associates.
Kim, T. K. (1998) *A History of Tuberculosis in Korea*, Seoul: Korean National Tuberculosis Association. (Korean)
Korean Statistical Information System (2006) Online. Available <http//kosis.nso.go.kr/> (accessed 30 March 2006).
Lee, M. Y. (2003) *A History of Christian Medical Work in Korea*, Seoul: Acanet. (Korean)
Lee, Y. T. (1954) 'Western Medical Theory Introduced First to Korea', *Journal of Seoul National University* (Natural Science), 1: 208–213. (Korean)
National Sorokdo Hospital (1996) *A History of Sorokdo Leper Hospital*, Sorokdo: National Sorokdo Hospital. (Korean)
Park, H. W. (2002) *Je Joong Won*, Seoul: Mommam. (Korean)
Park, K., Kim, D. S., Park, D. J. and Lee, S. K. (2004) 'Tobacco Control in Korea', *Medicine and Law*, 23(4): 759–780.
Park, Y. J. (1998) 'A Study on the Movement for Establishing a Private Isolation Hospital under the Rule of Japanese Imperialism', *Korean Journal of Medical History*, 7(1): 37–46. (Korean)
—— (2002) 'The Formation and Reorganization of the Modern Medical System in Late Great Han Empire and Early Japanese Colonial Period (1876–1919),' unpublished thesis, Yonsei University. (Korean)
—— (2003) 'From Regiment to Sanitation: Perception of Medicine by the Enlightenment Party and the Establishment of the Modern State', *Society and History*, 63: 30–50. (Korean)
Rosen, G. (1974) *From Medical Police to Social Medicine: Essays on the History of Health Care*, New York: Science History Publications.
Seo, H. G. (1992) 'Study on the Transition of Intestinal Parasites in Korea from 1913 to 1989', *Korean Journal of Medical History*, 1(1): 45–63. (Korean)
Shin, D. W. (1986) 'A Study on the Policy of Health Services and Korean's Health State in Japanese Colonial State', unpublished thesis, Seoul National University. (Korean)
—— (1997) *A History of the Modern Health Care System in Korea*, Seoul: Hanul Academy. (Korean)
Shin, J. S. (2000) 'The Policy of the United States Army Military Government in Korea toward Public Health and Medicine in Occupied South Korea', *Korean Journal of Medical History*, 9(2): 212–232. (Korean)
Son, A. H. K. (1998) 'Modernisation of the System of Traditional Medicine in Korea', *Health Policy*, 44: 261–281.
Underwood, L. H. (1908) *Fifteen Years among the Top-Knots*, Boston: American Tract Society.
Wilson, R. M. (1914) 'Report on Leper Work', *The Korean Mission Field*, 10(6): 65–66.
Yeo, I. S. (1993) 'The Medical Philosophy of Choe Han-ki', *Korean Journal of Medical History*, 2(1): 66–79. (Korean)
—— (1999) 'Herbal Doctors after 1876: The Transformation of Traditional Medicine in a Challenging Period', *Dong Bang Hak Chi (The Journal of Korean Studies)*, 104: 291–324. (Korean)
—— (2002) 'A History of Medical Licence in Korea', *Korean Journal of Medical History*, 11(2): 137–153. (Korean)
—— (2004) 'A History of the Research Department of the Severance Union Medical College', *Korean Journal of Medical History*, 13(2): 233–250. (Korean)

4 History of public health in modern India
1857–2005

Radhika Ramasubban

Introduction

Public health interventions and reforms, by their very nature as expensive and large-scale undertakings, have historically been the domain of governments. Their success depends upon a state's capacity to demonstrate a strong political will, based on enlightened understanding that financial resources and administrative competence invested in public health measures can produce long-term and self-multiplying economic and social gains.

The nineteenth and early twentieth centuries were a period when the developed countries of today successfully achieved control over preventable infectious diseases causing high and premature mortality. This they did through public health reform: state-led improvements in water supply, sewerage, drainage, air quality, housing and town planning backed by legislation, and accompanied by health education, often in response to public pressures. By the time the era of revolutionary clinical medicine based on antibiotics set in, these countries had virtually won the battle against killer communicable diseases. This transformation took place in, by and large, culturally homogeneous societies, in tandem with economic growth (urbanization, industrialization, a skilled and educated workforce, and rising incomes that facilitated improved nutrition) and considerable national wealth generated by an extensive engagement with overseas colonies.

It was during the peak of this phase in Britain's history that India became its flagship colony. It was inevitable that the rising tide of the new metropolitan sanitary science would have an impact on Britain's engagement with India. The challenge for the European constitution of coping with the Indian climate and its perceived propensity for generating disease had understandably been a preoccupation since the earliest days of the East India Company. This intensified during the nineteenth century when the Company's armies claimed new parts of the country. The colonizing project matured after the Sepoy Mutiny of 1857 – better known in India as the First Indian War of Independence – and the takeover of the country's administration by the Crown. The decision that Britain would relocate a third of all its armed forces in India, and not develop India as a Crown settlement colony but only exploit its natural resources for repatriation and international trade, set off economic, social and political currents that shaped the mix of public health solutions that evolved for the enclave community and the general population. For India – many times the size of Britain, geographically more heterogeneous, predominantly rural, socially highly stratified and culturally complex – the colonial encounter marked a unique moment in its public health history.

The first government of independent India had to contend with a precarious financial base, a burgeoning, predominantly poor population and high mortality rates from epidemic disease. It adopted an ambitious economic growth agenda whose emphasis on rapid industrial development was expected to have a trickle-down effect of wealth creation and improved standards of living. Its democratic constitution upheld the right of all citizens to good health. Among its first steps was the creation of a primary health-care apparatus to provide free services to its population. It also launched 'military' campaigns against epidemic diseases. In this, the State was seeking to right a major perceived historical wrong. The epidemiological transition agenda, however, was soon overtaken by a demographic transition agenda.

How did the country's colonial past impact upon the challenge of public health in independent India? What are the contradictions of the present? This chapter attempts to identify the continuities and discontinuities between the past and the present. In doing so, it sketches the main features of colonial public health policy and paints a broad brush picture of the evolution of health policy post-independence.

Colonial health policy

After 1857, the high direct costs of controlling India due to sickness and death from epidemic disease in the army assumed crucial importance. The dangers to the stability of British commerce and profits, from epidemics among the general population, constituted another worry. The potential of 'Asiatic cholera' to spread to Europe, and jeopardize Britain's international prestige as a scientifically advanced power, also acted as a consideration, as did Britain's status in the eyes of its Indian subjects as the bearer of a civilizing mission.

The focus on the army coincided with a closer scrutiny of British army health following the Crimean War, and the beginning of Britain's own period of thoroughgoing civilian sanitary reform. Sanitation, health and medicine as a 'tool of Empire' (Headrick 1981) acquired a clout that was to remain influential in British health policy in India until the end of colonial rule.

A Royal Commission appointed to enquire into the sanitary state of the army in India found that the leading recorded causes of death and sickness were 'fevers' (including malaria and typhoid) and cholera (including dysentery, diarrhoea and hepatitis) (*Royal Army Sanitary Commission Report* 1863: n.p.). Early nineteenth century observers had already noted that the spread of malaria was closely linked with major irrigation projects (revenues from agriculture being the mainstay of the colonial economy). The expansion of road and railway links for transporting primary produce from the rural hinterland to major ports, and attendant changes in the ecosystem without attention to drainage, also exacerbated malaria (*Annual Report of the Sanitary Commissioner with the Government of*

India 1900–1901: 125 [henceforth *Annual Sanitary Report*]; Klein 1972: 134; Nightingale 1874: 48). Another observable link during the political consolidation process through the first half of the century was between troop movements and the spread of cholera (Mackenzie Committee 1868: 22).

In the second half of the nineteenth century, epidemic cholera – decimating soldiers in India, and travelling to England and Europe through merchant, passenger and army ships – became a metaphor for all that was terrible and challenging about Britain's newest possession. Its mode of transmission excited scientific controversy within the colonial Indian Medical Service: was it the unique Indian climate that determined its virulence and the Englishman's susceptibility to it, or was it lack of attention to purity of water supply, sewage disposal and housing design, and/or individual behavioural practices? The controversy notwithstanding, prevention policies were implemented.

Sanitarians in the East India Company's army had already begun to compile medico-topographical reports on the climate, soil and environment, and their possible implications for disease, in different regions of the country that came under army occupation. Leading them was Sir James Ranald Martin, a Company surgeon who was influenced by the growing sanitary consciousness in England and who went on to serve the Royal Commission into the Sanitary State of the Army in India (Martin 1837). The findings were now combined with principles of town planning based on the new sanitary science to design residential spaces for army personnel and European civilians – army 'cantonments', 'civil lines' and 'hill stations' – resulting in physical and social/racial segregation (King 1976: 97–120), and to formulate sanitary legislation governing these enclaves (*Gazette of India [Supplement]* 1864). This approach also accommodated, to some extent, the climatic theory of disease causation.

The construction of better bungalows and barracks, arrangements for protected water and food supplies, efficient solid waste removal in cantonments, at camp sites and during marches and train journeys, and controls over entry of natives into these enclaves – 'sanitary cordons' – began to bring down sickness and mortality due to cholera. From an average of 3.09 per 1,000 of European troop strength in the decade 1860–1869, deaths fell steadily reaching 0.14 in the decade 1910–1914. Deaths due to enteric fever – which took severest form among younger recruits – proved more difficult to control, and hovered between 2 and 10 per 1,000 between 1877 (when they first came to be recorded as such) and 1909 (compiled from *Annual Sanitary Reports* for the years 1877 to 1909: n.p.). By 1899, army scientists in Britain had developed an anti-typhoid vaccine and conducted successful trials in India, and over the next decade a little over 90% of British soldiers in India were inoculated against enteric fever (Arnold 1993: 90). In 1910, typhoid deaths among European troops fell for the first time, to below 1 per 1,000 (*Annual Sanitary Reports* 1910 to 1929: n.p.).

Indian soldiers in the British army were not equal beneficiaries of the above reforms (Arnold 1993: 91–94). Even in 1914, when the Indian army was drawn into World War I, typhoid inoculation covered only a tenth of them. From an apparently superior position (attributed to their better acclimatization) vis-à-vis

European soldiers in the early nineteenth century – before the introduction of preventive medicine and sanitary works – Indian soldiers gradually became worse off, succumbing in much larger numbers than their European counterparts to the epidemic diseases sweeping the general population.

The potential of 'native health' to endanger European health and profits remained an ever-present source of concern. Periodic pronouncements about the inseparable links between army and civilian health pointed out the imperative of expanding sanitary administration to include the local population. There were also those from England (notably Florence Nightingale) who reminded the colonial government that it had a civilizing mission to perform (Nightingale 1874: 43). Accordingly, one sanitary commissioner was appointed to each presidency, and annual sanitary reports for each presidency – compiled into the Annual Report of the sanitary commissioner with the Government of India – began recording epidemic mortality in the European and Indian armies and in the general population.

Large cities and towns in close proximity to army cantonments were seen as the most immediate sources of danger. Starting in 1871, the former were encouraged to set up municipalities, each governed by its own Municipal Act. Separate Acts dealt with other (smaller) municipalities and 'notified areas'. The Acts contained health provisions, and towns and cities over a certain population could appoint medical officers of health, for which they were entitled to receive from the government a certain portion of the salary of these officers. But no legislation existed that actually *required* local authorities to do so (IOR: L/E/7/1110, File 559); sanitary improvements were left to the discretion of those who controlled the local bodies. This was different from contemporary developments in England where the State enacted public health legislation which was binding on local bodies.

Under the circumstances, only in the large towns and municipalities did there come to exist an executive authority for sanitation in the form of health officers; indeed, cities like Bombay had enlightened health officers. But funds were always inadequate and the local bodies proved to be apathetic about raising taxes to pay for sanitation (Harrison 1994: 166–201). Nor were funds readily forthcoming from the provincial governments. Each provincial sanitary commissioner – overseeing populations running into several millions – had only advisory powers, and was hopelessly understaffed, reflecting the low political priority given to general sanitation. The superior executive authority in the province was the Civil Surgeon who oversaw only curative health. This ambivalence towards prevention and absence of executive authority also plagued the sanitary commissioner with the Government of India, responsible for the entire civilian population of the country. This post was combined in 1880 with that of Surgeon General, restored in 1904 and relegated in 1911 to being a branch of the office of Director General of Medical Services. When World War I broke out, its abolition was advocated on the grounds that it was an unnecessary burden on the exchequer. The policy of vacillation around this post continued into the inter-war period (IOR: L/E/7/992, C and R 657; L/E/7/1071, C and R 2359).

In the absence of concerted sanitary interventions, cholera deaths among the general population continued unchecked. In the 1860s, cholera spread to Europe, resulting in successive pandemics. It spawned the first international sanitary conference in Constantinople in 1866, followed by three others in 1874, 1875 and 1885, where European powers pressured Britain to put its Indian colony in order. The first conference pointed to the movement of Hindu pilgrims to and from major fairs and festivals as the primary cause for the spread of cholera among the general population. It also held out the threat of embargoes on goods sailing out from Indian ports.

The immediate response of the government was to institute port quarantine. It also further secured the enclaves by extending the sanitary cordons around cantonments and civil lines to include Indian subordinate staff in closest contact with the enclave population and stricter surveillance over entry by outsiders. There were, understandably, limits to implementing 'land quarantine' beyond this to include social intercourse between Indian employees in the enclaves and their contacts in the 'black towns' or their kin in far-flung rural areas.

However, when it came to the question of regulating conditions of pilgrim train travel, and making sanitary improvements at pilgrimage sites, controversy and indecision took over. The lack of scientific consensus within the colonial medical community regarding the mode of cholera transmission became an excuse for continuing with a laissez-faire policy. Another reason cited was a possible political backlash arising out of an alien government's interference in the religion of its subjects (despite evidence that experimental sanitary measures at a major religious fair in Hardwar in 1867 had in fact resulted in positive responses from Indians and requests for more sanitary measures at pilgrim sites) (MacKenzie Committee 1868: 8).

The real obstacle was the perceived size of the financial commitments involved and the uncertain time frame over which this might be required to extend. For the British, reluctant to look beyond military and commercial matters, the task of extending public health measures to include the Indian population was rapidly beginning to look like an intractable problem. The pilgrim question remained in abeyance until the second decade of the twentieth century when, with a new focus on public health following the plague epidemic, committees were appointed and a few improvements instituted (Ramasubban 1982: 24). As the nineteenth century wore on, the colonial government's enthusiasm for remaking Indian society considerably declined (Hutchins 1967: xi, 170–178; Stokes 1959: 242, 269, 278–279, 288; Strachey 1961: 55). With segregation working well for the enclave population, the construction of India as a 'land of epidemics and cholera' and of Indians as a racially inferior mass and perennial reservoirs of disease was becoming a more acceptable approach The dominant policy now was that Indians should be left to develop a sanitary consciousness at their own pace.

The only large-scale intervention for which there had been some enthusiasm was smallpox vaccination using the Jennerian cowpox method. It was the only tried and tested prophylactic; a symbol of the efficacy of Western medicine, and Britain's benevolent governance (Arnold 1993: 135–136). The challenge was how to convey this message to the intended beneficiaries. India already had its own method of inoculation against smallpox. Both contemporary Sanskrit texts and early East India Company medical officers had commented on the relative efficacy of the method (Dharampal 1971: chapter 2).

In the eyes of the colonial government, this traditional system of inoculation was the principal enemy of its selective civilizing mission. Vaccination departments were set up in each province and inoculation banned. But the Vaccination Department was not able to play a convincing enough role to displace inoculation, leading several within the colonial medical establishment to question the wisdom of the ban on inoculation (Arnold 1993: 151).

The development of the colonial economy – promotion of commercial agriculture, growth of urban industrial and commercial centres, introduction of railways – was breaking down the isolation of disease strains. The unplanned and overcrowded 'native quarters' of the cities were becoming acutely vulnerable to epidemics, since famines were escalating rural-to-urban migration. Following the terrible epidemics in Bombay in the 1860s and 1870s, and pressures from some Indian quarters to make vaccination compulsory, the government passed the 1880 Vaccination Act. Much effort was put into impressing on urban elites and the upper castes the value of vaccination so that they would provide the leadership for the rest of the society.

Some of this must have borne fruit, as the 1870s and 1880s saw considerable improvement in the uptake of vaccination (Banthia and Dyson 1999: 34). However, little political will was put into the actual enforcement of the Vaccination Act among the mass of the population. Indeed, the growing Indian eagerness for government to extend the scope of its Vaccination department was becoming a source of alarm, as it would have meant a large-scale financial commitment (Arnold 1993: 145). Virtually until the end of British rule, the 'indifference of the people' towards the civilizing influence of the rulers and dangers of a 'religious backlash' were cited to justify inaction, despite there being no cultural resistance at all to smallpox vaccination. Smallpox remained a virulent epidemic disease until the compulsory programme of the 1950s and 1960s.

The period from 1870 to 1920 was a dark one. The decennial census instituted in 1870 and the annual sanitary reports together give us the picture of an unprecedentedly gloomy public health situation marked by a combination of epidemics, famines, migration and mass pauperization. The start of the period saw the onset of devastating famines. In 1896 a plague epidemic broke out in Bombay Presidency and spread to the rest of the country, causing consistently high mortality for over two decades; an estimated total of nearly 10 million deaths. The influenza epidemic of 1891 took a further 12 million lives. Malaria alone was estimated to have caused 20 million deaths in this period (Klein 1973: 643). Cholera continued to resurge in epidemic form around each famine. From a high of around 40 per 1,000 in 1881–1891, crude rates rose to around 46 per 1000 in 1911–1921. The 1920 census recorded the highest death rates ever (Dyson 2004: 20).

Plague deaths were most visible in cities such as Bombay. The years from 1896/97 to 1905 also witnessed a major famine, which was particularly severe in Bombay Presidency, causing a huge inflow of migrants – 300,000 in three months in 1897 – from the countryside (Bombay Plague Committee Report 1898: n.p.). Crude death rates which had hovered around 30 per 1,000 in the period 1891–1895 rose to an average of 65 in the years 1896 to 1906 before coming down to 40 in 1907. The epidemic highlighted as never before the class-driven nature of disease patterns. The effect of residential segregation of the elites was that the European population suffered a death rate of 1 per 1,000, Brahmins 13 per 1,000 and low caste Hindus 22 per 1,000 (Klein 1986: 724–754). The elites – European and Indian – responded to plague by moving out of the city for the peak years of the epidemic (Ramasubban and Crook 1995: 149). Not only did the plague draw attention to the drastically degraded environment of the city, there were serious dangers from other rampant diseases such as tuberculosis (TB) and cholera.

Plague evoked the first significant public health intervention. However, the measures that were carried out in the large cities – police-backed compulsory evacuation, fumigation and hospitalization, house searches and physical examinations, quarantine and isolation camps – were not only scientifically incorrect but so violent that they succeeded in antagonizing the nationalist political leadership and the common people alike (Arnold 1987: 203–218; Ramasubban 1982: 26–27). This was the first major organized political and cultural resistance to the government's public health proposals. The fact that almost all plague deaths were among Indians made the health of the people for the first time a concern of the nationalist movement.

Plague compelled the municipalities of the large cities to confront the issue of sanitary expenditures and re-housing schemes for the poor. In Bombay, however, there was confusion over who should take responsibility. In place of decisive municipal action, a Bombay Improvement Trust was set up in 1898 (City of Bombay Improvement Act [Bombay Act IV of 1898]) in the face of opposition from property owners who were hostile to any tax-based funding of improvement projects (Aibara n.d.), and from Indian members of the Governor-in-Council who contended that it was municipal corporation's responsibility and not that of a trust to tackle insanitation in the city (Boman-Behram 1983: 12). In the years that followed, some working-class housing came to be constructed, but the principal beneficiaries of the projects undertaken were the middle classes. Within two decades, the Bombay Improvement Trust was wound up and its functions transferred to the municipality, but pressures from the colonial government to cut provincial government and municipal budgets were never far away. In 1917, the president of the Bombay Municipal Corporation lamented that, 'The great majority of insanitary areas, the urgent necessity for improvement of which was the reason for the Trust's creation in 1898, continues to exist' (Sastry 1983: 15).

Plague prompted the Government of India to propose for the first time a Public Health Department and one sanitary officer for every district. Lord Curzon, governor general of India, couched the proposal in terms of the benefits that would accrue to the British soldier; but it was rejected as an unnecessary expense. Lord Hamilton, secretary of state for India wrote: 'It is a serious question of public policy whether the Indian Medical Service should continue to be augmented for the purpose of providing for the medical needs of the population at large'. He favoured, instead, an enhanced preventive medicine focus on British troop health, based on the new science of bacteriology (IOR: L/E/7/432, R and S 1127/1900). With the colonial government's expenditure per soldier being 130 times that per civilian, and army health reforms moving in step with metropolitan scientific developments, the general population was no longer seen as a threat (Megaw 1939).

The high mortality during World War I brought a new global focus to public health that was accentuated by the death toll from the worldwide influenza epidemic of 1918–1919. This focus went beyond the scope and objectives of the international sanitary conferences of the late nineteenth century that had acted merely as regulatory authorities. A significant actor was the Rockefeller Foundation which was already supporting the reform of medical education in the United States, inspired by German educational methods. In the period from 1913 to 1923, the International Health Board of the Foundation put into place a policy for both medical and public health education which divided the world into sectors. The aim was to create one or more strategically placed university centres of scientific medicine in each of the sectors. London, as the capital of the British empire, was an ideal location, and the School of Hygiene and Tropical Medicine was created within the University of London as a joint project of the Rockefeller Foundation and the British government (Fisher 1978: 27).

The Government of India subscribed to the costs of the London School. It also sanctioned a grant of 500,000 rupees as the nucleus of a proposed Public Health Fund for India. In 1918, a conference of experts met in Delhi to plan the use of this grant. The influenza epidemic had resulted in 6 million deaths thus far in India alone. One suggestion was the creation of something resembling a Public Health Ministry that would also work closely with similar bodies in the provinces. The Indian Medical Service (IMS) participants were unequivocal that any new policy must distance itself from the deadweight of the Sanitary Department which had a poor record of service to the mass of the Indian population (Bentley 1919: 15). The most serious indictment came from Dr C. A. Bentley, sanitary commissioner to the Government of Bengal: the Sanitary Department was a 'complete failure'. With the exception of the Presidency towns, there was practically no improvement in the health of the general population. On the other hand, since 1864, there had been a 'remarkable reduction' in sickness and mortality in the army – 90% and 80% among British and Indian troops, respectively – while among prisoners in jails (also a Government of India concern) mortality had gone down by two-thirds. The unpopularity of the Sanitary Department was evident from the fact that during the decade before World War I, only 12 IMS officers in all of India were willing to take up sanitary work (Bentley 1919: 16, 29).

A year later, a conference of medical experts met in Simla to again discuss how best to utilize the grant. The IMS participants proposed an 'elite corps' of mobile epidemiological units that would engage in research and also assist provincial and local bodies in dealing with epidemics – in keeping with the Rockefeller Foundation International Health Board's overseas operations (Report of Conference of Medical Experts 1919: 44). Despite the view that the provinces were the inescapable site for sanitary action, the vision was still a top-down one.

The last few decades of colonial rule saw some willingness to engage with some major public health problems. Committees were appointed to look into the conditions of pilgrim travel and sanitary conditions of pilgrim towns (Reports of the Bombay Pilgrim Committee 1916; Bihar and Orissa Pilgrim Committee 1913; Madras Pilgrim Committee 1915; U.P. Pilgrim Committee 1913). But in the case of the pilgrim issue, as with the Public Health Fund, the military preoccupations associated with the two World Wars and the financial stringency measures of the inter-war period blocked progress. Old arguments were resurrected: the need for economy; the size, complexity and culturally sensitive nature of the problem; the administrative inconvenience of initiating major public health interventions at the time; and the military orientation of the all-India Indian Medical Service.

In 1943, the government appointed the Joseph Bhore Committee to draw up a plan for health services for the general population. This step, as part of the planning process for the post-war period, was intended to convey the promise of a more proactive public health policy, broadly along the lines of the National Health Service being designed for Britain (Jeffrey 1996: 277). The Committee recommended a free curative health service, consisting of primary health centres with sub-centres each catering to 100,000 people, headed by medical officers and linked to district-level tertiary hospitals. Attached to each primary health centre would be a few sanitary inspectors to oversee vaccination, chlorinate wells and promote preventive measures, generally. The Bhore Committee also envisaged special disease control campaigns for malaria, smallpox, leprosy, TB, filariasis and sexually transmitted diseases along the lines of the Rockefeller Foundation International Health Board's approach (Report of the Health Survey and Development Committee 1946).

Health policy in independent India

When India emerged from 300 years of colonial servitude in 1947, the health situation in the country was one of a high general death rate (32 per 1,000) with considerable mortality due to epidemic disease. Life expectancy at birth was a mere 31 years (Dyson 2004: 20). Its population (around 360 million) was predominantly agrarian and lacking both preventive and curative services. Its health administration was tiny, financially starved and marginalized. A weak revenue base and considerable political instability completed the picture. None of this was compatible with fostering a radical public health policy departure.

The first few years were a period of uneasy coexistence between two approaches to the health of the mass of the people One was the rural-oriented and holistic Community Development Programme inspired by Mahatma Gandhi's thinking. This approach saw improvements in environmental sanitation and nutrition as the basis for improvements in individual and community health. The specific components were: controlling water and food-borne diseases through simple environmental sanitation methods; intensifying health and nutrition education; training women as health educators to promote family planning; maternity care and child welfare; and training local people to be paraprofessional health-care workers.

The other model of development was Jawaharlal Nehru's, with its focus on rapid modernization through a top-down, technology-led strategy, with the government in the driver's seat, and the emphasis on industrial growth and higher education and scientific research. Its assumption was that the benefits would trickle down to the mass of the people once they started moving from agriculture-based jobs to high productivity modern sector jobs in urbanizing areas, and acquired the incomes to purchase nutrition and health care, as had happened in the Western countries. The inculcation of modern norms and values would remove all cultural barriers to effective health services. This strategy favoured a family planning philosophy that stressed birth control using new technologies.

Political support for the Gandhian approach had declined to a mere trickle by the end of the 1950s. Impatience with the slow-moving Community Development Programme in general and the environmental sanitation component in particular – based on mass education and community participation – was high, and the 'growth-first-and-the-rest-will-follow' development strategy became the preferred option. The emphasis shifted from facilitating grassroots initiatives to creating a top-down, country-wide network of primary health-care centres, offering a single body of curative services without regional or sub-regional variations. The single-disease control programmes were also set in motion, administered by the central government and backed by international aid. However, the mechanisms for integrating these two sets of interventions were not spelt out, health education and community participation were missing, and the problem of how urban-oriented medical professionals could be induced to move to the rural areas was not addressed. Also, water, sanitation, nutrition and housing came under separate ministries and were not integrated with each other or with the health planning (Ramasubban and Rishyasringa 2002: 15–19).

The first two five-year plans (ending in 1961) allocated 3% of total public expenditure to medical and health services. In the subsequent Plans, this proportion declined to around 2%, although in absolute terms public health expenditure continued to increase. The declining trend continued until by the end of the twentieth century expenditure had fallen to 0.9% (Ramasubban 1984: 101–104; Government Of India (GOI) 2005: 3). As in the past, whenever governmental expenditures are reduced, it is the health sector – with the exception of family planning – that is the victim. Today, the central government allocation for health is only 1.3% of the total budget, while it is a mere 5.5% at the level of the states (GOI 2005: 3). The delivery of day-to-day primary health care is the responsibility of the individual states, just as it had been a provincial responsibility under the British Raj. The under-financing of health in a situation where the mass of the population is dependent on state services represents an unbroken historical tradition.

The grand design has proven unable to provide the free and universal care which might have transformed the health of the people. The states have failed to build the administrative capability within the health sector and have tolerated poor standards of quality, efficiency and accountability; in turn rendering the system unacceptable to its intended beneficiaries who prefer to access the ubiquitous private providers. The absence of public scrutiny have made it particularly vulnerable to political and bureaucratic manipulation and corruption. The neglect of community participation has left individuals unfit to undertake preventive measures. The result is that the public health services have steadily deteriorated, a decline that has been precipitous since in the 1980s, a policy orientation towards market reforms has emerged. The planning of the health system also remains unintegrated with related heath promotive programmes to do with drinking water, sanitation, hygiene and nutrition which are planned by different agencies. Only 10% of Indians have some form of health insurance, most of it inadequate (GOI 2005: 3). The inability of the poor to access good quality health services in the early stages of an illness often make hospitalization the only recourse. Every episode of hospitalization might absorb 60% of a family's annual expenditure. Families have to sell assets or risk indebtedness, leading to even greater pauperization.

The only preventive measures were in the form of the 'military' campaigns for disease control, launched in the early 1950s. Initially these enjoyed the financial and technical assistance of the Rockefeller Foundation; subsequently, considerable funding came from bilateral and multilateral agencies, in whose perception epidemic disease control was a key to the economic and political stability of the developing countries. Two of these programmes proved particularly effective. A massive vaccination and re-vaccination programme for smallpox eventually succeeded in eradicating the disease. In the case of malaria, powerful insecticides and drugs extensively used in combination – a method that had proved successful in malaria control in World War II – made for initially very optimistic results; between 1953 when the National Malaria Control Programme started and 1965, disease incidence and mortality fell from 100 million cases and 1 million deaths to 1 million cases and no deaths (GOI 1977: 22–23). Largely because of the success of these two programmes, the country's crude death rate more than halved from a high of 45.4 per 1,000 in 1911–1921 to 21.3 per 1,000 in 1961–1971 (Dyson 2004: 20–21). A control programme directed against epidemic cholera paid attention to provision of safe water and licensing of food stalls along major pilgrim train routes and at pilgrim centres, and inoculation and chemotherapeutic measures targeting pilgrims, again, unfinished tasks carried over from the colonial period. This brought down cholera deaths from 2.4% of all deaths towards the end of the colonial period to 0.4% by 1966–1967 (Cassen 1978: 84).

Although the national disease programmes were a commendable symbol of the new government's commitment to public health, with the exception of smallpox, they had several fatal flaws. The programmes were 'vertical': neither conceptually nor administratively were they connected with the curative health services at the state level, with any broader developmental policies, environmental prevention measures, or popular preventive health education. Where there was a financial and administrative link, as in the case of malaria where maintenance was the responsibility of the state health departments after the initial eradication phase, the states were entangled in uneasy financial relations with the central government.

Within a decade of the malaria programme's transfer to the states in 1965, the total number of cases had risen to an estimated 5.2 million. Subsequently, endemic malaria – complicated by pesticide and drug resistance – has become a major problem and India is now one of the leading applicants to the Global Fund for Malaria, TB and HIV/AIDS.

All these factors, together with mass poverty, sealed the fate of the National TB Control Programme, which was conceived in purely curative terms. The irregular inflow of TB drugs from abroad and their unreliable supply to patients depending on the free health centres, the high market cost of drugs for patients seeking alternatives to the state system, the pursuit of cheap cures by patients, haphazard treatment by inadequately trained and unregulated private providers and neglect of community education about treatment compliance have all contributed to the huge problem of multi-drug-resistant TB. The TB rates in India are among the highest in the world.

The aforesaid flaws notwithstanding, the combined effect of the disease control programmes and the availability of a wide range of curative services was that by the end of the 1950s the high epidemic mortalities that had marred the colonial government's record became a thing of the past. With the steady decline in death rates, population growth, which had already begun to accelerate after 1921, quickened its pace and the resulting population boom – a crude birth rate that hovered around 45 per 1,000 – set off alarm bells. The 1961 decennial census projected a very gloomy scenario. Soon after, a new national vertical programme – family planning – with considerable financial allocation and backed by foreign aid and international scientific and demographic research that supported a method-specific approach to fertility control began to displace public health and sanitation from their already precarious position on the political agenda. In the rural areas, the primary health centres (PHCs) and their sub-centres became the principal instruments, while in the urban areas the government hospitals and dedicated 'family planning centres' performed this role. The emphasis from 1965 on the import of intrauterine devices (IUDs) justified an even more intensive use of health centres, and with the creation in 1966 of a Department of Family Planning within the Ministry of Health to administer a 'target-oriented' programme for IUD insertion and sterilization, the field staff of the PHCs acquired a crucial role as 'motivators' of 'subjects'. The housing of family planning within health centres was to maximize the number of 'subjects' and make it acceptable. It was also presented as concern for the health of mother and child. Family planning along with infant immunization took centre stage even as the goal of malaria eradication receded after 1965 and the disease control programmes faded into obscurity. TB control was revived in the 1990s with the advent of the World Health Organization-led Direct Observed Treatment Scheme (DOTS) approach.

The resurgence of malaria and its appearance even in affluent areas of cities like Mumbai (formerly Bombay), the growing TB rates and the problem of co-infection with HIV/AIDS (most visible in urban slums), the periodic outbreaks of gastroenteritis and leptospirosis as a result of poor municipal governance, and the endemicity of a host of sexually transmitted and air-, water- and food-borne diseases have repeatedly brought health into the media spotlight. In response, health policy has lurched from one piecemeal intervention to another. In 1974, a Minimum Needs Programme (MNP), presented as a pro-poor, pro-women programme, purported to be a new approach to the contradictions plaguing the health system. It promised: a reorientation of the system in favour of the rural areas; better integration of promotive, preventive and curative services through their direction to specific 'target groups' in rural and tribal areas and urban slums, and removal of inter-group and inter-regional imbalances in the delivery of health services; extending the reach of the primary health-care services; integration of the delivery of various services – disease control and family planning – through the conversion of the vertical functionaries into multi-purpose workers; and community participation through the agency of volunteers and non-governmental organizations. In the years that followed, each new central government engaged in the same rhetoric, albeit with minor changes in emphasis.

However, the primary health-care system continued to be dragged by the wheels of history: vertically structured, bereft of a prevention philosophy and dominated by the family planning programme. The redesignated 'multi-purpose workers' at the PHCs remained multi-purpose only in name; their health promotion role never valued and their family planning duties overriding all their other work. The focus of the family planning programme was on female sterilization conducted by centrally-paid, female, family planning workers based in the PHCs. The community health volunteers, meant to promote prevention at the village level, quickly repositioned themselves as fee-charging 'doctors'; when they demanded they be made full-time government workers, abolition of the voluntary programme was considered (Ramasubban 1977: 25). The public health measures upon which the success of the Minimum Needs Programme rested – provision of safe drinking water and drainage and sanitation facilities in urban slums and rural areas plus nutrition programmes – remained ineffective (Ramasubban 1984: 111). When in the 1990s – the International Decade for Water and Sanitation – major rural drinking water schemes were launched across the country with soft aid from the World Bank, they established no horizontal linkages with the health system, nor indeed were they even accompanied by drainage and sanitation programmes until much later in the decade. Nutrition schemes begun in the 1980s became yet another national vertical programme; a direct feeding programme called the Integrated Child Development Scheme (with one state alone, Tamil Nadu, running a school lunch scheme covering older children), while the nutrition and immunization of pregnant women were covered by the Mother and Child Health component of the family planning programme.

A major factor in the picture of failure presented earlier has been the dominance of the central government. Planning for all health facilities is based on population norms and central government spending across states is fairly uniform; neither exercise reflects differences between states in terms of epidemiology, efficiency of the state services, political commitment to health as reflected in state financial allocation and presence of the private health sector (World Bank 1997: vii, 30–40; WHO 2006: 180–181). Equally, the states have preferred to remain dependent on the centre; although they account for over 75% of spending on health, the bulk of this is on salaries, with the result that they look to the centre even for drugs and other inputs (Peters, Rao and Fryatt 2003: 250). For this same reason, they have failed to take responsibility for disease surveillance and infectious diseases control at the grassroots. Today, there are major regional imbalances in the health status of the population (most poignantly evident in infant and maternal mortality rates that place India among the bottom-most countries on the Human Development Index) that reflect differences not only in performance of health systems but in governance and the degree of mass poverty. Despite constitutional amendments (dated 1993) that provide a legal basis for the financial independence of local governments (Panchayati Raj; local self-government in Hindi; literally 'rule of the elected five'), such change has yet to be reflected in the priority accorded to health at the local level.

The latest attempt to fulfil the original objectives of independent India's health policy is the National Rural Health Mission (2005–2012). It again speaks of universal access to public health services concerned with water, sanitation, hygiene, immunization and nutrition; prevention and control of communicable and non-communicable diseases; access to comprehensive and integrated primary health care; and reduction of infant and maternal mortality. It aims to 'undertake architectural correction' of the health system to enable it to deliver services effectively, integrate health services with provision of drinking water, sanitation and nutrition through district health plans, target poor people especially women and children, create a cadre of female health activists at the village level, regulate the private sector, involve non-governmental organizations (NGOs) and promote 'public-private partnerships' in the delivery of services (GOI 2005: 9). The scheme was announced in July 2005, so its future remains to be seen. The document outlining the scheme does not elaborate on how it will relate to the vertical disease control programmes, particularly the HIV/AIDS control programme. Nor does it indicate how it will tie in with the family planning programme which, since the late 1990s, has been reoriented from a female-sterilization programme into a women's reproductive and child health programme, both as a means for speeding up the demographic transition and a response to a worldwide movement for more gender-sensitive health policies. Nor does it discuss how it proposes to integrate the new rural health plan with planning for urban populations; rapid urbanization has prompted demographers to predict that over 50% of India's population growth will be living in cities by 2026, and some of these will be the most populous cities in the world (Dyson and Visaria 2004: 120–121).

Conclusion

We may discern several continuities between the colonial past and the post-independence present. On the one hand there is the continuing endemicity of water-, air-, food- and vector-borne diseases. Some have rebounded (notably TB and malaria and, briefly, plague, the defining epidemic disease at the beginning of the twentieth century), while new ones such as HIV/AIDS have emerged.

Infant and maternal mortality rates due to preventable causes – environmental and social – continue to remain high. The better-off sections of the population are able to buy themselves good housing, away from the teeming poor, and the new mantra of personal fitness has only accentuated this segregation. For the poor, who have little control over their micro or macro environment – urban slums come close to remote rural areas on indices of access to amenities like potable water and sanitary disposal of wastes, and infant mortality rates, and purchasing health care for episodes of sickness is the only resort.

Independent India's developmental goal of movement from poverty and infectious disease to affluence and health continues to elude it. It not only has one of the highest rates of TB (the classic disease of poverty), it is also among the countries with the highest rates of cardiovascular disease and diabetes (apparently diseases of affluence). But the latter are not to be only found among the relatively well-off sections of the population; ongoing research into prenatal causes of adult chronic disease shows that poverty and malnutrition of the mother during pregnancy, and the resulting low birthweight of infants, could be as much a foundation for adult diabetes and heart disease as affluent lifestyles (Barker, Olds and Wolfe 2003: 53).

As the country progresses through the first decades of the twenty-first century, it faces intermeshed epidemiological and demographic transitions. Both pose considerable challenges, given the country's aim of eradicating poverty. It is questionable whether a full-fledged 'epidemiological transition' can be achieved by public health programmes limited to water, sanitation and the environment, especially when poverty is a pervasive social reality. But this is probably the one set of public interventions that could have the most crucial impact upon the quality of life not only for the majority of the population that happen to be poor – for whom ill health has now become a major cause of further pauperization – but for society as a whole. For public action of this magnitude to happen, it is not enough to indulge in vague rhetoric about 'public-private partnerships' – the current global health buzzword. Such actions require efficient organizations in public ownership that are accountable to state-level bodies and monitored by strong local citizens groups with the statutory right to act as watchdogs.

Preoccupation with bringing down deaths and births has seen morbidity in India slip through the cracks. Ironically, until the later 1990s, even the World Health Organization accepted mortality as the measurement of health. There was a brief interregnum when primary health care for all became an international slogan; but the momentum was lost all too quickly. As the Government of India makes the old promises under a new set of slogans and commits itself to increasing expenditure on health from 0.9% of Gross Domestic Product (GDP) to 2 or 3%, and 'global health' becomes prominent again on the agenda of the developed countries, various efforts are being made to define health. Amartya Sen defines it as a 'capability' required for every person to fulfil his or her human potential, and global health theorists articulate it as a 'global public good' that is linked with considerations of equity both within and between countries (Bloom 2003: 17–18). There is an emerging 'people's' vision of health as a human right rather than a mere 'basic need', while 'patients' rights' movements in developed countries are attempting to reset the power balance between patient and health professional and make common cause with their counterparts in less developed countries as witnessed in the struggle for affordable anti-retroviral drugs for HIV patients.

As yet in India morbidity has been left to the tender mercies of the private medicine market. Private spending on health care accounts for about 75% of total health expenditure (WHO 2006: 180–181). India has a huge and unregulated private health market, ranging from the high end that is now being built into a health tourism sector to untrained but affordable 'hole-in-the-wall-doctors' on whom the poor depend. A greater role for the State in regulating private curative services and in reviving the moribund public health system is imperative. Recent research (Peters *et al*. 2002: 253) provides evidence that the Indian states supporting pro-poor services are also the states with better health outcomes. Global health concerns have as yet only produced a return to massive doses of international assistance for stand-alone control programmes, notably HIV/AIDS and the Reproductive and Child Health Programme. The Indian State itself is yet to pull together all the complex threads to fashion an effective health policy that can overcome the dualisms that presently plague the health system.

References

Aibara, A. (n.d.) 'Municipal Policies and Urban Development in Bombay City, 1880s to 1907', seminar presentation, Centre for South Asian Studies, School of Oriental and African Studies, University of London.

Annual Report of the Sanitary Commissioner with the Government of India (henceforth *Annual Sanitary Report*).

Annual Sanitary Reports for the years 1870–1929.

Arnold, D. (1987) 'Touching the Body: Perspectives on the Indian Plague, 1896–1900', in Ranajit Guha (ed.), *In Subaltern Studies, Volume V*, Delhi: Oxford University Press, 53–65.

—— (1993) *Colonising the Body: State Medicine and Epidemic Disease in Nineteenth Century India*, Berkeley: University of California Press.

Banthia, J. and Dyson, T. (1999) 'Smallpox in Nineteenth Century India', *Population and Development Review*, 25(4): 649–680.

Barker, D., Olds, D. and Wolfe, B. (2003) 'In the Beginning: The Events of Early Life and their Long-term Impact', in Barry Bloom with Phyllida Brown (eds), *The Future of Public Health*, Boston: Harvard School of Public Health, 53–65.

Bentley, C. A. (1919) 'Note on the Indian Sanitary Services', *Report of the Conference of Sanitary and Bacteriological Experts held at Delhi on 19 and 20 December 1918.* Appendix 2. London: India Office Library and Records: L/E/7/992/1920, R and S 2990/1919.

Bloom, B. (2003) 'Common Values: An Overview', in Barry Bloom with Phyllida Brown (eds), *The Future of Public Health*, Boston: Harvard School of Public Health, 7–19.

Boman-Behram, B. K. (1983) 'The Improvement Committee: A Retrospect', *Bombay Civic Journal*, xxx, October: 9–13.

Cassen, R. H. (1978) *India: Population, Economy and Society*, London: Macmillan.

Dharampal (1971) *Indian Science and Technology in the Eighteenth Century: Some Contemporary European Accounts*, Delhi: Impex Indica.
Dyson, T. (2004) 'India's Population: The Past', in Tim Dyson, Robert Cassen and Leela Visaria (eds), *Twenty-first Century India: Population, Economy, Human Development, and the Environment*, New Delhi: Oxford University Press, 15–31.
Dyson, T. and Visaria, P. (2004) 'Migration and Urbanisation: Retrospect and Prospects', in Tim Dyson, Robert Cassen and Leela Visaria (eds), *Twenty-first Century India: Population, Economy, Human Development, and the Environment*, New Delhi: Oxford University Press, 108–129.
Fisher, D. (1978) 'The Rockefeller Foundation and the Development of Scientific Medicine in Great Britain', *Minerva*, 16(1): 20–42.
Gazette of India [Supplement] (1864) Military Cantonments Bill. Papers Connected with the Formation of Sanitary Commissions in India, March.
Government of India (GOI) (1977) *Pocket Book of Health Statistics of India*, New Delhi: Ministry of Health.
—— (GOI) (2005) The National Rural Health Mission: 2005–2012 – Mission Document, New Delhi: Ministry of Health and Family Welfare.
Harrison, M. (1994) *Public Health in British India: Anglo-Indian Preventive Medicine 1859–1914*, Cambridge: Cambridge University Press.
Headrick, Daniel R. (1981) *The Tools of Empire: Technology and European Imperialism in the Nineteenth Century*, New York: Oxford University Press.
Hutchins, F. G. (1967) *The Illusion of Permanence: British Imperialism in India*, Princeton: Princeton University Press.
India Office Library and Records. IOR: L/E/7/1110, File 599.
IOR: L/E/7/432, R and S 1127/1900.
IOR: L/E/7/992, C and R 657/1920.
IOR: L/E/7/1071, C and R 2359/1923.
Jeffrey, R. (1996) 'Toward a Political Economy of Health Care: Comparison of India/Pakistan', in M. Das Gupta, L. C. Chen and T. N. Krishnan (eds), *Health, Poverty and Development in India*, Bombay: Oxford University Press, 270–294.
King, Anthony D. (1976) *Colonial Urban Development: Culture, Social Power and Environment*, London: Routledge and Kegan Paul.
Klein, I. (1972) 'Malaria and Mortality in Bengal, 1840–1921'. *The Indian Economic and Social History Review*, 9(2): 132–160.
—— (1973) 'Death in India'. *Journal of Asian Studies*, 32: 639–659.
—— (1986) 'Urban Development and Death: Bombay 1870–1914', *Modern Asian Studies*, 20(4): 725–754.
MacKenzie Committee (1868) Report and Order of the Madras Government Regarding the Control of Pilgrims in the Madras Presidency. Extract from Proceedings of the Sanitary Commissioner of the Government of Madras, London: India Office Library and Records.
Martin, James R. (1837) *Notes on the Medical Topography of Calcutta*, Calcutta: Huttman.
Megaw, J. (1939) 'Medicine and Public Health', in E. A. H. Blunt (ed.), *Social Service in India*, London: H.M.S.O, 97–116.
Nightingale, F. (1874) 'Life or Death by Irrigation', Appendix to paper 'Life or Death in India' read at the Meeting of the National Association for the Promotion of Social Science, Norwich, 1873. Appendix to India: *Annual Sanitary Report, 1873–1874*.

Peters, David H., Rao, Sujatha K. and Fryatt, R. (2003) 'Lumping and Splitting: The Health Policy Agenda in India', *Health Policy and Planning*, 18(3): 249–260.

Peters, David H., Yazbeck, A., Sharma, R. R., Ramana, G. N. V., Pritchett, L. H. and Wagstaff, A. (2002) *Better Health Systems for India's Poor: Findings, Analysis and Options*, Washington, DC: World Bank.

Ramasubban, R. (1977) 'Health Care for the People: The Empirics of the New Rural Health Scheme', Lucknow: Giri Institute of Development Studies, Technical paper.

—— (1982) *Public Health and Medical Research in India: Their Origins Under the Impact of British Colonial Policy*, Stockholm: SAREC.

—— (1984) 'The Development of Health Policy in India', in Tim Dyson and Nigel Crook (eds), *India's Demography: Essays on the Contemporary Population*, New Delhi: South Asian Publishers, 97–116.

—— (1988) 'Imperial Health in British India', in Roy MacLeod and Milton Lewis (eds), *Disease, Medicine and Empire: Perspectives on Western Medicine and the Experience of European Expansion*, London: Routledge, 38–60.

—— (1995) 'Policy Initiatives and External Assistance in Key Sectors in India: Focus on Child Development, Maternal Health, Drinking Water and Elementary Education', in Gosta Edgren (ed.), *Sharing Challenges: The Indo-Swedish Development Program*, Stockholm: Swedish Ministry of Foreign Affairs, 80–126.

Ramasubban, R. and Crook, N. (1995) 'Spatial Patterns of Health and Mortality', in Sujata Patel and Alice Thorner (eds), *Bombay: Metaphor for Modern India*, Bombay: Oxford University Press, 143–169.

Ramasubban, R. and Rishyasringa, B. (2002) *Sexuality and Reproductive Health and Rights: Fifty Years of the Ford Foundation's Population and Health Program in India*, New York: Ford Foundation.

Report of the Bihar and Orissa Pilgrim (Robertson) Committee (1913) Simla: Government Central Branch Press.

Report of the Bombay Pilgrim (Clemesha) Committee (1916) Simla: Government Monotype Press.

Report of the Bombay Plague Committee (1898) Appointed by Government Resolution– No. 1204/720 on the Plague in Bombay, July 1897–April 1898. Bombay: Times of India Stream Press (Bombay Plague Committee Report).

Report of the Cholera Committee (1868) Madras: Gantz Bros (Madras Cholera Committee Report).

Report of the Commissioners appointed to enquire into the Sanitary State of the Army in India (1863) British Parliamentary Papers, Cmd. 3184 (Henceforth Royal Army Sanitary Commission Report).

Report of the Conference of Medical Experts (1919) Simla, 23–24 May. India Office Library and Records: L/E/7/992 – 1920, R and S 6697/20.

Report of the Health Survey and Development Committee (1946) Vols. 1–4. Delhi: Manager of Publications (Bhore Committee).

Report of the Madras Pilgrim (Clemesha) Committee (1915) Simla: Government Monotype Press.

Report of the United Provinces Pilgrim (Robertson) Committee (1913) Simla: Central Branch Press.

Sastry, S. M. Y. (1983) 'Statutory Improvements Committee Comes into Being', *Bombay Civic Journal*, xxx(8), October: 15–24.

Stokes, E. (1959) *The English Utilitarians in India*, Oxford: Oxford University Press.

Strachey, J. (1961) *The End of Empire*, London: Victor Gollancz.
World Bank (1977) *India: New Directions in Health Sector Development at the State Level: An Operational Perspective*. Washington, DC: World Bank.
World Health Organization (2006) *The World Health Report, 2006*. Geneva: World Health Organization.

5 Public health in Thailand

Changing medical paradigms and disease patterns in political and economic context

Paul T. Cohen

Over the past two centuries public health in Thailand[1] has been transformed from a syncretic medical system centred on the body of the monarch – in a sense the sacred embodiment of the kingdom – to one that targeted the body of the population in an emergent modern nation state. The medical profession was charged with policing the new medicalized state and with popularizing scientific medicine. The discursive power of scientific medicine underpinned a form of medical dominance that either subordinated or excluded other aetiologies and modes of healing and promoted an elitist, urban-focused health system. The political struggle for democracy over the past several decades has developed synergistically with demands by reformist doctors and non-government organizations for a more equitable, decentralized public health system that fosters grassroots participation and self-reliance. The culmination of this struggle has been the formulation of a radically new health paradigm sanctioned by the State. In addition to outlining these discursive transformations this chapter will examine health status and epidemiological trends in relation to public health responses and in the context of economic and social changes linked to rapid modernization, industrialization and urbanization.

Thai traditional medicine in the nineteenth century

Before missionaries began to introduce the Thai elite to new Western medical concepts and practices in the nineteenth century, Thai royal medicine was centred on Ayurvedic medicine – a text-based, 'naturalistic' system in which the maintenance of bodily equilibrium (and good health) is through avoidance of upsetting the three 'morbid' humors (*tridosa*) of bile, wind and mucus. Disequilibrium and illness is related to factors such as climate, seasons, habitat and age; healing is predominantly oriented to herbal remedies. The 'Great Tradition' of Ayurvedic royal medicine in Thailand was controlled by court practitioners (*mor luang*). Interestingly the medical department to which these practitioners were attached came under the jurisdiction of the Palace Guards (Irvine 1982: 37). Thus, the 'policing' aspect of royal medicine was more concerned with the health and safety of the body of the king than with the body of the nation, though royalty did respond on occasions to epidemics that threatened the commoner population.

The response of the Thai king to the devastating cholera epidemic of 1820 was to hold a 'royal ceremony of illness destruction' comprising the chanting of Buddhist sutras and the firing of cannons to ward off evil forces (including malevolent spirits) (Davisakd 2003: 4; Terwiel 1987: 150). This underscores the syncretistic nature of court conceptions of illness at the time. The 'empirico-rational' medical tradition of Ayurveda (Zysk 1991: 5) was obviously considered inadequate protection against major pestilence.

The Thai tradition of Ayurveda took root in the countryside where it was preserved and practiced by male folk healers called *mor muang*. The arcane medical knowledge was transmitted orally from teacher to pupil and through texts (*tamra*). The basic concepts of Ayurveda were retained but the rural practitioners were much more eclectic than their court counterparts in both etiology and healing, combining with herbalism a wide range of beliefs and practices related to astrology, Buddhist spells, magic and manipulation of spirits. Further, villagers had access to a host of other types of healers, male and female, who had little connection with Ayurvedic medicine: soul doctors, exorcists, diviners, mediums and midwives. Many of these healers are still to be found in rural areas today (alongside modern medicine and facilities) though they are consulted in a much more limited way, either as a last resort for gravely ill patients or for mental problems less responsive to modern medical treatment.

Western and modern medicine

Davisakd Puaksom argues that most historical studies of medicine have tended to equate Western medicine with modern biomedicine (based on germ theory). Western medical practice dates back as early as the seventeenth century with the setting up of dispensaries by French missionaries, and a number of French physicians served the royal court at Ayutthaya (Davisakd 2003: 3). However, the key disseminator of Western medical theory and practice was the American missionary, Dan Beach Bradley (1804–1873). After he set up a dispensary in Bangkok in 1835, he published extensively on medical matters in his own newspaper, the *Bangkok Recorder*. His writings included advocacy of a range of public health measures, such as the regular cleaning of houses and the excavation of shallow canals (Davisakd 2003: 5). However, these recommendations were based on the theory of miasmas, popular in the West since the late eighteenth century, not on contagion and germ theory.

Miasmatic theory linked disease to the inhalation of vapours from rotting matter and other forms of filth. King Mongkut and King Chulalongkorn both issued decrees, in 1856 and 1870 respectively, to maintain the cleanliness of rivers and canals. This culminated in the creation of a sanitary system (*sukhaphiban*) in Bangkok in the 1890s including the formation, in 1898, of a department of sanitation responsible, among other things, for the building of public toilets. These measures were based on assumptions of miasmatic theory which underpinned government policy on public health until the end of the nineteenth century, well after it had been discredited in the West.

Germ theory (based on the discoveries of Koch and Pasteur) gradually won acceptance in the early twentieth century. In 1901 the Department of Sanitation set up a public health laboratory. The government's response to an outbreak of the plague in Bangkok and some provinces in late 1904 was based on acceptance of germ aetiology. A publication of the Department of Sanitation in early 1910 unequivocally attributes the cause of cholera to microbes, that is, 'tiny particles invisible to the eye' (*tua sat lek thi lae hen duai ta mai dai*). According to Davisakd, this signals that 'germ theory had taken a firm place in the Thai elites' thought' (Davisakd 2003: 23). He also asserts that the emergence of this new medical discourse laid the foundation for 'the marrying of state power and medical knowledge' (Davisakd 2003: 15).

Public health and the medical profession in the twentieth century

The evolution of public health in Thailand mirrored the earlier development of public health in Europe in the eighteenth century with 'the emergence of the health and physical well-being of the population in general as one of the essential objectives of political power' (Foucault 1984: 277). In twentieth-century Thailand there was an emergent view that 'national prosperity and progress' critically depended on a large, healthy and productive population. Prince Chainat (Director of the Department of Public Health, 1918–1925), in a speech in 1924, proclaimed that the strength of the nation depended on its population (*kamlang khong banmuang yu thi phonlamuang*) and that public health policy should be directed at improving the 'physical well-being' (*khwam suk kai*) of the population. Thus, we have the birth in Thailand of what Davisakd calls a 'medicalized state' (*rath wetchakam*) (Davisakd 2003: 23–27).

The medicalization of the state and accompanying medical 'policing' became even more pronounced under the influence of the nationalistic policies of the government of Field Marshal Phibun Songkhram.[2] Phibun Songkhram emphasized the need to combat the high mortality rate (caused by endemic diseases) as obstacles to the economic progress of the country. State-sponsored marriages, the institution of a Mothers Day and competitions to promote maternal reproduction aimed to increase population growth. Another key strategy of nation-building was the National Nutrition Project. Poor nutrition was viewed as a major cause of high mortality, particularly among children. Scientific information on nutrition was widely disseminated through schools, radio and newspapers. The importance accorded public health at this time is reflected in the establishment of a Ministry of Public Health in 1942. It is also noteworthy that the public health programmes for producing healthy bodies were combined with other state disciplinary techniques that targeted the populations 'everyday life practices' (*kit pracamwan khong khon Thai*) related to eating, working, recreation and clothing, and that aimed to create a civilized national culture (Davisakd 2003: 34).

Of course, national progress required the promotion of the health of the whole of the country's population, not just of Bangkok, which had been the focus of early public health measures in the nineteenth century. The establishment of a sanitary school in 1924 to train sanitary personnel facilitated the extension of public health measures to rural areas (Davisakd 2003: 24). In the 1930s, plans were made to construct hospitals and clinics and provide mobile medical units throughout the country to be serviced by physicians, nurses and midwives. They would be the agents for the rapid popularization of modern, scientific medicine in the provinces because 'The ultimate aim of the "medicalized" state was to encourage the popularity of modern medicine' (Davisakd 2003: 28).

The Rockefeller Foundation played a key role in the medicalization of Thai society. Beginning in 1923, it helped reorganize what was then Thailand's only medical school (Siriraj) by funding six chairs in basic and clinical sciences. The foundation was imbued with an unquestioning belief in the superiority of modern medicine. Thus, one of it representatives in Thailand advised that the problem was 'not to turn out hundreds of doctors yearly; it is how best to use the ones that are turned out in "selling" modern medicine to the people in the interior' (Donaldson 1982: 113).

The government's hospital-building programme proceeded apace after World War II. By 1961 there were already 80 hospitals; of these 68 were provincial hospitals (Yuwadi 2002: 78), compared to only 25 in the provinces in 1942. The hospital system became the foundation for the dissemination of modern medicine and also for promoting the status of the medical profession. In 1923–1924 medical doctors achieved the goal of licensing and in 1936 the Council of Medicine Bill was enacted to establish a professional supervisory body and legal professional authority for appropriately trained doctors (Chanet 1994: 142). Again, there are parallels with eighteenth-century Europe in that medicalization bestowed a 'surplus of power' on doctors as hygienists. Moreover, it was the doctor's function as hygienist, rather than as therapist, that assured him of a privileged position (Foucault 1984: 283–284). According to Donaldson, after the overthrow of absolute monarchy in 1932, Thai doctors became 'medical technocrats' co-opted by the bureaucratic elite of military and civil officials (Donaldson 1982: 121). This is supported by Maxwell's research that found that between 1934 and 1966 the proportion of medical students of elite-class origin fluctuated around the 90% level. Moreover three-quarters of the doctors in Thailand were employed in the bureaucracy and the majority were ranked in the top 1% of civil officials (Maxwell 1975: 483, 473). However, the salaries of even the highest ranked civil servants are relatively low. Thus, in order to earn an income commensurate with their high status and to recoup the great cost of medical training, doctors have been forced to work in the private sector – in private clinics or hospitals.

The Ministry of Public Health and the Board of Investment initiated the expansion of private hospitals in the early 1970s by granting special privileges to investors, such as exemptions on import duties on hospital equipment and from income tax during the first five years of operation. The justification for the policy was that more beds would be made available to the poor in government hospitals. However, one negative consequence was an 'internal brain drain', with a large number of doctors in the employ of public hospitals moonlighting for more lucrative work in private hospitals. The number of private hospitals increased from 23 in 1970 (with 236 full-time doctors) to a maximum of 473 in 1998 (with 3,567 full-time doctors). There was a corresponding decrease in the number of medical doctors in the public sector, declining from 93% in 1971 to 76% in1995. The growth of entrepreneurial medicine in Thailand centred on private hospitals is closely linked to expansion of the capitalist sector and free market policies of the government since the early 1970s (replacing earlier state capitalism). Predictably, the fastest rate of growth in private hospitals occurred in the economic boom period ('bubble economy') from 1988 to 1997.[3] It is noteworthy that during the economic boom, the Ministry of Public Health, by its own admission, had become 'a supporting agency for private care institutions' (Thailand Health Profile 1999–2000: 358).

Counter discourses; other voices

Over the past century, and especially since the early 1970s, alternative discourses have emerged to contest the hegemony of medical elitism (with its discursive roots in the biomedical paradigm). These counter discourses focused on two basic issues: first, the need to decentralize and democratize public health in Thailand; and second, the need to promote alternative medical paradigms and practices (based on traditional Thai medicine or modern holistic medicine).

The watershed of a more potent and enduring opposition to medical elitism was the student uprising of October 1973, which put an immediate end to military dictatorship and laid the foundations for parliamentary democracy in Thailand. The political philosophy of the student movement was syncretic – a mixture of democracy, populism, socialism and Buddhism, with a commitment to political and moral change rather than violent revolution. In early 1974 more than 4,000 student volunteers joined a Return to the Countryside Campaign and spent a month in rural villages investigating local problems. Many of the volunteers were idealistic medical students from Mahidol University. Not long after concerned doctors, public health workers, academics and students launched a Public Health for the Masses Campaign. Some conservative doctors criticized the campaign for having devalued the high status of the medical profession (Cohen 1989: 167).

The violent military backlash in October 1976 against the perceived threat of socialism and communism forced many radical students, who had by then graduated as doctors, to flee to the jungles to join the Communist Party of Thailand (Bamber 1997: 237). Most returned under amnesty in 1980 and eventually were able to resume their medical careers. After about a decade of parliamentary democracy, reform-minded doctors again became politically involved, following the military coup (of February 1991) that overthrew the elected government of Chartchai Choonhavan. Doctors and other health personnel were crucially involved in the so-called bloody Black May military massacre of civilian demonstrators (of 18–21 May): caring for the wounded (often in defiance of military orders), the dissemination of information by means of fax, hospital billboards, and the monitoring and taping of international satellite or TV broadcasts. After the fall of the military government (National Peacekeeping Council), health professionals continued political activities in support of the September 1992 elections including the establishment of the Health Assembly for Democracy in August that year (Bamber 1997: 241). The reformist doctors comprised a small minority within the medical profession. Nevertheless, they were politically committed, with a strong sense of obligation to take a leadership role in society. They were also adept at communicating their views through the mass media, and had links to both the poor and members of the political elite (in some cases the King himself).

The student uprising of 1973 provided a major impetus to the non-governmental organization (NGO) movement but the proliferation of NGOs occurred mainly after the return of parliamentary democracy in 1979. One reason is that the doctors who returned from the jungles under amnesty had to 'lie low and wait for the dust to settle'. NGOs provided a legitimate means for members of the medical profession to re-engage themselves in some of the reform activities which had previously led to accusations of being 'communist' (Bamber 1994: 6). By 1984, there were 113 development NGOs in the country; 17 of these were involved in various forms of primary health-care work.

The guiding principles of the primary health-care NGOs in Thailand can be summarized as follows: 'demystification' as a result of the 'medicalization of Thai society'; 'self-reliance' in health care; 'redistribution' of government funds for health to primary health care,[4] the redistribution of wealth as a means of improving the health of the rural poor, and integrated rural development for the fulfilment of 'basic needs'. These principles have no doubt been influenced by the writings of prominent critics of modern medicine (such as Ivan Illich), by participatory action research (PAR) philosophy, and the World Health Organization (WHO) Alma-Ata Declaration on Primary Health Care of 1978.[5] However, these principles also have deep roots in Thai political consciousness and have been given a distinctively Thai interpretation. This is especially evident in the writings and activities of Dr Prawase Wasi that reflect a consistently Buddhist perspective, emphasizing a holistic approach to health and self-reliance (Cohen 1995: 10).

The promotion of traditional medicine is one expression of self-reliance. One notable initiative was the founding of the Traditional Medicine for Self-Curing Project in 1980. This primary health-care NGO emphasized self-reliance through the use of traditional herbal medicine, collected information on local knowledge and Thai traditional texts, arranged clinical and laboratory tests on herbal medicines, and encouraged hospitals and villages to establish their own herbal gardens. This NGO also gave support to the Foundation for the Revival and Promotion of Traditional Medicine, which set up Ayurveda college in 1980.[6]

The movement for the revival and promotion of traditional medicine in Thailand to contest the dominance of the drug-oriented medical profession exemplifies what Foucault has called 'the insurrection of subjugated knowledges' – disqualified, popular knowledges – against 'the centralising powers which are linked to the institution and functioning of an organized scientific discourse' (Foucault 1980: 81, 84). The economic crisis of 1997 gave a significant impetus to this 'insurrection' in so far as the devalued Thai baht made the importation of Western pharmaceuticals increasingly expensive. The King's post-crisis pronouncement on the need for a 'self-sufficient economy' (*sethakhit phorphiang*) also gave a royal seal of approval to a movement that emphasizes self-reliance. The growing popularity and legitimacy of the movement is reflected in the fact that, by 2000, organizations involved with Thai traditional medicine included 19 registered associations, 9 registered foundations, 18 forums and centres and 2 networks of organizations (the National Federation of Thai Medicine and the Southern Federation of Thai Medicine). There were also 534 traditional health clinics and 2,366 traditional medicine pharmacies (Amara n.d.:1). Government support and funding has also increased substantially in recent years. Thus the Ministry of Public Health initiated a project called 'The Thai Traditional Medicine Decade' to be included in the Eighth Economic and Development Plan (1997–2001) and with the aim of promoting Thai traditional medicine as a substitute for high-cost imported medicine and equipment. In 1999, the government enacted the Thai Traditional Medicine and Local Knowledge Protection and Promotion Act and established a National Institute for Thai Traditional Medicine within the Ministry of Public Health.

While Thai traditional medicine has been promoted predominantly in rural areas, Western and foreign alternative medicines have become increasingly popular among well-educated middle-class urbanites, especially from Bangkok. Arguably, the best known of these modern alternative medicines has been Cheewajit (literally 'body and mind'), a Thai version of macrobiotics. The popularity of Cheewajit was partly a response to the limitations of biomedicine in treating the growth in Thailand (especially in urban areas) of modern chronic diseases such as cancer. The Cheewajit magazine became a forum for illness narratives that emphasized the 'feeling of despair of being disempowered and dehumanized in their encounters with modern conventional medicine' (Komatra 1999: 18). Cheewajit publications and organizational networks (including health rehabilitation camps) 'became an alternative discursive space in which counter discourses and differing views of medical reality could be expressed and shared with others' (Komatra 1999: 21).

The HIV/AIDS epidemic since the mid-to-late 1980s also led to a proliferation of self-help groups, especially in northern Thailand, which had the highest incidence of the disease. The groups were distinctive in that they were formed by lower-class day labourers, peddlers and small traders. The spread of these groups was a response to the fact that public health funding was directed almost exclusively to prevention, with little concern for those who had contracted the virus. HIV-infected persons were also subjected to severe social discrimination by families, communities and clinical institutions. By May, 1999, there were 209 HIV/AIDS self-help groups in six northern Thai provinces alone.[7] According to Tanabe, these self-help groups have formed a new type of 'community of practice' in which people with HIV infection 'acquire knowledge and organise practices for survival under social discrimination and overwhelming medical power and its discourse' (Tanabe 1999: 1). The practices for survival have included various 'holistic' forms of self-care such as meditation and use of herbal medicine (though without rejecting modern medicine entirely).

In addition to these small HIV/AIDS self-help groups there were by 2000 some 126 NGOs working in the field of AIDS, as well as a number of coordinating networks of AIDS organizations. At the same time there were 513 NGOs altogether with activities related to health promotion (Amara n.d.: 4). This is testimony to the spectacular growth of the NGO movement and of civil society in Thailand.

Health status and epidemiological trends

As a consequence of economic development and advances in public health, Thailand has recorded some significant improvements in health. Between 1960 and 1998, life-expectancy at birth increased from 52 to 68.9 years (Thailand Health Profile 1999–2000: 179–180). Infant mortality has declined from 84.3 per 1,000 live births in 1964 to 40.7 in 1984 to 26.1 in 1996, and maternal mortality has dropped from 374.3 per 100,000 live births in 1962 to a low 10.6 in 1997 (though with an increase to 12.9 in 2001) (Thailand Health Profile 1999–2000: 188). There has been a steady decline in first-degree (protein and calorie) malnutrition among pre-school children (from 20% in 1988 to 8.6% in 2001); the north and northeast regions have higher rates and in 2001 highland children (concentrated in the north) had three times the percentage of malnutrition of those of Bangkok in 2001 (14% compared to 4.5%) (Thailand Health Profile 1999–2000: 192–193). There have been marked improvements in vaccine-preventable diseases. From 1979 to 2001, the incidence of measles declined from 28.9 to 11.86 cases per 100,000 population, tetanus neonatorum from 70 to 0.36, diphtheria from 4.4 to 0.02, pertussis from 11.2 to 0.12 and polio from 2.3 to nil. However, hepatitis B increased from 0.09 to 2.80 cases per 100,000 population over the same period (Thailand Health Profile 1999–2000: 196). Encephalitis, leprosy and rabies have been reduced in incidence over the past 20 years or so to the point that they are no longer considered public health problems. There have also been significant advances in the fight against vector-borne diseases.

Historically malaria has long been a major health scourge. As recently as 1947 there were 52,034 deaths from malaria alone, giving a mortality rate of 297.1 per 100,000 population (Yuwadi 2002: 66). Since then the Ministry of Public Health (MOPH) has cooperated with the WHO and America to conduct widespread malaria eradication campaigns (including Dichloro-Diphenyl-Trichloroethane (DDT) spraying). By 1977, the mortality rate had been reduced to 10.9 per 100,000 population with a further steady decline to 1.2 in 2001. However, malaria still remains a serious problem in border areas as a consequence of highly efficient vectors (i.e., *Anopheles dirus* and *Anopheles minimus*) and human mobility such as seasonal agricultural migration of non-immune Thai into forested areas or cross-border movement of refugees or migrants from endemic areas such as Burma. The emergence of multi-drug resistant parasites continues to be a problem, particularly along the Thai–Cambodia and Thai–Burma borders.

Despite the significant public health achievements in the reduction of typical diseases found in developing countries, Thailand now has to contend with rather alarming increases in health problems—cancer, heart disease, road accidents, HIV/AIDS and mental disorders—linked to changing lifestyles. Rapid modernization, industrialization and urbanization, especially over the past 20 years or so, have led to rampant consumerism, changing nutritional habits, mental stress and air pollution. Non-communicable diseases, such as heart disease and cancer, are now leading causes of morbidity and mortality due to lack of physical exercise and unhealthy food consumption habits that cause high blood cholesterol and obesity. The prevalence rate for heart disease increased from 56.5 per 100,000 population in 1985 to 109.4 in 1994 and 285.4 in 2000. The prevalence of cancer has increased from 34.7 per 100,000 population in 1994 to 71.1 in 2000 (Thailand Health Profile 1999–2000: 213) and is now the major cause of death (66,956 deaths in 2002) (United Nations Development Programme (UNDP) 2004: 5). Between 1977 and 2001, liver diseases and cirrhosis, caused mainly by high levels of alcohol consumption, increased from 4.3 per 100,000 population, to 12.3. Alcohol is also a major causal factor in road accidents. Mortality caused by road accidents has skyrocketed, from a low 2,086 deaths in 1986 (3.94 per 100,000 population) to a peak of 16,727 at the height of the economic boom in 1995 (28.22 per 100,000 population) and then a decline to 11,652 deaths in 2001 (18.76 per 100,000 population) due to the economic crisis and reduced vehicular traffic. There has been a recent resurgence to 13,116 deaths in 2003 with the economic recovery (*Bangkok Post* 24 November 2004). About 80% of road accidents deaths are of those riding motor cycles (Thailand Health Profile 1999–2000: 223, 226).

Beginning in the mid-1980s the Thai economy was transformed from dependence on agricultural exports to export-led industrialization.[8] The subsequent economic boom made Thailand the fastest growing economy in the world. Rapid urbanization was a by-product of new economic policies and of the boom. From 1985 to 1995, the urban population doubled. A stagnant agriculture sector and rapid industrial growth (concentrated in the Greater Bangkok Region) provided a powerful stimulus to rural-to-urban migration. Urban expansion has been concentrated on the primate city of Bangkok. In the 1970s, migrants came mainly from nearby rural provinces, but in the 1980s, most migrated from more distant provinces, especially from the poor northeast (Pasuk and Baker 1998: 133). Rapid urbanization has created a range of health problems. The capacity of Greater Bangkok to absorb the influx of rural migrants has been limited; hence the proliferation of urban slums in this metropolis from 438 (in 1980) to 2,265 (in 2000) (Santhat 1995: 51; Thailand Health Profile 1999–2000: 127). Urban slums have created pathogenic urban environments with overcrowding, lack of protection against extreme heat, inadequate sewerage and drainage systems, residence near swamps, railway lines and canals, and proximity to polluting and hazardous industrial facilities. The health problems of the urban poor are exacerbated by inadequate public health-care services. Research reveals significantly higher rates of illness, hospitalization and mortality (especially child mortality) in the slums and poor housing areas of Bangkok than in suburban housing (Santhat 1995: 53).

HIV/AIDS has become a major public health threat to Thailand. In 2003, there were some 53,000 deaths due to AIDS. By this time the cumulative number of HIV/AIDS infections since the beginning of the epidemic was in excess of 1 million; the cumulative number of AIDS deaths was 460,000; and the total number of people living with AIDS was 604,000 (UNDP 2004: 1). From the late 1980s, the disease spread rapidly from homosexuals to injecting drug users, female commercial sex workers, their male clients and then from them to their wives and children. The rate of HIV infection is now highest among heterosexual women and the ratio of infected women to infected men could be 60:40 by 2005 (Dane 2002: 186).

The main impetus for the epidemic came from the expansion of the commercial sex industry, involving both sex tourism and domestic commercial sex. By the early 1990s, there was official acknowledgment of the existence of some 500,000 commercial sex workers (CSWs) in Thailand; some NGOs put the figure as high as 2 million (Gray 1995: 183). A large proportion of the CSWs came from upcountry, especially from the north (which is famous for the beauty of the women). Indeed, northern Thailand came to have the highest incidence of HIV infection, due to a combination of factors. These include return migration of HIV-infected CSWs from Bangkok, a cultural acceptance of male patronage of brothels (especially for sexual initiation), and an increasing disposable cash income with which to purchase sexual services. Another factor is the frequency of micro-mobility in the north of poor wage-labourers for temporary work in agriculture, construction (on roads and housing estates), and lorry driving. Micro-mobile workers 'stay overnight for periods of time in exclusively or largely male groups where peer pressure and local CSW activity promote risk behaviour' (Thiesmeyer 2001: 3).

However, the Thai Government has been remarkably successful in bringing the epidemic under control and in reversing the spread of HIV/AIDS. Despite initial apathy and denials, the government launched a massive education and information campaign in the early 1990s, using the country's extensive public communication infrastructure. 'Strong political leadership and commitment provided a powerful impetus for a broad-based response and led to a huge increase in domestic funding for HIV/AIDS programmes' (UNDP 2004: 1). New infections have been reduced from a peak of 143,000 in 1991 to only 19,000 in 2003 (UNDP 2004:1).

Yet there is no room for complacency and there is an ever-present danger of a resurgence of the disease within Thailand and its spread beyond Thailand's borders. Patronage of commercial sex has declined, but sexual permissiveness among Thai youth has encouraged more casual sex with minimal condom use (Lyttleton 2004: 5). Injecting drug users (IDUs) are another cause for concern. About a quarter of new infections are due to unsafe injecting drug use (UNDP 2004: 54) and, against the general trend, HIV prevalence among IDUs has increased from 35% in 1991 to 50% in 2001 (Thailand Health Profile 1999–2000: 209). Many IDUs are sexually active and therefore can spread the virus outside user groups. Prevention has been hampered by a punitive approach to drug use, exemplified by the government's 'war on drugs' in 2004. There is a continuing high rate of HIV infection among many highland minority communities in

Thailand due to a combination of female prostitution and male injecting drug use (Gray 1998: 1076–1077). Also, over the past 15 years or so, there has been a substantial increase in the trafficking of foreign girls and women for the sex industry in Thailand, especially from highland minority groups in Burma and Yunnan (China). Migrant women are especially vulnerable to HIV infection due to their illegal status, language difficulties, low education and little knowledge of HIV/AIDS, and limited access to health care.[9] They tend to concentrate at cross-border sites (such as Mae Sai in northern Thailand on the Thai side of the Burma-Thailand border), which become intersection points for foreign migrants, permanent residents, internal migrants and other mobile groups, and thus high-risk 'hot spots' for HIV infection (Beesey 2000: 39).

The link between HIV/AIDS and cross-border mobility underscores the regional dimension of the disease. The same can be said of new emerging diseases such as severe acute respiratory syndrome (SARS) and H5N1 avian (bird) flu. In response to the SARS epidemic of 2003 Thailand instituted effective systems of surveillance, infection control and public information and was able to limit the number of cases of infection to nine with only two deaths. However, the government's response to the following avian flu epidemic was subject to much criticism with Prime Minister Thaksin Shinawatra accused of an early cover-up to protect the poultry industry (Thailand is the world's fourth largest chicken exporter) and tourism. Eventually the government was forced to cull some 40 million birds. There were 12 reported deaths of humans by May 2005 and, ominously, there were some suspected cases of human-to-human transmission.

Public health reform: a new health paradigm

The growing influence of the NGO movement in Thailand is reflected in the fact that in recent years the oppositional discourses of NGOs have been mainstreamed and incorporated into government ideology, policies and institutions. Connors observes that ideas of 'civil society', of 'villagers' wisdom' and of participatory democracy 'are now signature tunes in the journals and public documents of the Thai state' (Connors 2003: 319). This development can be partly attributed to the progressive influence of NGOs since the 1970s and especially since the 'Black May' protests of 1992. However, the economic crisis of 1997 was the primary catalyst for change; it provided the opportunity for people to demand economic and social reform and to return to and advance some of the 'low cost, good health' policies introduced during the 1978–1987 recession.[10] According to Hewison, the crisis made 'rural localism' (with its emphasis on self-reliance, local wisdom and opposition to consumerism, urbanism and industrialization) a 'radical alternative'. The King's response to the crisis and his call for a 'self-sufficient economy', noted earlier, added legitimacy to this localism and also helped to bring conservatives and radicals together (Hewison 2002: 148–149).

State appropriation of NGO alternative, reformist discourses is particularly evident in the sphere of public health. On 9 May 2000, the Cabinet approved a national agenda for health systems and set up a National Health Systems Reform

Committee to draft a national health bill to be enacted by July 2003.[11] The Bill aims to establish 'a new health paradigm' for public health that is holistic, participatory and that promotes equity, efficiency, quality health care, consumer empowerment and self-reliance (Thailand Health Profile 1999–2000: 449). The strategy for reform is a 'triangle that moves mountains': creation of relevant knowledge, social movement and political involvement (Thailand Health Profile 1999–2000: 445; Wiput 2004: 14). The bill embodies the principles of the new 1997 Constitution that health is a basic human right to be protected by the state (Wiput 2004: 11). The process of drafting the Health Reform Bill provided a remarkable example of participatory democracy at work, with public hearings in 500 districts (involving 40,000 activists from 'grassroots communities') and another 20 public hearings on specific health issues. A summation of these hearings was presented for further discussion to provincial health assemblies in 76 provinces (with more than 40,000 people attending). In August 2002 a final draft of the National Health Bill was drawn up (based on a review of the conclusions of the provincial assemblies) and submitted for endorsement by the National Health Assembly (comprising some 4,000 academics and community representatives) (Wiput 2004: 24).[12]

Health reform also requires the decentralization of public health along with other public sectors. In 1999, Parliament passed the Act on Operationalization of Decentralization that required all ministries including the Ministry of Public Health to plan the devolution of their functions, facilities and personnel to the local administration within ten years. The legislation provides for the increase in the proportion of the revenue of local administration from 9% of total public revenue in 1999 to 20% in 2001 and 35% in 2006. For the Ministry of Public Health this could mean transferring as much as 80% of its annual budget and 90% of its staff to local administration units (Thailand Health Profile 1999–2000: 458). However, there is concern within the Ministry of Public Health that this could lead to a fragmentation and lack of coordination between local health units (e.g. health centres and district and provincial hospitals), corruption and insufficient management skills at the level of sub-district administration and loss of employment by current MOPH personnel (Thailand Health Profile 1999–2000: 456–458).

Another dimension for public health reform has been government funding of health NGOs, beginning with the post-May 1992 government of Anand Panyarachun. In 2000, 126 organizations (registered with the Ministry of Public Health) applied for financial support from the Ministry's Civil Society Organizations in Health Fund, with 157 projects funded for a total of THB 35 million (Amara n.d.: 20).[13] In addition, the government has provided major funding to the Thai Health Promotion Foundation (established in 2001) in the form of a 'sin tax' of 2% on liquor and cigarettes. The Foundation has programmes for tobacco and alcohol control, public exercise, traffic accident prevention and consumer protection.

The government has also adopted an innovative approach to distributing the national health budget through a THB 30 (USD 75 cents) per visit health-care scheme. By May 2003, 45.6 million people had registered at one thousand hospitals, with the hospitals receiving a per capita subsidy based on the number of people registered. The scheme has made basic health care more accessible to the poor and has been very popular (Pasuk and Baker 2004: 93–94).

Conclusion

In this chapter I have traced the evolution in Thailand of a medicalized state controlled by a medical elite with an entrenched belief in the superiority of modern biomedicine and increasingly oriented to urban-centred, curative, high-tech and entrepreneurial medicine. I have also described the rise of alternative discourses that advocate the revival of traditional medicine and the creation of a more equitable, decentralized and participatory public health system. The culmination of these institutional and discursive struggles has been the emergence of a new, government-sanctioned health paradigm. The public hearings for the drafting of the National Health Bill exemplify grassroots democracy at work and the THB 30 universal health-care scheme has realized a significant redistribution of health resources to the rural poor. Legislation has mandated the decentralization of public health administration. Some might, with good reason, view this change as a resounding victory for the democratic movement, for proponents of civil society and for NGOs. However, others point to countervailing political and economic tendencies that may serve to undermine health reform. Thus Connors contends that the new 'liberalising state' of Thailand has appropriated, influenced and developed progressive ideas 'in order to sideline radical projects and reconstruct national ideology' (Connors 2003: 320). The 'nation' has become an 'ideological straightjacket' in the sense that 'Citizenship and democracy are only to exist within the realm defined by national ideology' (Connors 2003: 322, 337). Furthermore, Hewison claims that government officials have co-opted localist ideas and transformed them into a 'top-down state development discourse' (Hewison 2002: 159). According to Pasuk and Baker, the main agenda of the present Thaksin government is to promote economic growth through economic nationalism and the creation of a strong central state to command and concentrate resources for big business (Pasuk and Baker 2004: 170). Populist policies have allowed the government to sidestep the bureaucracy and establish a direct relationship between the state and the citizen. However, the role of the 'people' is essentially passive in a society that is to be 'managed' both economically and socially (through social order and mass aerobics campaigns that are reminiscent of the Phibun Songkhram government). Furthermore, the priority accorded economic growth has led to government support for mega-projects that have the potential to damage the environment and health. The government's initial denial of the avian flu epidemic displays a willingness to place vested economic interests ahead of public health. This is a far cry from the ideals of the proponents of civil society who advocate the protections of individual rights and freedoms, participatory democracy and self-reliance.

Notes

1 Called Siam until 1939.
2 Phibun Songhram was prime minister from 1938 to 1944 and again from 1948 to 1957.
3 During the economic boom there was a rapid increase in the number of expensive CT scanners and MRI machines, heavily concentrated in Bangkok (Thailand Health Profile 1999–2000: 427).
4 In the early 1980s, about 80% of the government health budget was spent on hospitals and university medical schools.
5 The government PHC programme has been criticized as being top-down and lacking in grassroots participation. A MOPH public document itself acknowledges the programme has involved 'vertical manipulation by the state' (Thailand Health Profile 1999–2000: 470).
6 When Thailand's first medical school was established in 1889, Ayurvedic medicine was included in the curriculum on an equal footing with Western medicine. However, the teaching of Ayurvedic medicine was eliminated in 1913.
7 By early 2002 there were more than 400 such self-help groups in Thailand as a whole (Lyttleton 2004: 13).
8 In 1980 three-fifths of exports came from agriculture; in 1995 four-fifths derived from manufacturing (Pasuk and Baker 1998: 4).
9 In Mae Sai district (Chiang Rai province of the upper north) HIV prevalence among migrant girls from Burma ranged between 17% and 33% over the period 1995–1997 (UNDP 2004: 59).
10 The Thailand Health Profile 1999–2000 claims that public health actually improved during the recession due to more efficient health services delivery. For example between 1977–1987 the number of district hospitals was doubled and the number of beds quadrupled (Thailand Health Profile 1999–2000: 423 and 425).
11 By May 2004 the National Health Bill was still to be amended and finalized by cabinet and parliament (Wiput 2004: 28).
12 Another National Health Assembly was held in August 2003 in response to further meetings of provincial assemblies.
13 Contemporary MOPH funding of health NGOs could severely limit NGO autonomy and political activism, given that the conditions for funding include registration and eschewal of 'political affiliation or activities contradicting government policy' (Amara n.d.: 7).

References

Amara Pongsapich (n.d.) 'Current Status of Civil Society Organizations in the Health Sector in Thailand', unpublished manuscript, Chulalongkorn University Social Research Institute, Bangkok.

Bamber, S. (1997) 'The Thai Medical Profession and Political Activism', in K. Hewison (ed.), *Political Change in Thailand: Democracy and Participation*, London & New York: Routledge, 233–250.

Beesey, A. (2000) 'HIV Vulnerability and Mobile Populations: Thailand and its Borders', *Development Bulletin*, 52: 38–41.

Chanet Wallop Khumthong (1994) 'The Politics and Socio-Economic Transformation of the Thai Health Care System', in Komatra Cheungsatiansup (ed.), *Prawatsat Kan Phaet lae Satharanasuk Thai* (The History of Thai Medicine and Public Health), Bangkok: Rockefeller Foundation, 106–174.

Cohen, P. T. (1989) 'The Politics of Primary Health Care in Thailand, with Special Reference to Non-Government Organizations', in P. Cohen and J. Purcal (eds), *The Political Economy of Primary Health Care in Southeast Asia*, Canberra: Australian Development Studies Network, ANU, 159–176.

—— (1995) 'Buddhism, Health and Development in Thailand from the Reformist Perspective of Dr Prawase Wasi', in P. Cohen and J. Purcal (eds), *Health & Development in South East Asia*, Canberra: Australian Development Studies Network, ANU, 162–178.

Connors, M. K. (2003) 'The Reforming State: Security, Development and Culture in Democratic Times', in J. G. Ungpakorn (ed.), *Radicalising Thailand: New Political Perspectives*, Bangkok: Institute of Asian Studies, Chulalongkorn University, 319–343.

Dane, Barbara (2002) 'Disclosure: The Voices of Women Living with HIV/AIDS', *International Social Work*, 45(2): 185–204.

Davisakd Puaksom (2003) 'Modern Medicine in Thailand: Germ, Body, and the Medicalized State', paper presented at the Third International Convention of Asia Scholars, Singapore, 19–22 August.

Donaldson, P. J. (1982) 'Foreign Intervention in Medical Education: A Case Study of the Rockefeller Foundation's Involvement in a Thai Medical School', in V. Navarro (ed.), *Imperialism, Health and Medicine*, New York: Pluto Press, 107–126.

Foucault, Michel (1980) 'Two Lectures', in C. Gordon (ed.), *Power/Knowledge: Selected Interviews and Other Writings 1972–1977 by Michel Foucault*, Brighton: Harvester Press, 78–108.

—— (1984) 'The Politics of Health in the Eighteenth Century', in Paul Rabinow (ed.), *The Foucault Reader*, London: Peregrine Books, 273–259.

Gray, J. (1995) 'Sex for Sale: HIV/AIDS, Tourism and the Sex Industry in Thailand', in P. Cohen and J. Purcal (eds), *Health & Development in South East Asia*, Canberra: Australian Development Studies Network, ANU, 179–190.

—— (1998) 'Harm Reduction in the Hills of Northern Thailand', *Substance Use & Misuse* 33(5): 1075–1091.

Hewison K. (2003) 'Responding to Economic Crisis: Thailand's Localism', in D. McCargo (ed.), *Reforming Thai Politics*, Copenhagen: Nordic Institute of Asian Studies, 143–162.

Irvine, W. (1982) 'The Thai-Yuan "Madman", and the Modernizing, Developing Thai Nation: A Study in the Replication of a Single Image', unpublished thesis, University of London.

Komatra Cheungsatiansup (1999) 'Alternative Health, Alternative Sphere of Autonomy Cheewajit and the Emergence of a Critical Public in Thailand', paper presented at 7th International Conference on Thai Studies, Amsterdam, 4–8 July.

Lyttleton, C. (2004) 'Fleeing The Fire: Transformation and Gendered Belonging in Thai HIV/AIDS Support Groups', *Medical Anthropology*, 23: 1–40.

Maxwell, W. E. (1975) 'Modernization and Mobility into the Patrimonial Medical Elite in Thailand', *American Journal of Sociology*, 810(3): 465–490.

Pasuk Phongpaichit and Baker, C. (1998) *Thailand's Boom and Bust*, Chiang Mai: Silkworm Press.

—— (2004) *Thaksin: The Business of Politics in Thailand*, Chiang Mai: Silkworm Books.

Santhat Sermsri (1995) 'Health and the Urban Poor in Bangkok', in P. Cohen and J. Purcal (eds) *Health & Development in South East Asia*, Canberra: Australian Development Studies Network, ANU, pp. 49–58.

Tanabe, S. (1999) 'Practice and Self Governance: HIV/AIDS Self-Help Groups in Northern Thailand', paper presented at the 7th International Thai Studies Conference, Amsterdam, 3–7 July.

Terwiel, B. J. (1987) 'Asiatic Cholera in Siam: Its First Occurrence and the 1820 Epidemic', in N. G. Owen (ed.), *Death and Disease in Southeast Asia: Explorations in Social, Medical and Demographic History*, Singapore: Oxford University Press, 142–161.

Thailand Health Profile 1999–2000, Bangkok, Ministry of Public Health (MOPH), Online. Available <www.moph.go.th/ops/thealth_44/> (accessed December 2005).

Thiesmeyer, Lynn (2001) 'Mobility, Gender, and Hidden Costs of HIV Risk Households in Northern Thailand', Asia Pacific HIV Impact Research Tool/HIV Impact Assessment 2001, unpublished report.

UNDP (United Nations Development Programme) 2004 'Thailand's Response to HIV/AIDS: Progress and Challenges' Online. Available <http://www.undp.or.th/documents/HIV> (accessed December 2005).

Viroj Tangcharoensathien, Piya Harnvoravongchai, Siriwan Pitayarangsarit and Vijj Kasemsup (2000) 'Health Impacts of Rapid Economic Change in Thailand', *Social Science & Medicine*, 51: 789–807.

Wiput Phoolcharoen (2004) *Quantum Leap: The Reform of Thailand's Health System*, Bangkok: Health Systems Research Institute, Ministry of Public Health, Thailand.

Yuwadi Comphitak (2002) *Kanphaet Kan Satharansuk Muang Thai: Wiwathana Kan Khwam Pen Ma Cak Aidit* (Medicine and Public Health of Thailand: Progress from the Past), Bangkok: Odeon Store.

Zysk, K. G. (1991) *Asceticism and Healing in Ancient India: Medicine in the Buddhist Monastery*, New Delhi: Oxford University Press.

6 'Could confinement be humanised'?

A modern history of leprosy in Vietnam

Laurence Monnais

Oddly enough, it was in researching the history of pharmaceuticals in French Indochina (1858–1954) that I became interested in the history of leprosy in Vietnam. This is odd because leprosy was not even treated, much less cured, until the 1940s. Still, it was from this peripheral vantage point that I began to think about the relationship between public health – its policies and practices – and Hansen's disease, and to examine yet again the close association that most historians posit between medicalization and social control, in particular in the context of the management of leprosy, often seen as one of the worst symbols of the domination of Western biopower over the diseased body.

More specifically, this article re-examines the modern management of leprosy as a public health problem in Vietnam, beginning with the 1873 discovery of the bacterium which causes the disease. My particular concern is to demonstrate how the disorganized state of colonial health care limited the reach of medico-sanitary efforts in this arena. Looking beyond the colonial era, my research reveals a complex interaction among a wide range of factors – at once biomedical, economic and sociocultural – which accounts for the apparent neglect of lepers in the medicalization of Vietnam. I seek finally to participate in the emerging debate surrounding the World Health Organization's (WHO) confident promise of the imminent disappearance of leprosy 'as a public health problem' by explicitly addressing the burden of the various stigmas associated with the disease and its carriers.

The discovery of Hansen's bacillus and its impact on Vietnam

Leprosy is a chronic infectious disease of the skin and the mucus membranes that affects the peripheral nerves and upper respiratory tract. It is caused by the bacterium, *Mycobacterium leprae*, or Hansen's bacillus, named after its Norwegian discoverer (1873). Its seriousness is due to its tendency to result in disabilities (ranging from a loss of sensitivity to deformities of bodily extremities) in cases which are untreated or treated too late. The infection is propagated through nasal secretions and saliva, and perhaps also through skin-to-skin contact with the sores on a leper's body. While the appearance of skin lesions is among the first visible signs of the disease, these generally appear only years (sometimes as many as 20) after the moment of initial infection. Depending on the immune system's reaction to the bacillus, the disease can take on one of two forms: Paucibacillary (PB or tuberculoid) leprosy, the less contagious form, or Multibacillary (MB or lepromatous) leprosy, which is richer in bacilli and therefore more contagious. We now have convincing evidence, based on studies carried out by Doull and Guinto in the Philippines in the 1930s, that the disease is contagious only in the event of frequent and prolonged contact with a leper and affects no more than about 1% of the population worldwide.

While leprosy remained in many ways a mystery[1] at the moment that the French established their colony in Vietnam (1860–1890), the disease was certainly found in a number of Western countries as well as being considered an endemic disease typical of tropical regions. While the discovery of Hansen's bacillus coincided with the establishment of French control in Indochina, this discovery shed little light on the details of how leprosy spread. In fact, during roughly the same period, a policy of isolation of visibly infected individuals was (re)activated in Norway, Hawaii and Colombia by governments whose interventionism underscored the profound fears evoked by the disease even as it revealed trends in the institutionalization of public health at this point in history.

The construction and adaptation of a colonial health-care system

At the moment that Indochina came under French control, the field of public health was coming under the control of the sanitarians in Vietnam as in France. This new science was to endow modern medicine with a renewed social authority, and following the successes of Pasteurian bacteriology, modern medicine soon became an instrument of colonization (having already proved itself as an effective 'tool of pacification'). At this point, apart from the activities of certain religious orders, active in Indochina since the seventeenth century, Vietnam had no collective health-care system outside the imperial court at Hué where a medical corps, trained and organized in the Chinese style, served the Vietnamese aristocracy. In an effort to address the most urgent needs, the embryonic French administration of Cochinchina (the southern part of Vietnam) organized the first smallpox vaccination campaigns in the 1860s, and went on, with the help of a few military doctors and missionaries, to isolate those infected by cholera, plague and syphilis in makeshift quarantines (Monnais-Rousselot 1999: 121–152).

Efforts to build a health-care system for the colony as a whole began at the turn of the twentieth century, following the pacification of the region and its unification as the Union Indochinoise (1887)[2] under the sole authority of the governor general. In 1897, Governor General Paul Doumer created the position of local director of health in each of the five territories that made up the Union, and in Cochinchina began to enforce the metropolitan law of 1892 requiring a doctorate in medicine as a condition for practicing medicine. In 1902, as the Hanoi School of Medicine opened its doors to the first cohort of indigenous 'auxiliary doctors' to be trained according to French specifications, Doumer began to enforce yet another far-reaching law that had recently been passed in France: the basic law on the protection of public health (*Loi relative à la protection de la santé publique*). This law defined the responsibilities of the government in matters of disease prevention and in the provision of a healthy environment, while also establishing the list of contagious diseases which had to be declared to state authorities as well as the proper procedures to be followed in making such declarations.

Doumer's successor, Paul Beau, expanded on these policies by developing the idea of a health-care system geared towards the indigenous population: the Assistance Médicale Indigène (AMI). A genuine health-care system, the AMI had its own centralized administrative framework, the Inspection Générale de l'Hygiène et de la Santé Publique (IGHSP), and an independent budget; it was intended for the native population and in principle was meant to be free of charge (free treatment was provided for indigents; preventive measures were free for everyone). This generosity was meant to win over the Indochinese population even as it 'sanitized' them. It is perhaps not surprising that between 1905 and 1954, these initial plans were to undergo numerous modifications. Indeed in examining the successive five-year plans through which health-care policy was formulated, we see a passage from military to civilian control of the system as well as a certain oscillation between centralization and decentralization. The emphasis in health-care initiatives undertaken during this period was on preventive measures (vaccinations, public health education, urban sanitation and the provision of clean drinking water), together with the construction of an increasingly dense network of ever more effective hospitals. We also note a new focus, particularly marked after 1914, on the provision of essential medical services in rural areas, a mission entrusted to a mobile medical corps that was to undergo a process of indigenization (Monnais-Rousselot 1999: 269–314).

During the inter-war period, the French health-care system came to be better adapted to Vietnamese realities – pathological, geographical, economic and sociocultural. We see this adaptation in the increased attention afforded to the protection of mothers and children, and in the new campaigns against 'social diseases': infectious or hereditary conditions whose aetiology was believed to be linked to social and environmental conditions. Thus, lung disease, venereal disease, eye infections, skin infections – even cancers – were fought through campaigns to eliminate 'ignorance', poverty, poor sanitation, overcrowding, beggary and even immorality (prostitution). To fight these 'social plagues', a Service d'Assistance Sociale (Social Assistance Services), placed under the authority of the IGHSP in 1929, was given the mandate to ensure the liaison between public authorities and private charities. The creation of the AMI had required the separation of church and state and had — theoretically – relegated health-care provided by religious institutions to the margins. In reality, however, it seems that health-care authorities were willing to make use of any well-intentioned source of assistance (Monnais-Rousselot 2001: 511–540). Syphilis and tuberculosis ranked second and fourth, respectively, as the diseases most frequently treated in hospitals in 1930, which explains in part the authorities' concerns (Gaide 1931: 351).

Moreover, the expansion of health care into the rural areas had revealed the widespread threat of trachoma and intestinal parasites. Leprosy was ranked as the tenth cause of morbidity in the country despite the fact that the spread of the disease had supposedly been contained by the systematic internment of the infected for almost 20 years.

Where does leprosy fit in?

In fact, the religious orders had long been the sole groups providing care for lepers. In any event, this is the impression created by the silence of the documentary sources of the Indochinese health-care services on matters pertaining to the disease, and by scathing missionary reports accusing the colonial government of having done nothing for 'those poor wretches'.[3] It appears that around the turn of the twentieth century lepers could be 'treated' together with the indigent, the blind and the crippled in institutions managed by the *Missions étrangères de Paris*, the *Œuvre de la St-Enfance* or the *Sœurs de St Paul de Chartes*. In the village of Mui (11kms from Hanoi), for example, 400 lepers received minimal care: the dressing of their wounds and some pain relief. The main concern of the religious orders, however, was to encourage patients to convert to a religion that prized suffering, the expiation of sin, and sentiments of pity and charity towards others – values that were supposedly not taught in Buddhism. Preventive measures such as the protection of the inmate's family were nonetheless a minor preoccupation. Deaths were frequent and numerous in these 'asylums of extreme misery'.[4] As of 1908, 18 leprosaria, all run by religious orders, appear to have shared the task of caring for Vietnamese lepers, while the colonial administration dragged its heels, doing little beyond the occasional distribution of material assistance to victims of the disease or the institution of makeshift quarantines when lepers were diagnosed during the course of regular medical consultations.[5]

The colonial state could hardly plead ignorance in these matters. In 1897, the minister of colonies had commissioned the first large-scale epidemiological study of leprosy in Indochina, to be carried out by Dr Edouard Jeanselme (who was to become a famous dermatologist). The results of Jeanselme's work, published in 1900, were quite alarming: he estimated the number of cases to be between 12,000 and 15,000, concentrated in the deltas of the Red River (Tonkin) and of the Mekong (Cochinchina) (Jeanselme 1900: 3–4). As these were among the most densely populated areas, as well as the site of the principal urban concentrations and the scene of most colonial activities, we need to evaluate these assertions cautiously even if they would be confirmed 15 years later (Barbezieux 1914: 2). In any case, at the moment of their publication, these figures brought pressure on the colonial administration to consider the necessity of diagnostic screening and of health-care provisions for those infected by the disease. The idea of systematic and mandatory internment of lepers attained a certain credibility in Indochina at this time, coinciding as it did with the definitive acceptance of the contagionist theory of disease, and with the establishment of the AMI. One might note that this was consistent with the approach advocated by the first international conferences dedicated to this issue (Berlin in 1897 and Bergen in1906), and with what was done in other colonies.

In 1903, the governor of Cochinchina ordered the creation of a leprosarium and the isolation of lepers on Culao Rong (an island facing Mytho[6]). A second, broader order, issued on 15 September 1905 to protect the public health of the colony as a whole, forbade lepers from circulating on public byways and excluded them from certain professions including positions in the public service (December 1909). The law foresaw the state organization of leprosaria or of agricultural leper colonies and recognized as well the legitimacy of private leper villages under medical supervision. It also specified that internment would require the express order of local administrative authorities, contingent on the completion of full bacteriological and clinical tests. Finally, the law of 31 December 1912 prescribed the systematic isolation of lepers either in a leprosarium or an agricultural colony, or, under exceptional circumstances, in the home. Consistent with the principles enumerated at the conference in Bergen, infected individuals were prohibited from raising their own children; these were taken away at birth and placed in charitable institutions or foster families.

It was also in 1912 that a decree called for the creation of a pilot Service des Léproseries (Service of Leprosaria) in Tonkin. Placed under the direction of a civilian doctor of the AMI, Dr Georges Barbezieux, the service promised to build five leprosaria which would serve as 'laboratories for the study of all questions relating to the pathogenesis, treatment, aetiology and prevention of the disease'.[7] By 1913, nearly 2,400 lepers – of the 5,000 to be eventually interned – had already been relocated to the leprosaria: 732 in Van Môn, 685 in Tê Truong (the former village of Mui), 410 in Qua Câm, 310 in Huong Phong and 231 in Liêu Xa, in addition to 63 others in domiciliary isolation. Given the astonishingly rapid organization of these services and the high internment rate, it seems more than likely that pre-existing structures were incorporated into the implementation of the 1912 decree. In any event, Barbezieux was committed to an approach which we might call 'liberal'. He championed the principle of the agricultural colony, first tested on the site of Tê Truong, over that of the traditional leprosarium. The former, he argued, was less expensive in the long term, and created a lesser feeling of confinement. In these agricultural colonies, residents would receive a monthly allowance and would also enjoy the benefits of institutions resembling those of 'normal' villages, including: a *ly truong* (mayor), a council of notables in charge of local order, mechanisms to allow them to sell their farm and craft products, and places of worship.[8] Men and women were even allowed to intermingle (which was *not* the case in similar institutions in British India during the same period) (Kakar 2001: 198–201) but this relative freedom stopped at the well-guarded gates enclosing the village.

Barbezieux became an enthusiastic spokesman for his method from 1913 on, once the first results of his experiments became available. He admitted that there was still much to do: all such colonies should be headed by a doctor, they should have an infirmary, and a nursery to care for resident's children. To reach these goals, Barbezieux called for a substantial increase in funds to be allocated to the anti-leprosy campaign. And funding was doubled, going from 57,239 piastres to 99,753 in one year (representing about 3% of the total budget for the health services of Indochina), but this amount was still far from enough. In fact, in addition to the burden of the costs associated with the creation and upkeep of the villages, Barbezieux's colleagues had pointed out that the villages did not achieve the complete isolation of the infected population and that the financial compensation allocated to interns, inadequate to meet their needs and enable them to reach autonomy,[9] greatly exceeded budgetary capabilities.

As a result of such criticisms (together with budgetary restraints imposed by wartime necessities), the Service des Léproseries of Tonkin was abandoned by 1915, although the original plan had been to extend it to the rest of the Vietnamese territory.[10] Subsequently, the anti-leprosy campaign, entrusted to the AMI authorities of each province, entered a phase of decentralization.

'Colonial disarray' or the story of an aborted fight against leprosy

It is hard to know what to say about the fight against leprosy in Vietnam during the 1920s and 1930s. What stands out is the glaring contradiction between the stagnation of anti-leprosy activities on the ground on the one hand, and, on the other, the formulation of a project designed to rationalize such activities through three specific initiatives: the development of screening methods for the early detection of the disease (the earlier the better, even before the appearance of the first visible signs if possible); an increase of therapeutic experimentation so as to develop more effective treatments and eventually cures; and a realistic and 'humanizing' improvement in the conditions of the confinement of lepers. These three approaches were once again consistent with those fervently defended on the international scene by the Pasteurian Emile Marchoux (serving in French West Africa) and brought before the League of Nations by the Société Spéciale de la Lèpre (Bado 1996: 279–291).

Rationalizing the fight against leprosy: between theory and practice

In Vietnam, however, the development of the mobile services necessary to launch the new initiatives faced a shortage of resources at all levels. It is well known that decentralization brings increased financial strain on local budgets that in this case were already stretched thin. The personnel recruited to staff the mobile services, mostly local nurses, often had insufficient knowledge of the rules of screening – which were rather imprecise in any event – even when they had access to the required equipment. Nor was it possible for the Pasteurian-founded Service for the Research and Study of Leprosy, associated with the social hygiene laboratory of Saigon (1923), to provide the entire territory with technological resources. Shortages in financial and human resources were even more glaring when it came to tracing the identity of infected individuals and investigating their social backgrounds. In addition, there was the administrative conundrum of managing 'potential' patients – a procedure that was not only difficult but also lasted several months (Le Roy des Barres and Marcel 1927: 81–83) – or the transportation of reported cases to the appropriate leper colony when these cases had not already escaped from the hospital where they had undergone testing.[11] It is not surprising that this initiative never got off the ground.

It was in this context that therapeutic research seems to have become a priority in the anti-leprosy campaign during a time when trust in pharmaceuticals was growing. Following the success of arsenobenzenes (for the treatment of syphilis and several skin ailments), hopes were high for a miracle solution to leprosy, and these hopes were invested in chaulmoogra oil; extracted from the seeds of a tree belonging to the *Hydnocarpus* family. The use of chaulmoogra in the treatment of leprosy goes back to the dawn of time, or nearly, in the Far East. Discovered by Western doctors in the 1850s (Parascandola 2003: 47–57), and then put to the scientific test, the substance was considered to be effective but, at least through the 1920s, posed certain problems, particularly in terms of side effects (nausea, fever and severe pain). Although further work aiming to reduce these side effects was relatively successful, the discouraging outcome of therapeutic experiments dismissed hopes that chaulmoogra oil could cure leprosy. Furthermore, it came to be increasingly clear that treatment would have to be initiated very early in the development of the disease in order to be minimally effective in modifying its course. This brought therapists back to the shortcomings in the screening system.[12]

True enough, the range of experiments using chaulmoogra, alone or in combination with other substances (arsenic, mercury, methylene blue and synthetic medicines such as arsenical compounds including Salvarsan and Stovarsol and BCG[13]) is testimony to a vigorous local research initiative in which many colonial scientists, physicians, Pasteurians, pharmacists and chemists took part.[14] Still, after two decades of experimentation, the conclusions of the authorities were decidedly frank: 'All therapies yield temporary and disappointing results.... Our only choice is to await the discovery of a particular medicine which will revolutionize the current situation and enable us to treat a Hansenian with as much confidence as we would treat a syphilitic. When that time comes, we will shut down our agricultural colonies and will treat lepers on an out-patient basis'.[15]

The remaining question, posed by a number of colonial doctors, was how in the face of lack of treatment, obstacles to early diagnosis, and widespread ignorance about the condition, might we conceive of and implement a more humane method of confinement? As soon as colonial measures for segregation were taken, some physicians, Jeanselme among them, declared themselves sceptical of the applicability of such measures overseas (Delrieu *et al.* 1909: 166–175). Such voices insisted that while internment seemed necessary, it would, in order to be effective, have to be done on a voluntary basis, and be supported by the services of specialized medical personnel. And while it is true that, on paper, at least one native auxiliary doctor was to be assigned to each leper community of 100 or more, in reality, such communities were staffed by only a nurse or even an 'agent', himself a leper, charged with the surveillance of the group. Such an agent occupied an ambiguous position, one creating a power dynamic among the colonized peoples that has been shown, in other instances of colonial confinement, to carry negative social consequences (Kakar 2001: 198–207). The idea of expanding the agricultural colonies to eventually replace conventional leprosaria, with the hope of providing lepers with a certain quality of life, required an exorbitant investment in time, personnel and money. In the light of reigning conditions in Indochina, any talk of a 'humanization' of confinement or of a possible 'destigmatization' of the leper seems unforgivably utopian.[16]

The humanization of segregation: a pious vow?

The idea of the agricultural colony nevertheless gained some ground at the end of the 1920s, allowing for the achievement of a certain humanization: lepers were allowed regular visits by their relatives and their children were to be returned to them after being raised for ten years in a healthy family. Much attention was afforded to the selection of clean, spacious sites for the agricultural colony, but the rules of surveillance remained strict and the possibility of release distant (Le Roy des Barres and Marcel 1927: 100). We note as well isolated efforts to treat some lepers in traditional establishments in Saigon (Choquan hospital) and Hanoi (René Robin hospital), efforts which might have been part of an attempt to destigmatize leprosy although this hypothesis is difficult to verify. Only in Annam, a region with few lepers, was some success attained in experimenting with a regime of voluntary internment: between a third and a half of known cases (777) are reported to have been voluntarily confined in 1938, and attempts to escape were infrequent, at least according to the local director of health in his address to the Tenth Congress of the Far Eastern Association for Tropical Medicine held in Hanoi (Le Nestour 1938: 330).

As for institutions that we assume to have been under the control of religious orders, they do not appear in administrative statistics. As a result we know little about the public care afforded to inhabitants of isolated, mountainous regions that were populated mainly by minority ethnic groups.[17] The silence of official documents concerning the leper colony of Djiring, founded in the Central Highlands by Father Chassaigne of the foreign missions in 1929 to care for members of the Sré minority, is a telling example.

According to sources, in 1930 there were almost as many escaped lepers in Indochina (232) as there were under home confinement (255). One leprosarium (Culao Rong) and 15 agricultural colonies ministered to 3,287 lepers (Gaide 1931: 353). This accounts for roughly one-quarter of all lepers – even less if we take into account infection rates from later decades. In addition, we find no improvement in the prevalence or in the geographic distribution of the disease; particularly worrisome areas included the Red River delta (Nam Dinh, Ha Dong and Bac Ninh provinces). The scattered data we have been able to gather for Tonkin in the 1930s[18] show a linear progression in the number of interned cases (2,438 in 1931; 2,602 in 1934; 2,724 in 1935), while disparities in the provincial origins of the incoming residents underscores the uneven distribution of the disease as well as being probably related to screening problems. We note a high percentage of deaths (over 10% of the residents per year on average), and a rate of escape that decreases while remaining significant (6% in 1931; 4% in 1935), continuing low rates of home confinement (18% in 1931; 23% in 1935) but rising numbers of cases being released (5% of the isolated population in 1935) that might be explained by the recourse to chaulmoogra-based treatments which were increasingly effective, bringing about an increase of cases achieving 'remission'. The number of births is non-negligible and stable (around 60 per year), calling attention to the maintenance of spousal relations in the villages despite the persistence of a marked disproportion in the ratio between male and female residents (one woman for every three or four men).

If nothing else, these figures illustrate the application of a unilinear policy of confinement which by 1939 had led to the confinement of an important proportion of declared cases of leprosy among the Vietnamese. Those confined were essentially men, belonging to the dominant *Viêt* ethnic group, struggling with irreversible handicaps, living on a minimum of public welfare in makeshift shacks on the margins of society, with no hope of a cure, and even less of social rehabilitation.

Should we not be struck by the enduring silence of doctors and medical administrators on such topics as the potential methods to prevent the disease (there were already mechanisms in place for the diffusion of information concerning contagious diseases, health education in schools and in the maternity wards), and the management of the social consequences of the disease and its life course? Should we conclude that the absence of treatment reduces, in the minds of the medical community and in the budgets of colonial administrators, the importance of such efforts? Moreover, how and why should the management of leprosy be different from that of other infectious diseases – no other disease was ever treated in such a manner? Given that research had shown in the 1930s that the disease was not very contagious, should we not be all the more surprised that confinement remained the main strategy in the fight against leprosy, even as it continued to relegate lepers to the margins of medicalization, where they found themselves grouped together (tacitly) with the blind, the orphans, the Métis, the ethnic minorities and the mentally ill? What does this ambiguous 'omission' tell us about the policy of public health in Indochina, particularly its efforts in the area of social assistance through 1929?

This policy of confinement, increasingly unjustifiable, points us toward other dimensions of the modern history of leprosy which will be revealed all the more clearly, paradoxically, in the 1940s, following decolonization and the discovery of an effective cure.

From powerlessness to stigma: leprosy is (still) a social problem in Vietnam

According to the WHO, leprosy 'as a public health problem' is disappearing. Defined as having reached a national prevalence of less than 1 case per 10,000 population,[19] the disappearance of the disease will be the result of the massive application of Multidrug Therapy (MDT), made available without cost to governments throughout the world by the Nippon Foundation (1995) and by the pharmaceutical company Novartis (1999) under the supervision of the International Federation of Anti-Leprosy Associations (ILEP), an umbrella organization for non governmental organizations (NGOs) fighting leprosy. In the Western Pacific region (including Vietnam) the number of cases of leprosy has reportedly dropped from 600,000 in 1950 to 25,400 in 1997.

Toward a post-colonial history of Leprosy

In the 1940s, the introduction of sulfonamide antibacterials brought about a de facto revolution in the treatment of leprosy. In systematic use since the International Conference on Leprosy of Havana (1948), Dapsone had to be replaced in the 1970s when it was found that bacterial resistance to the drug had developed. A treatment combining Clofazimine, Dapsone and Rifampicin was then tested in various high prevalence countries in 1982, after which it came into general use in the 1990s (WHO 2004: 8). In the late 1950s, in response to the results achieved by sulfonamide treatment, the WHO issued the following recommendation: 'temporary isolation might still be necessary although for infectious cases only'. In the 1960s, the WHO Expert Committee on Leprosy suggested that ambulatory treatment could safely and satisfactorily be used on most patients. As a result, we note throughout the Western Pacific Region a general trend towards the incorporation of leprosy patients into general health services even if persistent problems with screening procedures in certain regions prompted the launching of certain initiatives (such as the Special Action Projects for the Elimination of Leprosy) which may have slowed the general trend toward integration in the 1995–2000 period (WHO 1999: 29–32).

Having seen its prevalence drop to 0.2 cases per 10,000 in 1995, leprosy in Vietnam is officially no longer classed as endemic. It is difficult to address the specific historical and national factors[20] that might be responsible for this 'success'. The available sources for the 1940–1970 period are few and understandably so: the divided country was at war and the battle against leprosy hardly constituted a priority for the governments in power.[21] Nevertheless, the distribution of sulfonamide drugs began, if slowly, in the 1950s, accompanied by an information campaign on leprosy carried out by the young Democratic Republic in the north. On the model established during the inter-war period, a few leprosaria, such as Van Môn, were converted into state-of-the-art research sites equipped with bacteriological laboratories and treatment facilities. But a full-fledged commitment to fight the disease had to await the reunification of the country in 1975 when the new government, estimating the number of lepers to be 200,000, decided to include the eradication of the disease among its ten top health-care priorities (which also included malaria and tuberculosis).

In 1981, the National Leprosy Control Program (NLCP) launched the strategy of 'area by area eradication'. From its inception, the NLCP has been fully integrated into basic public health services at the village level, overseen at the central level by the National Institute of Dermatology and Venereology in Hanoi (WHO 2003: 66–67).[22] Even after the privatization of the health-care system, beginning in 1989, lepers continued to receive free access to essential care as the Vietnamese government still fully funds its preventive programmes. In addition, the campaign has benefited from renewed international activity led by the Netherlands Leprosy Relief (NLR) that coordinates, on behalf of the ILEP, the activities of NGOs in Vietnam compensating for budgetary and technical deficiencies. A review of the *Bulletin* of the *Fraternité Viêt Nam* (FRVN), a Catholic NGO from Québec, reveals that its donors invest in the free distribution of MDT in a dozen leprosaria including the 'ex-colonial' sites of Ben San, Van Môn and Qua Cam in addition to contributing to the training of nurses among the patients and to the distribution of prostheses for the disabled.

In February 1996, following the meeting between the major actors in the anti-leprosy campaign, a directive from Prime Minister Vo Van Kiêt reemphasized the urgency of public–private collaboration even if, at the same time, several organizations complained of obstacles to their freedom of action, particularly with regard to the social rehabilitation of ex-lepers and the detection of new cases. Putting aside such problems, which could be linked to the Hanoi regime's mistrust of certain foreign and international organizations, four basic realities should command our attention. As we re-examine the elimination of leprosy, defined on the basis of epidemiological data, attention to these factors will allow us to continue our reflection on the modern history of leprosy in Vietnam and to examine in particular the linkages between policies of segregation and advances in treatment.

First, certain pockets of high endemic prevalence persist: in 1999, these were found in 16 provinces located in the High Plateaus of the centre and in northern mountainous regions, the areas already most affected by other endemic diseases such as malaria.[23] Second, the spread of the disease has not been arrested. In the last ten years, the Ministry of Health has detected some 1,000 new cases, the majority in poor, isolated regions. Further examination of the newly detected cases reveals a proportion of new infantile cases that has been stable since the 1980s (5–6% of the total), in addition to a rate of MB cases that is high and rising (40.6% in 1984; 62.2% in 2003). This profile should remind us that under-detection remains a critical issue. In particular, the rate of detection in women remains much lower than among men: 29.6% of new cases in 1984, 35.7% in 2003.[24] Third, it must be noted that Vietnam leads the world in the number of people disabled by the disease. In 1999, this number was somewhere between 20,000 and 50,000 (Kane 1999: 2–3) and the disability rate among new cases remains very high: in 2003, 31% disability Grade I and II, and 19% disability Grade II (NLR 2004: 3). Taken together, these statistical realities point to clear deficiencies in the Vietnamese screening system, including that of tardy intervention. More broadly, they reveal, if perhaps less immediately, the burden of exclusion, both physical and social, under which Vietnamese lepers continue to live.

Who is responsible for this enduring exclusion?

The political, economic and medical contexts of the colonial period can help to explain the confinement of lepers, even if the explanation cannot serve as a justification. But these conditions no longer prevail after 1945. Indeed, from the 1950s onward, the confinement of lepers was no longer obligatory (Tchou 1952: 5) and each leprosarium was to allow those whose disease had been arrested and who were no longer contagious to return home, even if they remained under the control of their provincial dermatological clinic. Even so, we have tangible proof that in the 1960s and 1970s, the number of state leprosaria increased to reach a total of 27 at the moment of reunification. The leprosarium of Quynh Lâp, opened in 1959 on an isolated coast of the Nghê An province, apparently accommodated over 5,000 lepers in five years, while releasing only 1,000; the leprosarium of Ben San counted 700 inmates in 1981 and 1,300 in 1987 (NLR 2004: 5). In fact, at least 4,000 'ex-patients' are apparently still living in leprosaria with their families. Such figures do not include the number of Hansenians living in self-imposed leper colonies.

Recently, the newspaper *Courrier du Viêt Nam* provided a compassionate account of the hardships faced by lepers in Quynh Lâp and in the leper village of Dông Lênh (Tuyên Quang) (Lê 2004; Vinh 2003). The account is of two healthy children – one in each village – born into these isolated areas and enduring with their families quite miserable socio-economic conditions. Even if the point of the story is to demonstrate that it is possible for young members of leper families to 'make it', even to receive a university education, the overall impression remains that social rehabilitation of 'cured' lepers remains difficult (for the entire community had supposedly been cured) even for their non-infected children.

The persistence of this institutionalized and/or voluntary physical and social separation compels us to examine the range of stigmas associated with leprosy in Vietnamese society and its history, in a perspective that looks beyond conventional chronological boundaries.

In 1886, Dr E. Hocquard, on mission in Tonkin, visited an 'indigenous leprosarium' (Hocquard 1999: 384–386). Putting aside his personal expression of disgust (which reminds us that doctors do not speak only as scientists), the physician described a miserable and overcrowded environment where sick and disfigured individuals lived alongside healthy ones. He also discusses certain local beliefs about leprosy (*phong*): the Vietnamese feared contagion and, for this reason, excluded from their village any leper bearing visible signs of the disease. In fact, in Buddhist countries, leprosy is seen as a karmic disease, a retribution for grave sins committed in a prior life. Living with the disease called for dedication to a rigorous spiritual practice and to the commitment of good deeds. At the same time, leprosy was considered a sort of pedagogical tool in the quest for enlightenment: by meditating on their painful disfigurement, lepers could prove that it was possible to liberate oneself from attachment to his body.

This dual vision – not so different after all from the Catholic interpretation of the disease – helps us understand the deeply ingrained local fear of the disease, as well as the fact that some lepers might refuse treatment. The same dual vision might account for the ambiguous range of social attitudes towards lepers, from demanding their exclusion to expressing compassion (Navon 1998: 97–98). In any case, according to Hocquard, common pre-colonial practices included supervised exclusion as well as the provision of subsistence to lepers. In fact, Emperor

Gia Long (1802–1820) was apparently following an ancient tradition when he institutionalized the management of leper villages and codified the rights of the lepers by placing prohibitions on marriage, on the exercise of certain professions and on raising their own children. As for the supposedly Western tendency, reinforced by the hygienist discourse, to link lepers to beggars and criminals, we find similar discourses in neighbouring territories that did not experience colonial rule (Chemouilli 2002: 3; Leung 2002; Navon 1998: 89–105). In addition, while the link between leprosy and beggary is clear in colonial discourse, that between leprosy and criminality is in any event less clear than in the case of venereal disease, especially infected women who were invariably judged to be prostitutes. Yet, none of these were targeted by programmes of systematic internment and instead continued to be treated in the hospitals and clinics of the AMI (Monnais-Rousselot 1999: 187–196).[25]

The de facto existence of leper communities segregated from Vietnamese society, as reported by several Western observers during the nineteenth century, reinforces the idea that there was an acceptance, on the part of infected individuals, of the discrimination of which they were the objects. Similar instances have been found in other Western colonies (Bargès 1996: 115–117). Even if it seems clear that this history of exclusion is not distinctively Vietnamese – to what extent, one might ask, did the long history of missionary presence in East Asia play a role in the acceptance of such practices (Leung 2002) – it remains nonetheless true that the reality of the pre-colonial experience must have had an impact on the implementation of a policy of systematic exclusion under French authority, and on its relative acceptance by the Vietnamese.

Confinement may have been expected as a solution, or even seen as a liberation in some instances, as hinted at by several colonial reports: confinement might offer an escape from the gaze of the others, from constant anxiety and from having to beg; it might also represent the beginning of a life in a place of calm, perhaps a pleasant life where one could enjoy the company of other lepers; confinement might eventually become a means to obtain a 'legal status'. Other reports speak of the hesitations expressed by some lepers to experiment with new treatments for fear of being released; still others note that even healthy people had tried to have themselves interned. Of course, not all of those interned would have shared this point of view. At least during the colonial period, official reports regularly decry the frequency of escape from leprosaria and leper colonies, even if once again this phenomenon can and must be interpreted in a variety of ways which might include the rejection of the very idea of internment, fear of being taken away from one's family, hesitation about testing new treatments, dissatisfaction with the upkeep of a particular leprosarium or even an attempt to reach a more modern institution (Kakar 2001: 188–190).

In fact, the strangely enduring practice of segregation owed its longevity to a range of (mis)representations drawn from a variety of factors: the physical malformities associated with the disease, traditional beliefs concerning its origins and the linkage of the disease to disturbing social conditions (poverty and disabilities) – factors that take us beyond usual social divisions such as the opposition between colonial and colonizer.[26] Lepers were a nuisance to the Nguyên administration and to colonial authorities, a nuisance to the construction of a unified Vietnam, and to the establishment of community harmony.[27] They were a nuisance wearing the visible signs of their sins on their own bodies which no one knew how to deal with and who cost a great deal and yielded little, especially when, seriously disabled, they had no choice but to rely on public (and private) charity. They were a nuisance in the form of the stigmatized individual who, even when cured, continues to suffer the after effects of the disease.

This underscores yet again the importance of early detection at the same time as it reveals the fact that leprosy is above all a still neglected social problem, treated via public health measures which depend on a private (religious) and foreign generosity and are thus not free of ambiguity. The recent history and the culture of Vietnam lend their own complexity to the situation, at the same time that leprosy itself is linked to other social problems, already symbolic of stigmatization and exclusion: the handicapped (the total number of disabled in Vietnam is estimated in 1999 to be between 2 and 6 million); the poor, especially women and children; and the discriminated ethnic minorities (the coincidence of high rates of leprosy with the regions inhabited by ethnic minorities speaks for itself).

Finally, and to underscore yet again the force of this complex link between social stigma and the internment – as a health-care measure – of Vietnamese carrying certain diseases, we should mention the recent, quiet internment of AIDS victims in several deserted leprosaria, as well as the forced confinement of intravenous drug users in detoxification camps; there were more than 75,000 of these latter 'social evils' in 2002 (Human Rights Watch 2003: 275). We find in this impulse the same slippage we saw in the case of leprosy. Under the contestable pretext of safeguarding public health, authorities endorse the internment of individuals guilty of behaviour thought to be reprehensible, of marginal individuals – even though no cure is in sight, even though access to antiretroviral tri-therapy is not a real option. How will interning those stricken with AIDS help to contain an epidemic in full expansion or its effects on Vietnamese mortality rates?[28]

There is room for discussion of the calculations and data behind the WHO's assertion that leprosy will soon be eliminated as a public health problem (Lockwood 2002: 1516–1518; Meima, Richardus and Habbema 2004: 28–30). But beyond these particular criticisms which target an arrogant biomedicine too sure of its therapeutic effectiveness, it is important to point out that the emphasis on national prevalence to determine the moment of 'victory' reveals a fundamental fact: that the WHO omits from its epidemiological objective the enduring negative effects of leprosy as a social problem, one that touches individuals, lepers and ex-lepers, their families, and communities who are still, by and large, stigmatized.

The superimposition of the modern history of leprosy in Vietnam on a longer history of continuing segregation constitutes one of the eloquent proofs of this omission, illustrating more broadly the limits of modern medicalization in the face of well-anchored sociocultural prejudices. In a country like Vietnam where the sick – the lepers, the HIV-positive and AIDS victims – are condemned as deviant or socially undesirable (the shame extending even to their friends and family), any public health policy will be limited in its effects insofar as it is not accompanied by a nationwide campaign of destigmatization designed to educate the public as to the social determinants of certain infectious and/or chronic diseases and of their resistance.

Notes

1. In many ways, leprosy is still a mysterious disease: its modes of contamination and transmission remain misunderstood. Besides our incomplete knowledge of the details of the incubation process, the diagnosis of leprosy and of its particular form still faces obstacles, while it remains impossible to develop a preventive treatment due to the impossibility of culturing *M. leprae in vitro*.
2. The *Union Indochinoise* was an administrative entity that encompassed five countries: Tonkin, Annam, Cochinchina, which form present day Vietnam, plus Cambodia and Laos.
3. Archives des Missions Etrangères de Paris (AMEP), Rapport annuel des évêques, Haut Tonkin, Mgr Ramond 1896; Tonkin maritime, Mgr Marcou 1906.
4. AMEP, Haut Tonkin, Mgr Ramond, 1906.
5. Centre des Archives d'Outre-mer, Aix-en-Provence (CAOM), Fonds du Gouvernement général (Gougal) 4465; Fonds de la Résidence Supérieure du Tonkin, Nouveau Fonds (RST NF) 8759; Archives Nationales du Viêt nam, Fonds 1, Hanoi, Gougal 2058.
6. CAOM, RST NF 34523.
7. CAOM RST NF 369.
8. CAOM RST NF 4016.
9. This allowance amounted to 2 piastres in 1913, 3.5 in 1927. At this time, the monthly salary of the least qualified indigenous labourers was estimated to lie between 4 and 7 piastres. In 1927, 135,121 piastres were allocated to the anti-leprosy campaign, of which 70% was distributed as allowances.
10. CAOM, RST NF 4016.
11. CAOM, RST NF 31958/ 47872/ 47879.
12. CAOM, RST NF 3823.
13. We now know that BCG provides immunity for at least a few years in 20% to 80% of treated individuals.
14. Several dozen articles in the *Bulletin de la Société Médico-chirurgicale de l'Indochine* and the *Archives des Instituts Pasteur d'Indochine* report on these therapeutic trials.
15. CAOM, RST NF 3685.
16. Interestingly, it was in the 1930s that a movement developed to suppress the use of the term 'leper' to replace it with more neutral terms such as 'leprosy sufferers' or 'Hansenians'.
17. There are 54 ethnic groups in Vietnam. The largest is the *Viêt*, representing 85% of the population. Besides the Chinese minority, the *Viêt* dominance over other ethnicities, who principally inhabit the mountainous regions, dates back to a march to the south (*Nam Tiên*) begun in the tenth century, colonizing the land of neighbouring empires.
18. CAOM, RST NF 3683–3685.
19. Only ten countries still form a zone of high endemic prevalence, the highest of which is in India with nearly a million new cases every year.
20. It would have been ideal to dispose of enough space to present a detailed comparison with India. Its colonial history, its tradition of segregation for leprosy and the range of stigmas that we find there would have made this a worthwhile endeavour.
21. I would like to thank the representatives of the NLR in Vietnam, Jan Robijn and Dinh Ngoc Han, for the information they shared with me.
22. Vietnam established a vertical health system that corresponded to the levels of government. The higher levels provided specialized services and supervised lower

levels. Vietnamese provinces organized training programmes and public health campaigns and ran modest hospitals. Most Vietnamese communes had a health facility with a small number of village health workers. This hierarchical management system made it possible to extend health services – especially preventive measures – rapidly to most localities.

23 In the 1960s, investigations directed by Hanoi estimated that in isolated regions the prevalence was as high as 10% of the population. In 1993, this figure, at least for the High Plateaux, has apparently fallen to 3%.

24 For the sake of comparison, in 2002, the rate of new infantile cases was 15% in India; the rate of MB was 35%, the rate among women was 35% and the proportion of cases with severe form of disabilities (Grade II) was 1.8% (OMS, 2004).

25 Of course, in the 1920s and 1930s, syphilis was being treated. However, the degree of contagiousness of the disease is not comparable to that of leprosy.

26 The fact that there is an ancient history of stigmatization and segregation of lepers in Vietnam casts doubt on the association made by certain historians between colonial anti-leprosy campaigns and social control or the more serious implications of the possibility that modern imperialism caused the non-Western stigmatization of the disease (Gussow 1989).

27 This is suggested by evidence that lepers were sometimes denounced to French authorities by the inhabitants of certain villages (CAOM, RST NF 31982/ 32010).

28 By the end of 2003, all 61 provinces in Vietnam had reported a total of 76,180 HIV-positive cases cumulatively. In 2003 alone, there were 16,980 newly detected infections, 2,866 newly diagnosed AIDS cases and 1,061 AIDS-related deaths reported nationwide (Nguyên *et al.* 2004: 141).

References

Bado, J-P. (1996) *Médecine coloniale et grandes endémies en Afrique*, Paris: Karthala.

Barbezieux, G. (1914) *Lèpre et lépreux au Tonkin. Prophylaxie et assistance*, Hanoi: Imprimerie d'Extrême-Orient.

Bargès, A. (1996) 'Entre conformismes et changements: le monde de la lèpre au Mali', in J. Benoist (ed), *Soigner au pluriel. Essai sur le pluralisme médical*, Paris: Editions Karthala, 280–313.

Chemouilli, P. (2002) 'Les anciens lépreux du Japon ont obtenu réparation. Aperçu historique d'une discrimination à contre-courant', *Bulletin de l'Association des Léprologues de Langue Française*, 14: 1–7.

Delrieu, Grall, Jeanselme, and Kermorgant, Drs (1909) 'Rapport de la Commission de la lèpre à la Société de Pathologie exotique, Paris, séance du 10 février', *Bulletin de la Société de Pathologie Exotique*, 2: 166–190.

Gaide, L. (1931) *L'Assistance médicale et la protection de la santé publique en Indochine*, Hanoi: Imprimerie d'Extrême-Orient.

Gussow, Z. (1989) *Leprosy, Racism, and Public Health: Social Policy in Chronic Disease Control*, Boulder, CO: Westview.

Hocquard, Dr (1999) *Une campagne au Tonkin, 1884–86*, Paris: Arléa.

Human Rights Watch (2003) 'Vietnam' in *World Report 2003. Events of 2002*, New York: Human Rights Watch.

Jeanselme, E. (1900) *Etude sur la lèpre dans la péninsule indochinoise et dans le Yunnan*, Paris: Carré & Naud.

Kakar, S. (2001) 'Medical Developments and Patient Unrest in the Leprosy Asylum, 1860 to 1940', in B. Pati and M. Harrison (eds), *Health, Medicine, and Empire. Perspectives on Colonial India*, Hyderabad: Orient Longman, 188–216.

Kane, T. (1999) *Disability in Vietnam in 1999. A Meta-analysis of the Data*, Washington: USAID.

Le Nestour, Dr (1938) 'Organisation de l'AMI en Annam', Rapports du Xe Congrès de la Far Eastern Association for Tropical Medicine, Hanoi: Imprimerie d'Extrême-Orient.

Lê Quê (2004) 'Une vie nouvelle pour les lépreux à Dông Lênh', Le Courrier du Vietnam, 31 March.

Le Roy des Barres, A. and Marcel, H. (1927) 'La lèpre au Tonkin', *Bulletin de la Société Médico-chirurgicale de l'Indochine*, 5(2–3): 72–112.

Leung, A. Ki-Che (2002) 'The Introduction of Segregation in China. The Case of Leper Houses in Southeastern Provinces in the Modern Period', paper presented at the Conference 'La diffusion des nouvelles pratiques de santé', Fondation Mérieux, St Julien-en-Beaujolais, 23–25 May.

Lockwood, D. (2002) 'Leprosy Elimination: A Virtual Phenomenon or a Reality?', *British Medical Journal*, 324: 1516–1518.

Meima, A., Richardus, J-H. and Habbema, J. D. (2004) 'Trends in Leprosy Case Detection Worldwide since 1985', *Leprosy Review*, 75: 19–33.

Monnais-Rousselot, L. (1999) *Médecine et colonisation. L'aventure indochinoise, 1860–1939*, Paris: CNRS Editions.

—— (2001) 'Colonisation et problèmes sociaux: une intervention médicale. L'expérience de l'Indochine française, 1860–1954', in H. Dorvil and R. Mayeur (eds), *Problèmes sociaux*, Sainte Foy: Presses de l'Université du Québec, 511–540.

Navon, L. (1998) 'Beggars, Metaphors and Stigma: A Missing Link in the Social History of Leprosy', *Social History of Medicine*, 11(1): 89–105.

Netherlands Leprosy Relief (2004) Leprosy Situation in Vietnam, Hanoi: NLR, unpublished paper.

Nguyên T. H., Nguyên T. L. and Trinh Q. H. (2004) 'HIV/AIDS Epidemics in Vietnam: Evolution and Responses', *AIDS Education and Prevention*, 16(suppl. A): 137–154.

Parascandola, J. (2003) 'Chaulmoogra Oil and the Treatment of Leprosy', *Pharmacy in History*, 45(2): 47–57.

Tchou Ping Kiun (1952) 'Contribution clinique à l'étude de la médication sulfonée dans les traitements ambulatoires des lépreux domiciliés au Sud-Vietnam', unpublished thesis, Faculté de médecine de Saigon.

Vinh Quang (2003) 'Des universitaires nés d'un village de lépreux au Nghê An', *Le Courrier du Vietnam*, 8 August.

World Health Organization (1999) 'Leprosy', in *Fifty Years of the WHO in the Western Pacific Region*, Report of the Regional Director the Regional Committee for the Western Pacific, Manila: WHO.

—— (2003) Leprosy: Overview and Epidemiological Review in the WHO Western Pacific Region, 1991–2001, Manila: WHO.

—— (2004) *Leprosy Elimination Project. Status Report (draft)*, Geneva: WHO.

7 Conflict and collaboration in public health

The Rockefeller Foundation and the Dutch colonial government in Indonesia

Terence H. Hull

The last century has been remarkable for the large and rapid decline in global mortality and the consequent improvement of the expectation of life virtually everywhere. Where rates of infant mortality had been uniformly above 100 per 1,000 live births in developed countries, and two to four times as high in colonies in the mid-nineteenth century, by the 1970s rich countries had rates below 20 per 1,000 and many poor countries had achieved rates below 100. The reasons for sustained mortality decline have been a matter for debate for many years. Medical professionals involved in the development of health care have claimed that advances in medical technology and particularly the development of an effective pharmacopoeia against infectious diseases are the key elements in the decline. McKeown (1976: 78) has systematically queried this notion and argued instead that the most important influence on mortality was improvements in nutrition and sanitation.[1] In addition, he contends, the improvement in conditions of hygiene was responsible for around a fifth of the reduction of the death rate in Britain between 1850 and 1950, but this was a product of the technological improvements of piped water, enclosed sewers and other modifications in the social and physical environments in which people lived.

Reduced to the most simple proposition, the opposition of 'medical technology' and 'environmental and nutritional conditions' is a perennial element in debates over the determinants of mortality decline. Evidence marshalled from the historical experience of Europe is frequently cited to justify particular strategies for improving the expectations of life in developing countries today. Some commentators have gone so far as to argue that investments in health-care programmes are of little use if priority is not given to maximizing the rate of economic growth in a nation (Bauer 1972: 60–68). In contrast, many national health plans confine investments to modern technologies in urban hospitals, ignoring the obvious nutritional and sanitary needs of poor rural populations. Over the course of the twentieth century the struggle to promote health often seemed to be a tug-of-war among people attempting to argue for single-strand solutions. Either investment in economic growth or hospital development; either primary health-care clinics or specialist facilities with the latest equipment; either public health prevention or provision of the best diagnostics and curative care – the nature of such arguments is to foster dichotomies.

This chapter argues that such debates are misguided in framing dichotomies and harmful in diverting attention away from the complex complementary nature of economic and medical measures required to address the health needs of people in developing nations. The case to be examined is the evolution of public health programmes in the Netherlands East Indies which became, after 1950, the Republic of Indonesia. The specific focus is on the role of the Rockefeller Foundation in promoting an educational approach to hygiene and the contrasting authoritarian approach of the Dutch colonial government. The political conflicts between these two institutions in the period up to World War II had a deleterious effect on the development of public health and the medical profession in Indonesia that has bequeathed effects right up to the present day. Yet the conflict, so full of passion, was based on the false dichotomy between medical technology and educational improvements. Then, as now, there was a need for both approaches to work together to address the public health problems of the majority of Indonesians, and the medical profession had a crucial, though not exclusive, role to play. Yet what characterized this struggle was not just the conflict of ideas between people who believed in different approaches to disease, but the irritation, mistrust and self-confidence felt by participants from contrasting cultures: Dutch colonial officials, American philanthropic pioneers and Javanese people who were developing a new national consciousness.

Seen from the vantage point of six to eight decades on, the story does appear most like a tragi-comic play, in which the roles of the characters were stereotypically defined. The plot is full of conflict and power plays, set against the backdrop of three very different cultural traditions: the European sense of superiority displayed by the Dutch, the American sense of a Manifest Destiny and the spiritual cultural traditions of the Javanese. The foreign actors appear to have played out their roles on separate sets of their own making, to scripts set down in classrooms, offices and cities half a world away, while the Javanese struggled to understand the unfolding drama, and from time to time step in to a bit part or a crowd scene. Elements of tragedy, including vital flaws of character, and the occasional rumblings of war and waves of economic depression in the background, create a rarefied atmosphere of sublime isolation, but this isolation is tempered by the constant presence and inexorability of death.

The hookworm campaign: a challenge and a response

In Indonesia the major impetus for hygiene education in the 1920s and 1930s came from the Rockefeller Foundation, following their successful promotion of interventions to overcome hookworm infestations. The hygiene activities were largely the work of Dr John Lee Hydrick, an American medical practitioner who worked in Java from 1924 to 1939. However, the foundation of this programme was laid down by Dr Victor Heiser, a remarkable physician who devoted much of his career to the circumnavigation of the globe in the service of the then very young Rockefeller Foundation. With a bravado built up over years of clinical practice and a commitment to the relatively new field of public health, Heiser was charged with the task of taking the successful model of fighting hookworm in

America to the poor nations of the world, first in the Caribbean and from there to major port capitals in the tropical regions. He recorded his travels in a book that became a bestseller in America (reaching number two on the non-fiction list of 1937) and an enduring record of public health activities (Heiser 1936).

Heiser visited Java regularly in the two decades between 1915 and the time of his retirement from the Rockefeller Foundation in 1934, but in all those visits he never lost his disdain for the Dutch nor gained an understanding of the Javanese. The original purpose of his missions was to negotiate a programme of assistance in the field of hookworm control. To carry this out he utilized the services of the US consul and the US Rubber Company to arrange transport and appointments. On his first visit in March 1915, his strategy for approaching the government was simple. First, he poked around some of the slum areas of Batavia getting a feel for the sanitary conditions, then he met with some of the medical personnel in the government laboratory to learn of their activities in promoting hygiene. On his third day in Java he went, 'arrayed in a redingote, heavy trousers, stiff shirt, patent leather shoes, [and] silk hat' to meet the Governor General in Buitenzorg (Bogor), there to explain the work of the International Health Commission of the Rockefeller Foundation, and request assistance in setting up a campaign against hookworm. In Heiser's words recorded in a letter back to the New York office, the eradication of hookworm was important for the 'lever which it gave toward other health reforms'. In response, the Governor General 'expressed great interest in the manner in which the International Health Commission (IHC) was going about tropical health problems' and indicated that he would want to discuss these issues with his chief medical officer.

Following an interview of half an hour, which included discussions of public health in the Philippines (where Heiser had been chief health officer in 1905), and the difficulties of the war then raging in Europe ('from the standpoint of hard suffering neutrals'), Heiser emerged with a promise of a letter of introduction to the chief medical officer and an agreement that if the latter so recommended, the Governor General would provide a government physician to assist any commission the Rockefeller Foundation might want to send to investigate hookworm in the Netherlands Indies. The promised letter arrived at Heiser's hotel within two hours of the end of the interview (Heiser 1915).

Two days later, as he was leaving Batavia for Singapore, Heiser noted in his diary that in the health field with 'educational work just beginning, the favourable attitude toward it and the general desire to reorganize, which is only held in check by the annual deficit, looks as if it would be a wonderful field for us in this country' (Heiser 1915: 64). This optimistic picture was offset by two factors: the rivalry between the Dutch petroleum industry and the Rockefeller family owned Standard Oil Co. which might give rise to suspicion of the motives of the Rockefeller Foundation, and the fact that the 'Dutch know very little about us Americans' (Heiser 1915: 64). On these grounds he concluded that the IHC would have to go slowly in promoting a study of hookworm.

Just over a year later Heiser was again in Java, and on this occasion travelled overland from Surabaya to Batavia, stopping on the way to observe tourist sites and examine people encountered on the street for signs of hookworm infestation. During his 12-day stay he concluded that the Javanese were 'as industrious as Chinamen, and far more cheerful' (Heiser 1916: 256–257) but continued to be frustrated by the Dutch bureaucracy and amused by Dutch spelling and eating habits. At the end of this visit agreement was reached that Dr Samuel T. Darling of the foundation would return later in the year to carry out a study of the hookworm situation.

The Darling Commission Report established that hookworm was indeed a major problem with very high rates of infestation found in 12 sample areas, and concluded that 'at least 90 per cent of all the inhabitants of Java are infected with hookworm disease... The heaviest infection was recorded in densely populated Mid-Java'. The reasons for these high rates were said to be the 'insanitary habits of the natives' and the system of irrigation which allowed the rapid spread of the infection from one area of the country to another (Darling 1918: 23). The report provided an analysis of the relative impact of hookworm and malaria on the health of Javanese, concluding that the greatest risks occurred in malarial regions where the severity of anaemia among inhabitants was greater than if they suffered only malaria or hookworm alone. This made the need for broadly based environmental sanitation programmes all the more urgent, to address such a dual threat to health.

Following the submission of the Darling Report it appeared that the foundation and the Netherlands Indies government would begin cooperative work on health issues, and a representative of the foundation was selected and dispatched to Batavia. When his ship reached Ceylon (Sri Lanka) he found a telegram waiting for him, saying that the Java post had fallen through and that he had been transferred to another position. The reason for this abrupt change of plans was that officers of the Public Health Service (Burgerlijk Geneeskundige Dienst) raised serious objections to the Darling Commission Report, citing in particular a photo of a labourer with the caption: 'In the great struggle for subsistence in the beautiful island of Java, men and women become beasts of burden' (Hydrick 1935). This tweaking of colonial sensitivities caused 'a very unpleasant reaction', and delayed for eight years the issuance of another invitation for the foundation to work in Java. The sensitivity over the photo was likely just a catalyst for Dutch officials' objections to Heiser's plans. As Darling records, the chief medical inspector in 1916 had said that he would prefer to have his own staff undertake a hookworm campaign. 'This is the thing I have long wished to do', he declared, 'and now it is to be done by others. But I have no men – no men'. (Darling 1918: 23). This was something of a setback for Heiser, but he was persistent, and continued to press the foundation and the Dutch to accept a mission to set up hygiene work.

On 10 April 1924, two representatives of the Rockefeller Foundation finally arrived in Java to undertake the demonstration project on hookworm control first mooted by Heiser nearly a decade earlier. Dr John Lee Hydrick and Dr van Noort were not a happy pair. The former, an American from South Carolina of Dutch descent, was the senior of the two, having worked for the foundation in the southern part of the United States and the Caribbean, while the latter, a 'Hollander', had been recruited specifically to work on the project in Java, in the hope that he would be able to smooth over the difficulties the foundation had encountered with the Dutch government. Their mission started out badly, with Hydrick being embarrassed by an incident provoked by van Noort in Holland, and irritated by his attitudes and behaviour on the long sea voyage to Batavia. By 8 December, Hydrick had lost patience, and sent a letter to Heiser stating that 'in addition to rendering unsatisfactory service he [van Noort] refuses to listen to the hints given him by government officials concerning the use of the name of the Rockefeller Foundation and his criticisms of government officers' (Hydrick 1924b). In short order the officer ostensibly responsible for establishing good relations with the Dutch government was sent packing.

With the departure of van Noort, Hydrick was able to concentrate on the work of setting up a demonstration of the value of educational approaches to the control of hookworm infestation. In November 1924 he wrote a letter to Heiser reporting that the conditions of east, central and west Java were so different that the Dutch suggested working first in the west, and then setting up stations in central and east Java for comparative purposes (Hydrick 1924a). Further, the foundation would take prime responsibility in Bantam, an area to the west of Batavia, inhabited by Sundanese people, and the Health Service would work in central Java. This seemed a reasonable plan to Heiser and Hydrick.

In many ways the story of the comparison is a classic in the history of public health interventions. On the one side was the educational approach advocated by Heiser and Hydrick. On the other stood the more authoritarian approach of the Public Health Service of the Dutch colonial government, which insisted that provision of chenopodium (a worm medicine) through dispensaries and mandatory enforcement of regulations to build latrines were necessary to force the essentially 'lazy' Javanese into action. The competition was joined in 1924. By directing them to Serang [Tjifroes, about 60 miles west of Jakarta], the chief health officer of the Netherlands Indies, Dr J. J. van Lonkhuyzen, had essentially challenged the foundation to test their methods in a district noted for anti-government unrest. In contrast the Service would work in Kroja, central Java, where the ethnic Javanese residents were noted for compliance with government directives.

On the basis of their experience in America and other countries, the foundation considered that the demonstration of the efficacy of hookworm preventive measures should normally take only a few months, but the Dutch argued that at least 18 months would be needed to do a good job. Hydrick accepted their arguments, but Heiser was impatient and wanted to see the work speeded along. The whole of 1925 was taken up with the establishment of demonstration areas.

Finally, in early January 1926, Heiser steamed into Tanjung Priok harbour to be met at dockside by Hydrick and Dr J. J. van Lonkhuyzen, who, said Heiser, 'in the usual Dutch way offered no assistance in landing or in passing through the customs. Often I have an intense longing to speak Dutch. Perhaps then one could judge whether they are stupid or discourteous' (Heiser 1925: 266).[2] The trip was obviously off to a bad start.

Later, a further hitch arose when it was announced that Dr J. J. van Lonkhuyzen would not be able to accompany them to Serang to examine the Rockefeller demonstration site. Heiser and Hydrick thus set off on the trip accompanied by Dr Tuyter of the sub-district and Dr Mollinger, the medical director for west Java. These two officials appeared quite proud of their cooperative work with the foundation in Serang since it represented 'practically the first time in the history of Java that a large scale undertaking has been undertaken by persuasion instead of by order' (Heiser 1925: 267). The education campaign was carried out by *mandoers* who gave large public lectures attracting large crowds of people seeking information and treatment. Instructions were given on techniques of building latrines, and as a result, 800 latrines were voluntarily constructed in a district which had 1,100 houses.

On their return to Batavia, the team found that their enthusiasm for the results in the demonstration area was not shared by central officials. The latrines, Dr van Lonkhuyzen declared, were substandard. They were made of poor materials, and did not reach the government's criteria for hygiene. He paid little attention to the accomplishment of health workers who had conducted the education campaign, and in any case, he said, the methods were too slow to be applied to the major problems of hookworm among Java's large, densely settled population.

On 12 January 1925, the team went on to Kroja. There they found a series of latrines, standing 'new and trim'. Heiser and Hydrick were indeed impressed at the solid brick construction. They were also amazed at the report that 150,000 such latrines had been built under government order. Then Heiser went over to the first latrine, lit a piece of paper and dropped it through the hole. 'This latrine', he announced to the onlookers, 'has never been used'. So with the second, the third and on through the hot and dusty day. As recorded in Heiser's diary and his later memoirs, Dr van Lonkhuyzen first questioned his own officials closely, and then turned to Heiser and Hydrick and declared 'I surrender...I'm convinced now. We must have public health education in Java' (Heiser 1936: 477). Back at the guest house that evening they mapped out a strategy for the development of a Public Health Education unit, and arranged the commitment of Rockefeller Foundation funds, and Hydrick's services, to this activity. This was the start of what eventually became the Hygiene Propaganda Unit, an innovative attempt to use mass media techniques and an educative approach to encourage Indonesians to take an active part in preventive health measures. Heiser and Hydrick were very pleased with their achievement.

As recorded by Heiser, this dramatic episode had produced a thoroughly satisfactory climax: the Dutch had capitulated, the foundation's international mission would expand into one of the largest colonies in the world and the Javanese had demonstrated a responsive attitude to the educational approach advocated by the medical enthusiasts of the foundation. His later autobiography portrays this as a definitive event (Heiser 1936: 476–479) but his 1926 diary recorded some remaining doubts (Heiser 1926: 275ff).

The hygiene propaganda unit

Heiser's pleasure at having staged such a convincing demonstration of the shortcomings of the authoritarian approach did not reduce his basic suspicion of

Dutch motives, and over the next few days, as the team travelled east to Wonosobo and Karangkobar to inspect various health programmes, he had occasion to reflect on the basic approach of the Dutch to health care in Java. 'Everywhere we stopped we were surrounded by a curious multitude... The cringing of the natives and never standing in the presence of the officials is most impressive... the well trained Residents and Civil Service are no doubt largely responsible [for this]' (Heiser 1925: 276). As they travelled on, they moved into regions where the bubonic plague was active (Hull 1987: 220–225) and Heiser had the opportunity to discuss the strategy of plague control with the chief officers of the plague service. He found their approach very disturbing:

> The plague view is more or less typical of the Dutch attitude toward all health problems. They wait until something happens, then concentrate heavily on the infection itself, thus avoiding the expense of guarding the many places where nothing happens. They say it is their duty to keep their population happy, and as it never wants anything done, they feel that in attacking infection after its appearance they are interfering about as much with the habits and customs of the people as circumstances warrant.
> (Heiser 1925: 281)

Disturbed by what he had seen, Heiser confronted van Lonkhuyzen to ask point blank whether the Dutch government really wanted the foundation to work in Java on hygiene education, and if so, on what basis. The latter 'stated in very positive terms' that he welcomed the participation of the foundation and agreed to a four-point plan for the establishment of the work:

1. The International Health Board (of the Rockefeller Foundation) was to conduct the programme of public health education.
2. The foundation and the government should cooperate in the establishment of carefully designed test demonstrations to work out plans suitable to Java.
3. Dr Hydrick 'not only in name but in reality' should act as chief of this unit and be the official advisor to Dr van Lonkhuyzen in hookworm control.
4. The government should pay all expenses for latrines and treatments, while the foundation should pay for the development of health education. Because of the growing demand for hookworm treatment, local governments should be involved in the payment of extension work (Heiser 1925: 282).

The structure agreed upon, Hydrick prepared himself for his new work of developing a full-blown health education unit. On 16 January 1926, he and Heiser discussed these plans over lunch and then he drove Heiser to the docks, where the latter boarded the *S. S. Plancius* to continue his circumnavigation on behalf of the foundation.

The Division of Health Education was largely concerned with the control of the spread of parasitic infection. The strategy was to establish field stations across Java, and eventually throughout Indonesia. At each station, programmes of public lectures, treatment of worm infestations and encouragement of the construction of latrines were to replicate the successes of the Serang experiment. To support this an automobile was modified to carry film and slide projectors into remote villages. Called the Healthmobile, it attracted a great deal of interest among villagers, who were particularly attracted by the lantern slides showing local subjects related to the hookworm campaign.

The slides and films were followed up by house-to-house visits of a trained *mantri* (health worker) who talked to groups of three to ten people in a household courtyard, showing them enlarged photographs of parasites, briefly explaining the purpose of proper hygiene and then questioning them to confirm that they understood his presentation (International Health Board, *Quarterly Report* 1926: 6).

Mantris were recruited from a very small section of the population. Initially all males, they were to be literate, have a good speaking voice and good personal appearance. They could not be too young, since the people would not respect a callow youth, nor too old, since the duties were onerous. Further, 'the *mantri* must be polite and yet not servile, he must not be shy and yet not too aggressive, and most important of all, he must be patient with those he is trying to teach, and not easily discouraged' (International Health Board, *Annual Report* 1926: 6). Once selected the *mantris* underwent both office and intensive field training before being sent out to the villages. However, Hydrick noted that training essentially never ceased, because, while the hookworm campaign was the entry point of the campaign, and as success was achieved there, the *mantri* would be expected to master new subjects to improve the hygiene conditions of his region.

Throughout the 1930s, the Division of Health Education followed the strategy set out by Heiser in 1915 and moved steadily from hookworm eradication through an array of other diseases and conditions that were thought to be caused by poor hygiene or poor nutrition. Starting off with imported films for educational meetings, they soon started producing their own films in a small studio in Jakarta. Unfortunately, a disastrous fire in the Gang Kwini office of the unit on 25 June 1928 destroyed practically all the negatives as well as the copies of the films they had made on hookworm disease, framboesia, latrine construction and other topics. Again, showing the persistence that was typical of the International Health Board, Hydrick was given support to rebuild, and a few months later the unit moved to 67/70 Jalan Kebon Sirih, Weltevreden, where they began, with new equipment, to rebuild their collection of films. At that time their emphasis was on participation in the annual fairs held in the major cities. Like fairs all over the world, these events brought tens of thousands of curious people to the central squares where they had the chance to see acrobats, strange animals and, courtesy of Hydrick and his teams, silent films about health topics accompanied by lectures. The films and photo displays were hugely popular. Recently an American researcher following the Hydrick story carried out interviews with elderly villagers in central Java. These octogenarians told of the delight they had as young people when the health educators would put on their displays. They could even remember some of the details of the messages. Perhaps this is not surprising given that health officials have ever since been repeating the admonitions to wash hands, boil water and eat a balanced diet, but the events they were remembering were literally the first time such villagers had ever heard of the link between such practices and good health (Stein 2005: 108 ff).

Despite the apparent success of the health education activities of the unit, there was still an undercurrent of conflict. Hydrick was contending with another rival, Dr P. Peverelli. The latter had been assigned as his 'counterpart' with the expectation that he would eventually take over Hydrick's work. This is an arrangement that is still very common in development projects carried out throughout the region when donors send consultants to assist developing countries. In the case of Hydrick and Peverelli, the complaints started at the outset with the Dutch doctor requesting a monthly bonus from his government employers to put him on a comparable income to that enjoyed by the American. The bonus was paid for a while, but was soon dropped. The foundation also offered Peverelli a fellowship to carry out further studies, but this was refused because it was not equal to Hydrick's salary. The bickering went on continuously even after Peverelli was removed from the unit by the Director of the Public Health Service. When the Director was replaced in 1931 and Hydrick took his home leave (then involving a long ocean voyage), Peverelli urged the new Director to write to the Rockefeller Foundation to tell them that Hydrick's services were no longer needed. At the same time he sold Hydrick's official car that had been provided by the foundation. When Hydrick returned later in the year he found himself caught in a squabble that took months to resolve.

Meanwhile Peverelli, perhaps inspired by youth brigades being organized across Europe in the early 1930s, set up his own health brigades in cities across Java, as an alternative to the intensive school work that Hydrick was pursuing in the unit. Hydrick's position had changed in 1930 when the government took over the full costs of the hygiene education work, thus 'mainstreaming' all the activities within the central bureaucracy. The contest of paradigms meant that there were no clear winners or losers – changes came to Java, and to some extent they involved education, but they also involved top-down commands. What determined the outcomes at each stage were the complex patterns of the unfolding politics of the colony.

The Hygiene Mantri School in Purwokerto

In 1932, on his return from an extended home leave, Hydrick turned to the development of general rural health programmes based on the regencies. Essentially this was an acknowledgement of the need for a decentralized approach to medical development in Java. Experience with a purely educational approach gradually convinced Hydrick and his Dutch and Indonesian colleagues that there was a need for a broader range of health services to be provided on a permanent basis close to the people. Health units, the forerunners of modern clinics, were designed to meet this need.

By 1936 the activities of the health units had led to the establishment of a Hygiene Mantri School in Purwokerto to train cadres who would take the lessons of preventive health measures into villages. The school was opened on 1 April and an 18-month course was designed for the students, who were drawn from all over the archipelago. The government and Hydrick had requested that the foundation should provide some seed money for this innovation, but in 1935 this request was refused.

Part of the programme Hydrick was building was an attempt to improve the safety of births by giving basic hygiene training to the traditional birth attendants (TBAs or *dukun bayi*), who assisted in the vast majority of deliveries in rural areas. This was not a new idea. The Dutch had trained TBAs as early as 1807 – before the time of Raffles – but had not conducted formal training programmes to upgrade these traditional healers on a widespread basis, preferring instead to promote the concept of professional midwives. This strategy proved to be very slow and resulted in very few graduates from the government programmes. In 1907, it was decided to rely on private foundations for the training of professional midwives. This was also a slow, uncoordinated process, which in any case failed to provide services to village areas, where they were most needed.

Hydrick's innovation was to formalize the structure of training using experienced midwives based in hygiene demonstration units. The *dukun* were then to be trained routinely in small groups, concentrating on demonstrations using dolls and encouraging peer criticisms of the actions of each trainee. In Hydrick's later description of the training (1937: 44–45), it was emphasized that the midwife could not have a private practice or else she would be seen as a competitor, and the *dukun* would not trust her. It should be remembered that in 1938 there were only 158 professional midwives in all of Java. Of these, just over 100 were in government service (Hanifa 1987: 27).

At about the same time, in a hospital in Cianjur, west Java, Dr Poorwo Soedarmo[3] was grappling with the question of how to rapidly and efficiently extend modern obstetrical services to the vast population of his regency. He specifically rejected the idea of training the TBAs on the grounds that they were too old, too uneducated and too set in their ways to adopt hygienic practices. But there were problems with trying to expand the numbers of midwives quickly. The government required a midwife to have two years of basic nursing training, followed by two years of practical residential training and a further year of obstetrical training and practice. For young women, most of whom were encouraged to marry early by their parents, and who would then bear their own children fairly quickly, this was a daunting educational programme. Instead, Poorwo and his midwife assistant proposed that women with basic nursing training should be given a short period of practical obstetrics training so they could serve as 'midwife helpers'. These women could then act as part-time workers to extend the coverage of the maternity services by carrying out antenatal care and early referral of difficult cases.

Around 1937, these two approaches came into conflict when Hydrick and the head of the National Health Services visited Dr Poorwo to try to convince him to train TBAs. The events precipitating this visit were related to a *sandiwara* or folk play that Poorwo, the midwife and the trainees had written and performed to educate rural Sundanese families on the danger signs of difficult pregnancies. In addition to performances in Cianjur, the group visited neighbouring regencies where increasingly enthusiastic officials and audiences called for assistance in training midwife helpers.

Remembering back 60 years to the fateful meeting, Poorwo tells of his concern over the words of the head of Health Services and his lack of any strong impression of the conversation or personality of Hydrick. The head talked long and categorically of the need to train the TBAs, and argued that it was too slow and too expensive to train midwife helpers. Poorwo countered that there was nothing quick about teaching hygiene to old women whose entire lives had been spent surrounded by unsanitary conditions and practices. In his hospital, he declared, it was often difficult to train young doctors in hygienic practices. Despite constant reminders and strong discipline, it might be a year or more before hand-washing became second nature to them. What could you expect from a TBA brought in for a short course, and then returned home to a virtually unsupervised setting?

The head rejected these arguments and ordered that Poorwo and his team not stray beyond their territory in promoting the midwife-helper programme.[4] In essence this meant that by the late 1930s there were three competing models of programmes to reduce maternal mortality (Hanifa 1987: 8). In Cianjur, Poorwo and colleagues concentrated on the training of midwife helpers. In Purwokerto, Hydrick and colleagues trained and supervised TBAs under the Hygiene Propaganda programme. Finally, in Yogyakarta, a programme was devised to train male nurses to become male midwives, thus ensuring workers who would be able to go anywhere, would not have their careers interrupted by marital obligations or childbearing, and who could eventually head a polyclinic (Hanifa 1987: 8).

Lest it be thought that these events were somehow the exclusive province of the Dutch and other foreigners, it is important to note the major showdown among competing strategies which took place in Semarang in December 1938. The occasion was the first congress of the Vereniging van Indonesische Geneeskundigen (Association of Indonesian Doctors). A debate was held between men who were later to be acknowledged as giants of the Indonesian medical scene: Dr Poorwo and Dr Mochtar, with Dr Sarjito as moderator. Nearly six decades later the event is remembered with some bitterness by Dr Poorwo. As he was presenting his case for training *pembantu bidan*, Dr Sarjito frequently interrupted to tell him to hurry, and as a result he was unable to complete his prepared presentation. Dr Mochtar's arguments, though longer, were unhindered, and he swiftly and devastatingly attacked Dr Poorwo's case, including arguments which the latter had been unable to present. Suspicious about the course of the debate, Dr Poorwo was hurt and angry when the delegates voted for a resolution to reject the *pembantu bidan* programme; to promote the training of fully qualified and certified *bidan*; and to support the Purwokerto efforts to train *dukun bayi*, as a temporary measure.

The indigenous Indonesian medical profession thus determined the decision which was to shape obstetric training for the next 50 years, until the *bidan di desa* programme in 1989 resurrected the form and structure of Dr Poorwo's original innovation. Perhaps, to paraphrase the old saying, even those who remember history are doomed to relive it, in endless cycles of reincarnated debate.

The departure of the Rockefeller Foundation

From the outset of its cooperation with the Dutch the stance of the Rockefeller Foundation had always been that it should design its projects for eventual withdrawal, and in reports and correspondence the question was frequently asked: 'When will the government take over the activity?' For Hydrick this was a dilemma, for he was constantly trying to impress upon his superiors and colleagues in the Colonial Health Service that he and the foundation were fully committed to working with them on the complex programme of hygiene education activities, while at the same time he was engaged in regular correspondence with the New York office, acknowledging the need for eventual self-sufficiency in Java, but arguing that there were special circumstances, new difficulties or unusual opportunities which justified the foundation staying on in the Netherlands Indies.

Finally, however, on 18 July 1939, Hydrick boarded a ship in Tandjung Priok and sailed away from Batavia. The foundation's patience had run out, and he was being transferred. Hydrick was confident in the hope that the hygiene work that he had pursued for the previous 15 years would be carried on and expanded by the colonial government. On 10 May 1940 Holland was overrun by the German army, and on 8 March 1942 the government of the Netherlands Indies fell to invading Japanese forces. Soon after, the medical schools in Jakarta and Surabaya were closed and the Dutch doctors still in the country were interned. Years of war and revolution followed. By the time relative stability returned to a newly independent Indonesia, and work could resume to improve the public health conditions of the people, the world had developed new notions of how such work could be carried out. Mass campaigns became the dominant mode to attack the continuing problems of yaws, malaria, smallpox and the immunizable childhood diseases, and the hygiene work pioneered by Hydrick was either forgotten or dismissed as being too tedious. Programmes of continuous education and the application of local technologies appeared to governments to be too expensive in the era of cheap and near 'magical' antibiotics ushered in during the war. A syringe and a briefly trained paramedic appeared to conquer a wide range of infectious diseases.

Hydrick retired from the Rockefeller Foundation in 1953 at age 65, and died five years later in Arizona, leaving behind only his one book *Intensive Rural Hygiene Work* (1937), but no recollection or summary of the meaning of the foundation's three-decade involvement in Java. It was, with surprising finality, the close of an era.

Notes

1 See also the opinion of Dr W. R. Aykroyd, Director of the Nutrition Research Laboratory in South India, who contended: 'one finds that, in a strange manner, diseases which have been ascribed to this or that parasitic or microbic agent simply disappear as a result of a little more food of the right kind to eat'.. Quoted by A. S. Haynes (1938) 'The Hygiene Conference in Java: Some of the Leading Personalities'. *Asiatic Review*, 34: 342.
2 Heiser did not include initials for any names in his original diary entries.
3 I interviewed Dr Poorwo Soedarmo in 1994 when he had just turned 90 years of age. His memory of detailed dates and events was remarkable, as was the passion that came into his description of old battles and career disappointments.
4 For a brief record of the debate and its resolution, see Hanifa Wiknjosastro (1987) *Pelayanan Kebidanan Tempo Doeloe, Kini dan Kelak di Indonesia*, speech given at the Seventh Congress of the Association of Obstetrics and Gynaecology, Semarang 5–10 July 1987 (printed in both Indonesian and English).

References

Bauer, Peter (1972) *Dissent on Development*, Cambridge: Harvard University Press.
Darling, Samuel T. (1916) 'Letter to Drs Rose and Heiser', 12 December 1916. Tarrytown, New York: Rockefeller Archive Center.
—— (1918) 'Hookworm Infection Survey of Java From 15 August to 18 November 1916', New York: International Health Board, Rockefeller Foundation.
Hanifa Wiknjosastro (1987) *Pelayanan Kebidanan Tempo Doeloe, Kini dan Kelak di Indonesia* (Obstetric Services Past, Present and Future in Indonesia), Keynote speech to the Seventh Congress of Obstetrics and Gynaecology in Semarang, Central Java, Indonesia, 5–10 July 1987.
Heiser, Victor J. (1915–1916 and 1925–1926) 'Trip Diary, 26 March 1915–1 April 1915, 44–64; May 1916, 256–257; 17 September 1925–8 June 1926. 266ff. Tarrytown, New York: Rockefeller Archive Center.
—— (1936) *An American Doctor's Odyssey*, New York: W. W. Norton & Co.
Hull, Terence H. (1987) 'Plague in Java', in N. G. Owen (ed.), *Death and Disease in Southeast Asia: Explorations in Social, Medical and Demographic History*, Singapore: Oxford University Press, 210–234.
Hydrick, John Lee (1924a) 'Letter to Dr Sawyer, November, 1924', File 655. Rockefeller Archive Center.
—— (1924b) 'Letter to Dr Heiser, 8 December, 1924', File 655. Rockefeller Archive Center.
—— (1935) 'Letter to Dr Sawyer, 17 December, 1935', RF/220. File 655. Rockefeller Archive Center.
—— (1936) *Intensief Hygiene Werk en Medische-Hygienische Propaganda van den Deinst Der Volksgezondheid in Nederlandsch-Indie*, Batavia-Centrum, Java, Netherlands India.
—— (1937) *Intensive Rural Hygiene Work and Public Health Education of the Public Health Service of Netherlands India*, Batavia-Centrum, Java, Netherlands India. Republished in 1942 with minor revisions. New York: The Netherlands Information Bureau.
International Health Board (1926) *Annual Report*, New York.

International Health Board (1926) *Quarterly Report, Second*, Second Quarter, New York.

McKeown, Thomas (1976) *The Role of Medicine: Dream, Mirage or Nemesis*, London: Nuffield Provincial Hospitals Trust.

Mesters, Han (1996) 'J. L. Hydrick in the Netherlands Indies: An American View of Dutch Public Health Policy', in P. Boomgaard, R. Sciortino and I. Smyth (eds), *Health Care in Java: Past and Present*, Leiden: KITLV Press, 51–62.

Stein, E. A. (2005) 'Vital Times: Power, Public Health and Memory in Rural Java', unpublished thesis, University of Michigan.

van Heteren, G. M., A. de Knecht-Van Eekelen, M. J. D. Poulissen and A. M. Luyendijk-Elshout (eds) (1989) *Dutch Medicine in the Malay Archipelago 1816–1942: Articles Presented at a Symposium Held in Honor of D. de Moulin on the Occasion of his Retirement from the Professorship of the History of Medicine at the Catholic University of Nijmegen 30 September 1989*, Amsterdam: Rodopi B. V.

8 The political determinants of public health in Timor-Leste

Foreign domination and the path to independence

Sue Ingram

Introduction

On 20 May 2002, Timor-Leste (formerly East Timor) became the world's newest nation after almost 300 years of colonial rule by Portugal, 24 years as an unwilling and internationally unrecognized province of Indonesia and two and a half years under United Nations administration. The country's complex history of colonization and conflict has played out in the patterns of disease and population health.

Timor-Leste sits at the cusp of Asia and the Pacific, between Indonesia and Papua New Guinea, and its geography is reflected in its mixed linguistic and cultural heritage of Melanesian and proto-Malay. At independence, it was estimated to be the poorest country globally in terms of per capita income (UNDP 2002: 23), with a predominantly rural population living by subsistence agriculture. Two years on, it remained well behind the rest of the Asia-Pacific region in terms of human development, with a GDP per capita of USD 497 and an overall human development rating that places it amongst the world's 20 most disadvantaged countries, flanked by Senegal and Rwanda (UNDP 2004: 187).

This plays out in the health status of its people, with widespread undernutrition and stunting, an infant mortality rate of 8.9% of live births, and an under-five mortality rate of 12.6%. For every 151 births, one woman dies. Average life expectancy at birth is 49.5 years (UNDP 2004: 171), lower than for any country outside sub-Saharan Africa where AIDS is taking a huge toll in terms of premature mortality. This is not a factor in Timor where poverty and underdevelopment alone account for the disturbing mortality rate. Malaria, dengue, leprosy and filariasis are endemic, tuberculosis is a major public health problem and diarrhoeal and respiratory tract infections account for much of the burden of disease and child mortality. For the people of Timor-Leste, the epidemiological transition is still a long way off.

The colonial period

Timor's high-grade sandalwood was a magnet for foreign interests over the centuries. The first recorded contacts are of Javanese and Chinese traders who regularly visited the island from around AD 1000. The Portuguese followed in their wake, finding their way to Timor sometime around 1512–1514, although settlement and colonization came somewhat later. An initial Portuguese toehold was established on the neighbouring island of Solor by Dominican friars in 1566, acting under the protection of the Portuguese crown; a fort was built, and a community formed around it which traded with, and progressively began to settle in, Timor.

Through the next century, the territory was notionally administered by the viceroys of Goa although their influence was never strong, and effective control was in the hands of the traders and Dominican friars. It was not until 1702 that the Portuguese crown assumed the formal administration of Timor and appointed a governor, under the jurisdiction of the viceroy of Goa, who established a base at Lifau in West Timor. Under increasing pressure from the Dutch, in 1769 the Portuguese governor shifted his headquarters and some 2000 people east to Dili, which became and remains the capital of East Timor. 'Dili was little better than a malarial swamp but it was safe from attack and there, amidst squalor, deprivation and death the administrative foundations of Portuguese Timor slowly took shape' (Hastings 1975: 21).

While the Portuguese administration had a toehold on the coast, colonial policy and strong resistance in some of the Timorese kingdoms slowed the development of administrative and military posts in the interior for a further century. Towards the end of the nineteenth century, policy shifted and a concerted effort was made to establish effective control across the colony and turn it to economic benefit (Taylor 1999: 10). The changed political and economic conditions triggered a series of rebellions from 1893 to 1912, when the last major uprising was put down, with 16,000 killed and injured on the Timorese side and 900 on the Portuguese side.

The final Portuguese conquest of Timor, coordinated by a colonial administration headquartered in Macao until the end of the nineteenth century and drawing heavily on troops from Portugal's African colonies for combat and garrison functions, introduced a dangerous cocktail of new pathogens from across the Portuguese empire to a susceptible indigenous population. The use of Timor during the last century as a place of deportation for political dissidents and criminals from other Portuguese territories and Portugal itself added to the infusion of new pathogens. Reports from the colonial period suggest an explosion of new diseases in the late nineteenth and early twentieth century as a result of immigration and subjugation of the interior of the territory.

The introduction of leprosy and tuberculosis, both now endemic in East Timor, is attributed to soldiers from Africa (Carvalho 1946: 328–330). In the late nineteenth century, tuberculosis was reportedly rare but after the widescale use of African troops to pacify the interior of Timor, the incidence of the disease rose sharply. Leprosy is reported to have entered at much the same time, with the first case identified in 1914 in an African soldier, and a second case in 1916. By 1917, the first case was diagnosed in the indigenous population. Cohabitation between African troops and Timorese women accelerated the spread of disease into the indigenous population. Reports of amoebic dysentery in 1914–1916 are also linked with the presence of African troops or infection from Macau, where the disease was endemic (Carvalho 1946: 321). Both these elements are captured in the colonial records of 1888 from Macau, which report nine Mozambiquan soldiers en route to Timor being hospitalized in Macau with dysentery, of whom three died (Governo da Provincia de Macau e Timor 1888: 330).

While syphilis was evident in both the Portuguese and the Chinese communities (Carvalho 1946: 331), its spread into the Timorese population appears to have been contained by the widespread incidence of yaws. Most of the several hundred deportees sent to Timor in 1927 and 1931 were reportedly infected with syphilis (Correa 1935: 13–14). An outbreak of cerebrospinal meningitis in 1923 is also attributed to deportees – in this case Chinese pirates who had been convicted in Macau and sent to Timor for punishment (Felgas 1956: 365). A smallpox epidemic in 1900 which killed more than 5,000 people may not have been the first. While a medical report from 1886 suggested that the disease was rare in Timor, there are references to a massive outbreak in 1731 that killed more than 30,000 (Carvalho 1946: 313). The global influenza pandemic reached Timor in 1918, killing huge numbers (Carvalho 1946: 320).

In the early twentieth century, tuberculosis spread out along the road network that was developed by the colonial power for political control of the interior and the export of cash crops, just as in other parts of the world in the late twentieth century the spread of the HIV infection followed the major road transport routes. An observer in the 1930s, criticizing the Portuguese administration's preoccupation with roadbuilding, wrote caustically of the consequential effect of 'tubercularizing' the country and accomplishing in a short space of time what otherwise would have taken significantly longer (Braga 1936: 22).

Foreign conflict again brought disease and death to Timor when the country was pitched abruptly into World War II. The landing of a small Australian and Dutch expeditionary force in Dili within days of the attack on Pearl Harbour provoked a full-scale occupation of the territory by the Japanese (Australian Senate 2000: 113). When the allied troops withdrew in January 1943, the Timorese, who had provided significant assistance to them, fought on for several months. Over the course of the war, Timor's towns and centres were severely damaged by allied bombing, while villages seen to support the allies were destroyed and villagers executed by the Japanese. Populations were forced to relocate, and food supplies were ruthlessly appropriated (Hastings 1975: 24). By the end of the war some 60,000 people – around 13% of the population – were estimated to have died as a direct result of fighting or, far more numerously, from the starvation and disease that followed in its wake (Dunn 1996: 22).

Timor's colonial history destined it to be a developmental backwater.

> On the eve of the outbreak of World War I, Portuguese Timor was undoubtedly the most economically backward colony in southeast Asia, its living conditions often a subject of derision to the few who ventured to it.
>
> (Dunn 1996: 17)

Over the course of the next 60 years, until its abrupt transition from Portuguese colony to Indonesian territory in 1975, Timor continued to stagnate, as Portugal's own development was retarded under a 50-year dictatorship that left it the poorest country in Western Europe when a military coup in 1974 overthrew the ultra-conservative regime and opened the path to political pluralism. Timor's underdevelopment was mirrored in its demography. A colonial report from 1956 referred to the abnormal stagnation in population growth, reflecting the poor health status of much of the population. In some areas of the country, population numbers were actually falling (Felgas 1956: 359–360). Twenty years later, the population was only growing by around 6,000 persons per annum (Aldeia 1973: 87), or under 1%.[1] The death rate for children under five at this time was around 50% (Taylor 1999: 18).

Malaria, tuberculosis, respiratory tract infections and diarrhoeal disease, compounded by undernutrition, were taking a huge toll on the population. 'Intermittent daily fever' dominates the Dili hospital admission records throughout the 1880s, with smaller numbers of admissions for tuberculosis, syphilis, ulcers and respiratory tract infections. Portuguese, Chinese and Africans account for a large majority of the admissions, giving little direct insight into the epidemiology of the Timorese population. Admissions data from Dili hospital in the early 1950s show much the same pattern, with malaria and tuberculosis dominating, followed by pneumonia, anaemia, intestinal infections and bronchitis.

Some limited public health measures were introduced to tackle major communicable diseases. The colonial bulletins of the late nineteenth century chronicle the mounting frustration of colonial officials seeking public works funding to drain the swampy ground on which Dili was built and to relocate the soldiers and Portuguese civilians and the hospital to higher ground above the town, 'beyond the range of the terrible focal point of malaria that calls itself Dili' (Governo da Provincia de Macau e Timor 1892: 29). Permission to build the new hospital was finally given in 1893 and it was eventually opened in 1906.

Health services gradually spread out into the districts and by the late 1930s clinics had been set up in four districts supporting a larger network of health posts. In 1937, a training programme for indigenous nurses was introduced, with a focus on child health, and in 1938 an isolation ward for tuberculosis patients was opened in Dili hospital (Felgas 1956: 362). Immunization programmes beginning in the early 1900s eventually eliminated smallpox and the incidence of yaws was significantly reduced by the 1960s through the use of penicillin.

In the reconstruction after World War II, there was a further expansion of health services with the opening of regional hospitals in two districts, and health clinics in several others. By 1956, the primary care network had expanded to a health centre in Dili, six district sub-centres and 47 health posts. In 1957, a Permanent Mission for the Study and Combat of Endemic Diseases in Timor was established under the supervision of the Portuguese Institute of Tropical Medicine. Gubernatorial reports to the Legislative Assembly through the last decade of the colonial period track the Mission's efforts to contain yaws, leprosy, tuberculosis, filariasis and malaria.

In the last decade of its colonial administration Portugal made some effort to strengthen basic health and education services in Timor. By 1972, hospitals had been established in 11 of the 13 districts, and there were 12 health centres, 12 maternity facilities, 48 health posts and two diagnostic laboratories. While there were only three civilian doctors and two dentists for a population of around 670,000, 19 army medical officers were providing part-time services in rural areas. Health posts were staffed by Timorese nurses, and nurse training expanded significantly in the 1960s as part of a wider boost to secondary and technical education. Despite this expansion, primary health care barely penetrated into the villages beyond the sub-district centres where the health posts were located. While there were regular vaccination programmes, little was available in the way of treatment for the overwhelming burden of disease borne by the rural villagers who made up the bulk of Timor's population.

The greater investment in health did translate into observable improvements in population health.

> there was evidence that the health and appearance of the population had improved markedly in the ten years prior to mid-1974. ... It might be pointed out that, whatever the shortcomings of the Portuguese system, health and nutrition conditions appear to have been no worse than in the adjacent Indonesian islands.
>
> (Dunn 1996: 41)

The Indonesian period

The military overthrow of the Portuguese dictatorship in 1974 was the culmination of 13 years of debilitating conflict in Portugal's African colonies that sapped the resources and the spirit of the country. The central plank of the new leadership in Portugal was an immediate and rapid process of decolonization across the Portuguese empire. Timor, which had slumbered through the political turbulence in Lusophone Africa, had little in the way of popular political organizations but rapidly made up for lost time. Within weeks of the coup in Lisbon, the three major political parties – União Democrática Timorense (UDT), Associação Social Democrática Timor (subsequently renamed Fretilin) and Apodeti – had emerged.

In the following months, as both Fretilin grew more radical and the government in Portugal shifted to the left, the prospect of an unpredictable leftist government in an imminently independent Timor was causing growing unease both in the neighbourhood and in wider international circles. A coup in Timor in August 1975, led by UDT and Apodeti in an attempt to outmanoeuvre Fretilin, resulted after several weeks of fighting in Fretilin's victory. At the outset of the fighting, Portuguese civilians were evacuated by boat to Darwin and most of the military followed them at the end of the month, leaving only a small core of paratroopers and the governor who withdrew to Atauro – a large island to the north of Dili – whence they too were eventually evacuated to Portugal.

The leadership of the vanquished parties sought refuge in Indonesia, which under cover of a partisan struggle, intensified its military action along its common border with East Timor. On 7 December 1975 Indonesia launched a full-scale invasion of Timor, ironically on the anniversary of the Japanese attack on Pearl Harbour. And just as that attack had propelled Timor into years of conflict that decimated its population, so Indonesia's invasion dragged Timor into a brutal conflict that was to last for almost a quarter of a century and lead to the deaths of one-third of its population (Dunn 1996: 283–285).

Armed conflict is a major public health issue, and the victims are predominantly civilians. For each death directly due to conflict, an estimated nine people die indirectly as a consequence of the conflict (Murray *et al.* 2002: 347). And for each death in the aftermath of conflict, many more people suffer serious ill health. Conflict produces massive social and economic upheavals: populations are displaced, infrastructure destroyed and livelihoods lost. This translates into severely compromised population health from malnourishment, exposure, overcrowding, contamination of the water supply, trauma, injury, sexual violence and epidemic diseases that thrive in these conditions. Displaced populations are particularly vulnerable. During recent periods of conflict in several African states, the mortality rates for internally displaced persons ranged between 4 and 70 times the rates for non-displaced persons in the same country (Rehn and Sirleaf 2002: 33).

All of these conditions were present in Timor in the years following the Indonesian takeover. As the Indonesian military pushed outwards from its coastal landing points, encountering stiff resistance from the Fretilin guerrilla forces, much of the population evaporated from the small towns and villages into the rugged hinterland behind Fretilin lines where many remained until 1978 when they were forced by military action and hunger to move back into Indonesian-controlled areas.

Frustrated militarily, and determined to choke off support to the guerrillas, the Indonesian forces systematically destroyed villages and crops and moved those left behind into resettlement camps. Violence against the civilian population was systematic and even UDT and Apodeti leaders who had collaborated with the Indonesian government condemned the widespread killing (Taylor 1999: 71). By December 1978, the majority of the surviving population of Timor was no longer living in their own villages but had been moved into makeshift camps (Taylor 1999: 90). In 1979, when the first international aid workers were permitted into the country, around 20,000 people were found to be close to death from malnutrition and another one-third of the population at serious risk (Dunn 1996: 290). Epidemic diseases flourished, tuberculosis was a major problem, and infant mortality soared.

From the camps, people were ultimately resettled in strategic villages strung out along roads for ease of supervision and remote from areas where Fretilin was active.

> This often resulted in villages being built in lowland areas which traditionally had been avoided by Timorese, since they were infected with malaria, had poor water supplies and a much hotter climate than the mountain areas.
> (Taylor 1999: 93)

For security reasons, villagers were restricted from developing fields at any distance from their villages, compounding food shortages and the cycle of undernutrition and disease.

Malnutrition and disease were intensified by operations mounted over several years from the late 1970s to flush out the guerrilla forces. For these operations, known as the 'fence of legs', thousands of villagers were conscripted to march in lines ahead of Indonesian units. The first largescale operation, in 1981, involved 80,000 men and boys, many of whom died of starvation and disease on the march (Taylor 1999: 117–119). As the operation coincided with the harvest and planting seasons, severe food shortages followed.

Indonesian rule was consolidated in the early 1980s, underwritten by aggressive military tactics and close supervision of the civilian population. Despite ongoing military action, the guerrilla forces were never completely crushed, and continued to harry the Indonesian military until its final withdrawal in 1999. They had solid backup from the civilian population which was organized into an effective clandestine movement in support of the independence struggle.

With the collapse of the Portuguese administration in August 1975, public health services also disintegrated, to be only slowly rebuilt as the Indonesian administration moved in behind the military. In the vacuum, new service providers emerged. In the last months of 1975 in the hiatus between Portuguese and Indonesian administrations, Fretilin organized the remaining health workforce into a new health administration divided into five zones across the country. Only one doctor – a long-term resident from India – remained in the territory, and the Australian Red Cross visited three times weekly with a medical team working out of Dili hospital. As the security threat grew, many health workers fled to Australia or to the border, reducing the original nursing cadre of 190 to 120.[2]

Following the Indonesian invasion, Fretilin attempted to maintain a basic health-care structure. However medical supplies were rapidly exhausted, and health workers turned back to traditional medicine. Training in basic health care was set up behind Fretilin lines, and traditional medicines produced and distributed for malaria, wounds and pain relief.

After the surrender of most of the civilian population in 1978, health care was organized for the guerrilla fighters through the clandestine movement. Like the movement itself, health care was organized on a regional basis, and involved both traditional and modern medicine. Initial reliance on traditional medicine fell away as it became easier to access modern medicine with the reopening of primary health-care services for the general population. Health workers were able to both supply and treat the guerrilla forces. Wounded fighters would be brought to safe houses or to churches, and health workers would themselves travel into the mountains to provide supplies and services.[3]

Publicly provided health-care services gradually resumed from the late 1970s although they took another decade to normalize.[4] Progressively, the government introduced a comprehensive primary health-care system modelled on that provided in all other Indonesian provinces. It offered a far broader geographic and service coverage than that available under the Portuguese administration.

By 1999, a network of 309 health posts radiated out into the villages, linked to health centres in all 67 sub-districts which in turn linked to 8 district hospitals and a provincial referral hospital. A health workforce of 160 doctors and some 1,600 nurses and midwives delivered health services at the community level (World Bank 1999: 18).

During the Indonesian period, the Catholic Church emerged as a parallel provider of health services – a function which, in the Portuguese period, it had left largely to the government. When Portugal abandoned Timor in 1975, the Church had still not penetrated deeply into Timorese cultural and spiritual life. Although some 30% of the population was 'at least nominally' Catholic (UN 1976: 4), the people beyond the towns and the chiefly class (whose status was contingent on embracing Portuguese language and religion) were predominantly animist. During the Portuguese period, the Church's principal social role was in education, deriving from a 1940 Concordat between Portugal and the Vatican which assigned the prime responsibility for education in the colonies to the Church, as a principal agent of Portugal's 'civilising mission' (Smythe 2004: 35).

The functions and standing of the Church expanded rapidly after the Indonesian occupation. The Church, as the one institution able to stand up to Indonesian authority, became the rallying point for the people.

> As the sole institution to function independently of the Indonesian State it enjoyed the special confidence and loyalty of the native people. Church membership became a symbol of Timorese identity to such an extent that there was a fusion of the religious and the secular, a merging of Catholicism and nationalism. ... The institutional Church's corporate link with the Universal Church also afforded it significant (but not complete) protection against the malevolence of the occupying forces and helped it to be the sole 'moral force' capable of critical comment on the Indonesian administration.
> (Smythe 2004: 48)

Another factor, perhaps, was that the Church came to fill the spiritual vacuum of a people torn from the land of their ancestors and their sacred places.

The Church moved into the provision of health services for the people in 1977, following a call from the bishop in March that year to provide assistance at the parish level.[5]

> The reality was that people were coming in from the bush, sick, and living in stark conditions. The military was everywhere. It was logical for the church to step in. At this point the church was the only credible institution and it was in touch with the world outside, which in turn sent medicines and humanitarian assistance through the church. Language was another factor – people did not speak Bahasa. So they would go to the priests who had medicines. Also people coming in from the bush were very fearful. This led the church to create mechanisms for providing health care.[6]

By 1999, 22 Catholic polyclinics were operating across the country providing curative services, a national tuberculosis programme and some health education at the village level (Araujo 2001: 14).

A major public health issue which put the government, the Catholic Church and the people of East Timor on a collision course was the national family planning programme, known by its Indonesian acronym Keluarga Berencana (KB) and introduced into Timor in 1980. The programme is a central plank of Indonesian social policy, and has its own dedicated department of state, separate from the health department. Outside Timor, the programme was generally well received and, in 1989, the Indonesian President Suharto was awarded the UN Fund for Population Activities prize in recognition of his government's efforts to promote family planning and improve population health.

In Timor, the programme encountered strong moral and political resistance led by a young Timorese priest, Carlos Belo, who was appointed in 1983 to head the Church after a succession of Portuguese bishops. Appointed by the Vatican's envoy to Jakarta without proper consultation with the clergy in Timor, and initially not well received by them, he quickly emerged as a courageous critic of the abuses of the Indonesian administration.[7] In March 1985, and again in 1993, Bishop Belo issued pastoral letters criticizing the family planning policy in uncompromising terms.

The Church's opposition was taken up by the people.

> Many Catholics... would argue against KB the fact that the Catholic religion taught how Jesus Christ had said 'grow and multiply', and also because they had lost many children in the war. They would say that while the number of children lost in the war wasn't replaced by an equal number of other children they wouldn't stop having them. This type of resistance would be found amongst the urban population. They were aggressive, and they would even glue to the church walls posters saying 'Indonesians, baby killers'.[8]

Making a link with other radical demographic changes – the deaths through conflict, the massively high infant mortality rate and the transmigration programme that was bringing settlers to Timor from other parts of Indonesia – the Timorese portrayed KB as *a way of terminating our people, using our active cooperation and agreement.*[9]

Feared and bitterly resisted, KB had far less reach in Timor than in other Indonesian provinces where the message of a two-child family was generally embraced as good civic conduct. In Timor, the programme consistently failed to meet the targets set by the central government, despite their progressive reduction over time. In the late 1990s, only 20.7% of currently married women were reportedly using any contraception, the lowest rate of usage in Indonesia (Sissons 1997: 13).

This low result defied the programme's aggressive promotion. Throughout Indonesia, mass recruitment drives referred to as *safaris* were used to enlist women into the programme. While the same approach was employed in Timor, civilian and military officials worked in tandem, adding to the sense of coercion and resistance. The programme in Timor also differed from that in other parts of Indonesia because of the unusually high usage of Depo-Provera: 72% of all new users in 1993/94 (Sissons 1997: 22). Health workers report that no explanation of contraceptive methods or side effects was given. In this environment, women became fearful of using public health services lest they be tricked or coerced into contraception, possibly contributing to the broad preference for Catholic health-care services.[10]

As with the Portuguese, the Indonesian influx appears to have added to the disease mix in Timor. Dengue, which is now endemic, seems to be a late arrival. Although it was reported amongst Japanese soldiers in Timor during World War II, infection was thought to have occurred outside Timor (Carvalho 1946: 320). While not significant during the Portuguese period, it represented a major public health threat in 1999 when the UN established its peacekeeping presence in Timor, and its spread has been attributed to the mass population movement from Indonesia to Timor (Pinto 1999: 4).

HIV may also have been introduced from elsewhere in Indonesia. The first case of HIV infection in Timor was reportedly identified in 1996 in a sex worker from East Java who had been working in Timor for around three months,[11] and Indonesian data reported at least one suspected death due to AIDS (WHO 2001: 10). The prospect of HIV finding its way into the indigenous population would have been high given the high underlying rate of sexually transmitted infections and the large number of military deployed across Timor. Military personnel around the world have elevated levels of sexually transmitted infections – up to 2 to 5 times the rate for civilians (Rehn and Sirleaf 2002: 40) – placing the civilian populations with whom they come into contact at risk.

The UN transitional administration

Under intense international pressure over East Timor, and weakened domestically by the economic crisis that swept through Asia in 1997 and the subsequent resignation of its president of 32 years, Indonesia offered in June 1998 to give East Timor wide-ranging autonomy. As pressure continued for a more generous formula, the Indonesian government formally agreed in May1999 to a UN-sponsored popular consultation to allow the people of East Timor to vote for continued integration with Indonesia or for independence. Despite violence and intimidation in the months leading up to the ballot, the people of East Timor voted overwhelmingly for independence on 30 August 1999.

By the time of the popular consultation, the population was projected to have grown to around 900,000 (UNICEF 2003: 4), an increase of only 230,000 over 24 years, over half of which reflected migration from other parts of Indonesia (Dunn 1996: 306). Despite higher government expenditure on health in East Timor than in other provinces (Araujo 2001:17), health outcomes lagged well behind. Compared with the other provinces of Indonesia, East Timor consistently had the worst health conditions, more akin to those found in poor African countries than among its Asian neighbours (United Nations 2000: 52).

The weeks following the announcement of the results of the popular consultation, which overwhelmingly supported independence, saw an explosion of violence. Timor's infrastructure was systematically and comprehensively destroyed by rampaging pro-Indonesian militias, backed by the military, and one-third of the population fled or was pushed into West Timor. Many of those who remained in Timor fled their homes. As the violence continued unchecked, the UN Security Council on 15 September mandated a multinational peacekeeping force to restore peace and security and facilitate humanitarian assistance operations. The first deployment occurred only five days later, but in the few weeks that it took the force to re-establish security almost all public buildings, between half and two-thirds of all housing, and water, electricity and telecommunications systems in the capital and across the countryside had been destroyed.

This situation had all the makings of a humanitarian disaster: from malnutrition, exposure and disease. The flight of the population occurred in the lead-up to the wet season, when fields are cleared and planted. By the time that many of those displaced returned to their villages, the annual planting cycle had passed and the population was reliant on emergency food distribution for several months. The destruction of domestic housing left people crowded into makeshift shelters at the beginning of the wet season when the incidence of diarrhoeal diseases and respiratory tract infections traditionally rises. Uncleared rubble multiplied the breeding grounds for mosquitos, and damaged water reticulation systems further reduced access to safe drinking water. Many people were severely traumatized or disoriented. These factors added to the poor underlying health status of the population.

The health sector itself was, literally, in ruins: the network of village clinics and district hospitals had been razed, equipment trashed or stolen, and records destroyed; the Ministry of Health had been sacked; and the clinical and administrative workforce had scattered. This experience was replicated across all sectors. With the exodus of the Indonesian administration, the destruction of government buildings and records and the massive population displacement, central government had simply disappeared and all government services had ceased.

Confronting this extraordinary conjunction of humanitarian crisis and governmental vacuum, the UN Security Council established the UN Transitional Administration in East Timor (UNTAET) on 22 October to maintain security, coordinate humanitarian assistance and – in an unprecedented first for a peacekeeping mission – to govern the country through to the formation of a national government and the formal transition of the country to independence.

In February 2000, almost six months after the popular consultation, an Interim Health Authority made up of seven UN personnel and sixteen East Timorese health professionals was formed under the UN Transitional Administration to begin the process of rebuilding a health administration and a national public health-care system. At this time, primary health care was being provided by a patchwork of emergency non-governmental organizations (NGOs) and some still-functioning church clinics, leaving significant gaps in coverage. Villages isolated by terrain or distance from the small towns in each district were affected most. Hospitals were operating in the two major towns, managed by Médecins Sans

Frontières and the International Committee of the Red Cross, and other NGOs were managing a handful of smaller facilities with a few beds in the districts. Of 160 doctors in East Timor before the conflict, fewer than 30 remained; there was one specialist, and no dentists.

A major challenge for the Interim Health Authority was an effective transition from NGO-provided services to a public health system. Early priorities were the recruitment of a temporary health workforce at the district level, the procurement and distribution of essential pharmaceuticals and the restoration of basic laboratory services; in parallel, the authority was planning the longer-term rehabilitation and development of the health sector. Within weeks of its formation, the authority joined the World Bank-led Joint Donor Mission to design the programme for health sector rehabilitation. This had two main components: restoring access to basic services for the entire population and development of the health policy and system for the future. The Interim Health Authority, the forerunner to the future Ministry of Health, led the implementation of what became a sector-wide approach to health system reconstruction and development.

A fundamental component of the transition strategy from NGO to government service provision was to bring the NGOs into formal partnership with the authority to work within an agreed planning model. The aim was to ensure a basic standard and coverage of primary health care across all districts. In each district, one or sometimes two NGOs took the lead in coordinating service provision, and supporting the temporary public health workforce. This was expressed in terms of an agreed district health plan. A major concern of the authority in negotiating the plans was to secure the sustainability of the future health system by ensuring that the large network of overstaffed, underfunded and underutilized facilities which had characterized the previous primary health-care system was not simply put back in place (Tulloch *et al.* 2003: 11–12).

Progressively, over the next year, NGO services contracted as the public system developed. By late 2001 over 800 health staff had been recruited and a fully East Timorese Ministry of Health was in place and had assumed full responsibility for the management and delivery of the national public health system. Importantly, the foundations laid during the transition stage had ensured that the basic infrastructure and policy framework were appropriate and affordable.

Inevitably the donors, the NGOs and the UN itself influenced the public health agenda, at times in ways that were antithetical to elements of the Timorese leadership. As with the KB programme of the Indonesian administration, the clash was most evident in the sensitive area of reproductive health. This came to a head within months of the arrival of UNTAET, when Bishop Belo became aware that several NGOs were distributing condoms. For the NGOs, this was a basic public health measure in the context of a high incidence of STDs and the known risk factors associated with a post-conflict environment. For the Church, it threatened a fundamental tenet and in June the Bishop forcefully directed that UN agencies and health providers involved in reproductive health to cease providing condoms or other forms of birth control. Church and State were on a collision course in a complex environment where the Church exercised enormous moral authority and the UN's role was essentially custodial pending the formation of a Timorese government.

Another prominent element of the international public health agenda, initiated by, and in part a response to, the international presence, was the development of an HIV/AIDS policy for East Timor. While there was little evidence of HIV in the local population, the post-conflict setting presented a number of factors which could contribute to an epidemic developing: the massive social dislocation of 1999, a lack of information about what constitutes risky sexual behaviour and the character of sexually transmitted infections, a low level of HIV and sexually transmitted infection (STI) awareness, poverty and large numbers of young people in neither the educational system nor employment (WHO 2001: 10).

This dangerous cocktail was compounded by the presence of over 10,000 UN peacekeeping personnel, including some 8,000 military and 1,400 civilian police, some from countries with a high HIV prevalence. The majority were under 40 and male, and all were unaccompanied. The garrison lifestyle, increased earnings, absence of family and an asymmetric relationship with the local population increased the probability of sexual contact. For precisely these reasons, the UN now builds an HIV adviser into the core staff of all peacekeeping missions.

Early in the term of the UN administration, evidence emerged of a low level of HIV infection in the general population. Screening of blood donors at Dili hospital beginning in February 2000 through to mid-2001 showed up an infection rate of 1.3% of 531 people tested. In 2003, 12 cases (0.07% infection rate) were identified through testing at Dili hospital, and in the first five months of 2004 a further 6 cases were identified (4% of those tested). A survey of at-risk groups conducted in late 2003 suggested a relatively low HIV infection rate, with 3% of sex workers and 1% of men who have sex with men testing positive. All those infected reported previous sexual contact with foreigners. An examination of the HIV positive specimens in the survey found them to belong to two sub-types: one common mostly in West Africa and the other common in Africa but also circulating in the Indian subcontinent. This was consistent with the partnerships reported by the infected respondents (Family Health International 2004: 26) and with the composition of the peacekeeping mission.

Independence

East Timor became the independent nation of Timor-Leste on 20 May 2002, although a pared-down UN peacekeeping mission stayed on, at the request of the new government, to support the maintenance of security and stability. The foundations of public policy had been laid in the months leading up to independence through the formulation of the National Development Plan, a wide-ranging vision for all sectors directed towards the dual goals of poverty reduction and economic growth. The plan drew on broad-based consultations across the country led by the future President, Xanana Gusmão. The president had himself set out a realistic strategy for health three years before in the planning leading up to the ballot for independence

> Let us not be tempted to build and develop modern hospitals that are costly and in which only half a dozen people benefit from good treatment. Let us

concentrate above all on planning intensive campaigns of sanitation, prevention, and treatment of epidemic and endemic diseases for the whole population.
(Ministry of Health 2002: 2)

Less than a year after independence, the Council of Ministers approved the Health Policy Framework for East Timor, the strategic approach for which is comprehensive primary health care. The framework sets out a basic package of services that aims to ensure the greatest coverage and impact for the majority of people within the available funding of USD 8 per capita per year. It consists of essential health services and cost effective interventions to prevent and control or treat problems causing the highest burden of disease in the country. The Ministry of Health believes that the rehabilitation of the health system is still in its very early stages and is not expected to produce sound health outcomes in the near future, in particular given the range of factors outside the health sector that are reinforcing the low health status of the community (Ministry of Health 2002: 23). A further serious challenge for the public health system is the progressive contraction in donor funding after the significant injection of funds in the immediate post-conflict period, including budget support in the initial years after independence. As a result, the ministry is projecting a fall in real per capita government on spending in the coming decade.

Family planning is one of the priority areas of health policy for the ministry. Timor's birth rate of 7.5 per woman puts it close to the highest in the world. This is coupled with an alarmingly high under-five mortality rate – up to 15% in rural areas – and moderate to severe stunting and underweight in half of all surviving children (UNICEF 2003). In March 2004, the Council of Ministers of the Timorese government approved a family planning policy which commits to providing family planning information, counselling and services, and a secure supply of a wide range of contraceptives, at all levels of the public health system.

Importantly, the Catholic Church was formally consulted in the development of the policy and, while emphasizing the importance of natural methods, recognized that the responsibility of the Ministry of Health to guarantee the health of the nation required professional counselling and services which would cover the diverse methods of family planning, both natural and artificial. Thus, the focus of the national discourse on family planning has shifted from nationalism and resistance under the Indonesian administration and the assertion of Timorese cultural values during the UN administration to the centrality of the health of the family in an independent Timor-Leste.

Timor's political history has been acted out in the public health of its people, with colonization and conflict exacting a huge toll. The test for the new nation will be a peace dividend measured – in part – in significantly improved levels of population health.[12]

Acknowledgement

This chapter is the product of many collaborators: Kevin Sherlock whose archive of materials on East Timor was invaluable in reconstructing the colonial period; and Rui de Maria Araujo, minister for health, Emilia Pires, former head of the Planning Commission and the many, many East Timorese in Australia and Timor-Leste who generously shared their experience with me.

Notes

1 In a speech to the Legislative Assembly of Timor the outgoing governor referred to a birth rate of 23 per 1,000 and a death rate of 12.5 per 1,000, translating into a population increase of around 6,000 per year. The total population estimate for Timor used by the Portuguese in 1974 was around 670,000.
2 Personal communicaton from Antonio Calaeres Jr, the current director of Dili Hospital, who was chief of health for Ainaro district in 1975.
3 I am indebted to Brig. Gen. Taur Matan Ruak, head of the East Timor Defense Force, Luis Lobato, vice-minister for health, and Antonio Calares Jr, director of Dili Hospital, for their accounts of the provision of health care to displaced populations and Falintil fighters during the period of Indonesian occupation. Further accounts are available in the records of hearing of the Reception, Truth and Reconciliation Commission.
4 Personal communication from Antonio Calaeres Jr.
5 Personal communication from Padre Monteiro, Dili Diocese.
6 Personal communication from Padre Jovito Araujo do Rego, deputy chairperson, Reception, Truth and Reconciliation Commission, Dili.
7 Bishop Belo was awarded the Nobel Peace Prize in 1996 jointly with Jose Ramos Horta.
8 Evidence of former Governor Mario Carrascalão to the Reception, Truth and Reconciliation Commission in 2003.
9 Ibid.
10 I am indebted to Sister Dorothy (Mary Knoll Sisters, Aileu) and Isabel Guterres (commissioner, Reception, Truth and Reconciliation Commission) for their accounts of the KB programme in Timor. Other material is contained in the reports of the Commission's public hearing on women and conflict.
11 *Jakarta Post* 14 February 1997.
12 Since the time of writing this chapter, Timor-Leste has been hit by a new wave of civil unrest triggered by disaffection within the security forces and a consequential crisis in political leadership. Widescale violence and destruction of property in the capital peaked in late May to early June 2006 and some two-thirds of the population fled to makeshift camps or into the mountains. Weak governance and institutional failures contributed directly to the crisis (United Nations Security Council 2006: 8) and a new UN intervention was mounted in August 2006 which focuses not only on the immediate security issues but also on the underlying issues of institution-building and economic and social development. The mandate for the new UN mission includes support to the government to design poverty reduction and economic growth strategies to achieve the Millenium Development Goals enshrined in Timor's National Development Plan. Improved public health is an important component of both.

References

Aldeia, F. A. (1973) 'Na Hora do Arranque', speech to the Legislative Assembly of Timor, Lisbon: Agencia-Geral do Ultramar.
Araujo, R. de M. (2001) 'A Suitable Medium-to-long Term National Health System for East Timor: An East Timorese Perspective', unpublished thesis, University of Otago.

Australia Parliament Senate Foreign Affairs, Defence and Trade References Committee (December 2000) *East Timor: Final Report of the Senate Foreign Affairs, Defence and Trade References Committee*, Canberra, ACT: The Senate.

Braga, P. (1936) 'Dili-Bázar tete Sintese da vide timorense *Cadernas Coloniais* No. 14, Lisboa: Editorial Cosmos.

Carvalho, J. (1946) 'Estudos Medicos Timorenses', unpublished manuscript (Kevin Sherlock archive, Darwin).

Correa, A. P. (1935) *Gentio de Timor*, Lisboa: A. P. Correa (Kevin Sherlock archive, Darwin).

Dunn, J. (1996) *Timor: A People Betrayed*, Sydney: ABC Books.

Family Health International (2004) 'HIV, STIs and Risk Behaviour in East Timor: An Historic Opportunity for Effective Action', Dili.

Felgas, H. A. E. (1956) *Timor Português*, Lisboa: Agência Geral do Ultramar, Divisão de Publicações e Biblioteca.

Governo da Provincia de Macau e Timor (1888) *Boletim da Provincia de Macau e Timor*, XXXIV (supplemento ao No. 38): 329–330.

—— (1892) *Boletim da Provincia de Macau e Timor*, XXXVIII (supplemento ao No. 3): 29–32.

Hastings, P. (1975) 'The Timor Problem-I', *Australian Outlook*, 29(1): 18–33.

Ministry of Health, Democratic Republic of Timor-Leste (2002) 'East Timor's Health Policy Framework', unpublished government policy paper in possession of author.

—— (2004) 'Política Nacional de Planeamento Familiar', unpublished government policy paper in possession of author.

Murray, C. J. L., King, G., Lopez, A. D., Tomijima, N. and Krug, E. G. (2002) 'Armed Conflict as a Public Health Problem', *British Medical Journal*, 324: 346–349.

Pinto, C. A. (1999) 'Análise Geral do Sistema de Saúde em Timor-Leste e Perspectivas de Desenvolvimento', paper presented at the International Conference on East Timor, Melbourne, 1999.

Planning Commission, United Nations Transitional Administration in East Timor (2002) *National Development Plan*, Dili.

Rehn, E. and Sirleaf, E. J. (2002) *Women, War and Peace: The Independent Experts' Assessment on the Impact of Armed Conflict on Women and Women's Role in Peacekeeping*, New York: United Nations Development Fund for Women.

Sissons, M. E. (1997) *From One Day to Another: Violations of Women's Reproductive and Sexual Rights in East Timor*, Melbourne: East Timor Human Rights Centre.

Smythe, P. (2004) *The Heaviest Blow – : The Catholic Church and the East Timor Issue'*, Münster: LitVerlag.

Taylor, J. (1999) *East Timor: The Price of Freedom*, London: Zed Books.

Tulloch, J., Saadah, F., de Araujo, R. M., de Jesus, R. P., Lobo, S., Hemming, I., Nassim, J. and Morris, I. (2003) *Initial Steps in Rebuilding the Health Sector in East Timor*, Washington: The National Academies Press.

UNDP (2002) *East Timor Human Development Report 2002: Ukun Rasik A'an. East Timor – the Way Ahead*, Dili: United Nations Development Programme.

—— (2004) *Human Development Report 2004: Cultural Liberty in Today's Diverse World*, New York: United Nations.

UNICEF (2003) *Multiple Indicator Cluster Survey (MICS) Timor-Leste 2002*.

United Nations Country Team (2000) *Common Country Assessment for East Timor: Building Blocks for a Nation*, East Timor.

United Nations Department of Political Affairs, Trusteeship and Decolonization (1976) 'Issue on East Timor', *Decolonization*, 7: 1–70.

United Nations Security Council (2006) *Report of the Secretary-General on Timor-Leste pursuant to Security Council resolution 1690(2006)*, S/2006/628, 8 August.

World Bank Joint Assessment Mission to East Timor (1999) *Health and Education Background Paper*, unpublished report in possession of author.

World Health Organization (2001) 'WHO's Contribution to Health Sector Development in East Timor', Dili, unpublished report in possession of author.

9 From colonial economy to social equity

History of public health in Malaysia

Kai Hong Phua and Mary Lai Lin Wong

Introduction

The development of public health services in Malaysia is here traced from their historical roots under British colonial rule to the present. An historical approach throws light on the heritage of a centralized bureaucratic organization with a strong paternalistic orientation financed mainly from taxation. During the colonial period a combination of enlightened British self-interest and firm administration of a compliant and industrious population appears to have achieved relatively good health and promoted wealth, although at a high, initial, social cost (Phua 1987: 366–367). Public health services and health standards reflected the socio-economic disparities and racial inequalities of a colonial society.

In the post-colonial period, public health services were extended as part of the national development plans. The primary health-care infrastructure was built around the district health services to allow access to a multitiered, referral system of community clinics, health centres and hospitals. In all the successive national development plans following the implementation of the New Economic Policy (after 1969), emphasis was given to the political objectives of equity and income redistribution across racial lines. Massive expenditure on infrastructural development in rural areas was intended to reduce the imbalances between regions and population groups. However, the growing disparities between the public and private health sectors in terms of equity and efficiency continue to pose challenges to public health development (Wong 2006: 214). This problem is compounded by recent privatization policies and attempts to introduce a national health-care financing plan amidst a growing demand for higher-quality health services by an increasingly affluent population.

Early historical background

The history of modern health services in Malaysia dates back to the colonial period. The presence of the West began when the Portuguese conquered and settled in Malacca in 1511, followed by the Dutch in 1641. In 1786, the British settled first on the island of Penang and replaced the Dutch in Malacca in 1795. The colonial powers established small military hospitals and infirmaries to serve mainly European officials and their families. It was not until 1867 when the British formed the Straits Settlements of Malacca, Penang and Singapore, under the direct control of the British Colonial Office, that medical services were organized for the general population.

Prior to British colonization, peninsular Malaya was one of the unhealthiest parts of the tropics with very heavy mortality among the local population as well as the European settlers. The principal causes of death were malaria and 'unspecified fevers', tuberculosis, pneumonia and the 'dirt' diseases such as dysentery, enteric fever, typhus and anklylostomiasis. Singapore, being an entrepôt and centre of immigration, was subject to epidemic diseases such as smallpox and plague, while malaria produced a large death rate in Penang (Mills 1942: 297–298).

Development of medical and health services under British rule

In the early nineteenth century, Chinese migrated to Malaya in large numbers after tin was discovered. They were housed in unhygienic conditions which led to outbreaks of disease. Similarly, with the introduction of rubber plants, Indian labour was brought into the country to work on the plantations in the late 1800s. There were major outbreaks of beriberi (Vitamin B1 deficiency) among the miners and periodic outbreaks of malaria on the plantations.

The British established the first general hospital in 1872, and by 1895, there were 14 hospitals in Selangor, four in Negeri Sembilan and two in Pahang. By 1910, there was a general hospital in the capital city of each state. However, health was given low priority as shown in the small expenditures on hospitals in the early budgets: for example, in 1877, Perak hospitals accounted for 0.7% of the total budget and in Selangor it was 0.4% (Phua 1987: 44). In 1875, the colonial government took control of all pauper institutions and public hospitals that were established initially as military hospitals. The pauper hospitals had been built by the Chinese to meet the needs of their own communities. The Chinese in 1880 built in Kuala Lumpur a 28-bed hospital providing traditional medicine. The colonial government supported curative medicine in hospitals but public health measures to prevent diseases were given minimal attention. The first government dispensary was started in Singapore in 1882 and later dispensaries were established in the other Straits Settlements. The first medical school was established in 1905 following various earlier, unsuccessful attempts to have the government meet local needs by providing locally trained doctors.

A massive increase in population (from about 2.2 million in 1911 to 3.8 million in 1931 due to immigration), and lack of proper sanitation, a safe water supply and public health measures, saw an upsurge in disease. A cholera epidemic in 1851 led to the building of waterworks in place of town wells in Singapore. Sanitary boards were set up in larger towns to regulate sanitation, the water supply, drainage, roads, housing, public markets and slaughter houses. Many sanitary regulations were introduced from 1869–1870, among which was a requirement for proper sanitation on the rubber plantations. In 1887, a Municipal Health

Department was established. Other public health activities included port health work to identify infected ships and the establishment of a quarantine station on St John's Island as a result of a cholera epidemic in 1873. A port health officer, appointed in 1901 in Singapore, inspected ships as well as supervised the quarantine station. The result of these measures was a steady decline in the number of outbreaks of smallpox, cholera and plague (Mills 1942: 297–298).

Other preventive work included research on endemic diseases. In 1900, the Institute of Medical Research was set up in Kuala Lumpur where research was done in collaboration with the London and Liverpool Schools of Tropical Medicine. It earned an international reputation for investigation of tropical diseases like malaria, beriberi, Japanese yellow fever and tropical typhus. The institute also prepared vaccines for rabies, cholera and other diseases and carried out analyses required by the hospitals in the Federated Malay States and by health and veterinary officers and the police (Mills 1942: 311).

In 1910, the government established a separate Health Branch in the Medical Department to control antimalarial and other public health work on estates and in mines and rural areas. Gradually, health officers were appointed in the towns and their duties included anti-malaria measures, inspection of water supplies, enforcement of sanitary regulations, supervision of public health aspects of building regulations, licensing of premises and the testing of foodstuffs offered for sale. Other responsibilities such as medical inspection of schools and maternity and infant welfare followed. Among the public health activities, campaigns against malaria had been more successful after the creation of the Malaria Advisory Board in 1911. The death rate from malaria was reduced from 17.47 per 1,000 population in 1911 to 15.24 in 1920 (Mills 1942: 301). The growing network of health facilities and close cooperation with village heads, the police and the post office greatly helped in the distribution of quinine to the kampongs. By 1920 there were 51 government hospitals, 60 dispensaries, 151 estate hospitals and 18 ambulances doing dispensary work in rural areas in the Federated Malay States.

In 1921, an Infant Welfare Advisory Board was established to combat the high infant mortality rate. Among the causes were the ignorance of the mothers as to proper methods of feeding, neglect of sick children and insanitary living conditions. During 1911–1920, the average infant mortality rate had been as high as 195.62 per 1,000 children under the age of one year (Mills 1942: 302). In its campaign against hookworm, the government began building latrines in rural schools and other government buildings and more strictly enforced the Labour Code requirements on the estates. Insanitary village latrines were being replaced by bore-hole and 'bucket' latrines and limited numbers of septic tanks. Sanitary inspectors carried out regular inspections to enforce stricter regulations. Piped water was also being supplied to the towns, larger estates and some villages, although many still depended on wells.

Tuberculosis was one of the major causes of death and was especially prevalent among the urban Chinese due to overcrowded dwellings without adequate ventilation and their refusal to attend hospital for treatment. House-to-house inspections had to be made regularly by sanitary inspectors. Venereal disease was also a serious problem especially among immigrants. The Social Hygiene Branch of the Medical Department was created to carry out educational campaigns. Maternity, infant welfare and school health work also expanded. Infant welfare centres were started with 3 in the principal towns in 1922 and 14 by 1937 (Mills 1942: 326). Their staff provided antenatal and postnatal care, vaccinations, dental work, treated minor ailments and gave childcare lectures and demonstration to mothers.

The colonial government was successful in transforming peninsular Malaya from one of the unhealthiest regions in the world to one of the most productive economies in the tropics. Thus in the Federated Malay States, an infant mortality rate of 218.45 per 1,000 births in 1917 was reduced to 203.11 in 1927 and further reduced to 147 per 1,000 in 1937. Annual death rates on the early rubber plantations were as high as a fifth of the labour force, but in 1942, many of these same estates had large hospitals that were nearly empty. Many towns were now free from malaria, while dysentery and hookworm had almost disappeared. The high death rates due to communicable diseases such as tuberculosis and cholera had decreased tremendously due to preventive measures.

The colonial government regarded health services as an investment to raise the productivity of its labour force and so health services were provided in major towns and then on estates and in tin mines where the conditions were particularly bad, but the vast majority of people in the subsistence sectors was ignored (Fong 1989: 14–15, 43). The two major export earners – the rubber and tin industries – were located on the west coast of the Malay Peninsula where the Straits Settlements and most of the Federated Malay States were situated. It was not surprising that the upsurge of economic development there had brought about a parallel expansion of health-care services. Although the health services were developed initially to serve the economic interests of the colonialists and concentrated more on curative medicine, there was a relatively well-developed basic network of public health services established in each state.

But the rural health services and those in the poorer Unfederated Malay States were given much less attention. This problem of equity deepened during the period of the Emergency which began in 1948 as a guerrilla war against a Communist movement and resulted in a major resettlement of rural Chinese in New Villages between 1950 and 1953. The Chinese were provided with midwifery clinics or small, first-aid facilities in an attempt to win them over. Many voluntary and religious organizations also seized the opportunities for social and welfare work. During the Emergency, the colonial government began to recognize that the rural Malay kampongs also had similar needs. A series of national programmes was started, focusing on improving the conditions of the rural areas, and these led to the formulation of the Rural Health Services Scheme in 1953.

The British realized that provision of medical services could also be used to win the loyalty of aborigines. So basic health care was introduced with regular visits to the jungle posts and air support to fly out those who needed further treatment. The medical services for the aborigines were managed not by the health authorities but by the Department of Orang Asli Affairs within the Ministry of Home Affairs because of problems of geographical access, communications and sociocultural barriers in addition to security issues.

Pre-independence development planning

The British government passed the Colonial Development and Welfare Act in 1945 which provided for comprehensive ten-year plans to encourage centrally administered schemes for development. It ensured that GBP 120 million would be provided for development and welfare in colonial territories over ten years. The Federation of Malaya government submitted a plan of development.

Draft development plan 1950–1955

The Draft Development Plan was an attempt to define the objectives of social and economic policy and to plan them within the range of resources available. Priority was given to economic services and infrastructure projects to attract overseas investment in order to broaden the country's economic base. Communications, transport and public utilities were accorded highest priority, receiving two-thirds of the funding. Next was agriculture and land development which received 22%. Social services were only allocated 11% and medical services was only one of the components of social services. At the end of 1951, the plan was revised and the allocation for medical services was reduced from 7.9% to 2.2% of total funds (Phua 1987: 264). The shortage of staff was most acute in the medical department where there were 228 vacancies in 1950 and 259 in 1952 (Progress Report 1953: 8–9).

The government recognized the need to develop social services as part of the effort to counter the insurgency. The urban areas continued to be favoured in the allocation of resources. Capital expenditure proposed for rural health amounted to under 10% of the entire medical programme while the recurrent expenditure was less than 20%. The main development projects proposed under the Medical Programme for 1950–1955 were the construction of a training school, rural health centres, tuberculosis clinics, sanatoria and other facilities, with the bulk earmarked for the improvement of hospitals. By 1956, there were 50 district hospitals and 10 general hospitals. Static dispensaries were mushrooming in the towns and some additional travelling dispensaries in rural areas were organized. Maternal and child health clinics were established in scores of cities and towns.

The Federation government invited the International Bank for Reconstruction and Development (IBRD) to send an Economic Survey Mission to give independent advice regarding priorities and economic policies in relation to development in 1954. The knowledge gained from the Draft Development Plan and the IBRD Mission Report formed the foundation of the Federation of Malaya's first five-year plan. At the macro level, the priorities for development were concentrated on economic services. Health services were seen as less important. Except for emergencies, this had been the pattern throughout the colonial period.

Post-independence development planning

The first five-year plan 1956–1960

After independence in 1957, responsibility for health and medical services was transferred from the states to the federal government. The new Malayan government decided that of the total allocation for capital expenditure (excluding requirements related to the Emergency and the armed forces), 60% would go to the economic sector, 30% to the social sector and 10% to the government sector (Report of Economic Planning in the Federation of Malaya in 1956, 1957: 3–4). Within social services, the plan specifically mentioned that education and health jointly were to be given second priority. But actual expenditure for education was more than 60% and on housing 97%, whereas on health only 25% of what was planned was spent (see Table 9.1).

When the federal government took over from the British, the distribution of health services was inequitable – 70% were concentrated in the urban and suburban areas that had 40% of the population. Rectification of this imbalance was given priority by the new government. For every 50,000 population, there would be a main rural health centre; for every 10,000 population, a rural sub-centre and for every 2,000 population, a midwifery clinic. There was a growing tendency for the population to use hospital facilities and the review of the plan revealed a 20% increase in government hospital patients. The rapid rate of population growth also contributed to this. Although the expenditure for security remained high, there was an increased proportion of allocation to health and other social services as spending on the Emergency declined.

Table 9.1 Public investment for social services 1956–1960

Sector	Plan target (millions of dollars)		Percentage of target
	Approximate	Actual	
Social services	212.7	138.8	65
Education	95.4	60.9	64
Health	50.0	12.7	25
Housing	67.3	65.2	97
Total public investment[1]	1,148.7	971.7	85

Source: Malaya (1961: 8).

Note
1 Not including investment on defence.

The second five-year plan 1961–1965

In the second five-year plan, a total of 25.4% of capital investment was allocated to the social sector compared to 14% in the first plan. Expansion of health services to rural areas remained the priority. The aim was to establish 37 main rural health centres, 148 sub-centres and 652 midwifery clinics to serve another 2 million rural population. The total planned expenditure amounted to USD 151 million including social welfare which was allocated USD 6 million. The government made a larger allocation to the public health services. The preventive measures were focused on control of communicable diseases such as tuberculosis and malaria, and promotion of health and sanitation through the rural health service. Curative measures were concentrated on the expansion of existing hospitals and building new ones.

The first Malaysia plan 1966–1970

After a decade of independence, the government recognized that there was a marked disparity in health-care provision between the more developed states in west Malaysia and the less developed in east Malaysia and also between the rural and urban areas within the states. Therefore, one of the four main objectives of the first Malaysia plan was to improve further health facilities in rural areas. The other objectives were to provide facilities for training, to promote the general health of the population through preventive measures and to establish a family planning programme.

The network of rural health facilities was extended even in Sabah and Sarawak, with linkages to major hospitals. At the same time curative services were expanded. Six new hospitals were to be built during the plan period in Peninsula Malaya, six treatment centres and expansion of one general hospital in Sarawak, and one hospital and four cottage hospitals in Sabah. Preventive services were focused on the control of tuberculosis through vaccination programmes and disease surveillance, the leprosy control programme and the malaria eradication programme. A national family planning programme was adopted. At the end of the plan period, only USD 114.2 million (76%) was spent in Malaya, USD 19.4 million (92%) in Sabah and USD 13 million (72%) in Sarawak. However, no reason for these shortfalls was given in the review of the plan.

National development policies and plans 1970–2000

The new economic policy

After the race riots in May 1969, it was felt that past government policies had failed to reduce socio-economic disparities between the predominant *Bumiputra* (Malay and indigenous population) and other races, in particular the Chinese. In order to correct these imbalances, the New Economic Policy was drawn up with the aim of eradicating poverty and restructuring society to eliminate the identification of race with economic function. Resources were redirected to underdeveloped rural areas to benefit the Malays.

The Outline Perspective Plans (OPP)

Changes in the health-care system were planned using three types of planning horizon, namely, the five-year socio-economic development plan, the medium-term plan and the long-term plan. The medium-term plan was also known as the Outline Perspective Plan (OPP). The objectives of the first OPP, for the period 1971–1990, were to restructure the community and to eradicate poverty. The second OPP (1991–2000) was implemented through the National Development Policy to achieve the objective of growth with equity. Currently Malaysia is in the third OPP (2001–2010), also known as the National Vision Policy, and its objectives are achieving national unity and the development of a knowledge-based economy.

Vision 2020 and Vision for Health

Malaysia aims to be an economically developed country by the year 2020. This 30-year planning horizon is also known as Vision 2020:

> By the year 2020, Malaysia is to be a united nation, with a confident Malaysian society infused by strong moral and ethical values, living in a society that is democratic, liberal and tolerant, caring, economically just and equitable, progressive and prosperous, and in full possession of an economy that is competitive, dynamic, robust and resilient.
> (Malaysia (1991) Second Outline Perspective Plan 1991–2000: 4)

Vision 2020 sets the framework of action for all sectors including health. The Vision Statement of the Ministry of Health states that

> Malaysia is to be a nation of healthy individuals, families and communities, through a health system that is equitable, affordable, efficient, technologically appropriate, environmentally adaptable and consumer-friendly, with emphasis on quality, innovation, health promotion and respect for human dignity, and which promotes individual responsibility and community participation towards an enhanced quality of life.
> (Ministry of Health (1999) Policies in Health: 11)

Health sector reforms: privatization and corporatization

In the mid-1980s, the Malaysian government initiated a programme of economic liberalization that included a comprehensive privatization policy. With government encouragement in the 1980s, there had been a steady rise in the number of private hospitals and private clinics. It has been claimed that private health care has resulted in inequitable distribution of medical and health resources and in poorer quality of care (Economic Planning Unit 1996: n.p.). In the seventh Malaysia plan (1996–2000), it was re-stated that the government 'will gradually reduce its role in the provision of health services and increase its regulatory and enforcement functions' (Malaysia 1996: 544).

Corporatization meant that while a public entity was owned by government, it was operated like a private organization. This would allow for greater use of private resources, and flexibility and autonomy throughout the public sector. From 1991 to 1995, 204 projects (non-health-care services) were privatized and 11.4% of civil servants were transferred to the private sector (Wong 2006: 207).

In 1992, the National Heart Institute (IJN) became the first health institution to be corporatized. One of the reasons for the move was to retain highly trained personnel within the public sector through better terms and conditions. Also, many people were opting for heart surgery overseas or in the private sector. With corporatization, revenue could come from fees from private patients and subsidies from the government for civil servants, pensioners and the poor. However, the reimbursements by the government were high, increasing from MYR 31.3 million in 1992 to MYR 65.5 million in 1997. In terms of equity, private patients were given priority while the public or subsidized patients were on longer waiting lists. The proportion of private patients increased. To counter this problem, the government has set up three regional cardiothoracic units which cater for the poor.

In 1999, there was another attempt to privatize health care by corporatizing the 14 general hospitals in the country. There was much opposition to the scheme, with accusations of lack of transparency and accountability on the part of the government. Significant sections of Malaysian civil society were critical of the policy changes (Barraclough 2000: 356). Just before the 1999 general elections, the Minister of Health announced that the policy had been scrapped and any future privatization programme would be transparent, competitively tendered and involve shorter terms of contract.

Under the eighth Malaysia plan (2001–2005), the government was to implement the concept of cost sharing through a health-care financing scheme that will give the public more choice about using the public or the private sector (Malaysia 2001: 495). Moreover, the government has allowed managed care organizations and private health insurance companies to operate so that the private sector has expanded, especially in the urban areas.

The health-care system

The federal government through the Ministry of Health (MOH) has been the main provider of health services since independence and their primary functions include curative, preventive, rehabilitative, promotive and regulatory aspects. The health-care system is currently a mixed system with a public sector and a private sector; the former takes care of those who cannot afford to pay for medical care whereas the latter caters mainly for the urban rich. The public health-care services have three levels: primary, secondary and tertiary care. The first point of contact is the community clinic (in the rural areas), urban health centres, outpatient clinics in hospitals or mobile health units. The rural clinics are easily accessible. Primary care providers serve as the gatekeepers to the more costly secondary and tertiary care.

Primary health-care includes outpatient medical services, dental services, health promotion and education activities, maternal and child health, and more recently, geriatric care, adolescent, mental and occupational health, rehabilitative services and family specialist services. There has been a gradual shift from a three-tier to a two-tier referral system at the primary care level. Thus a health centre is designed to serve a population of 15,000 to 20,000 while a *Klinic Desa* (community clinic) covers a population of 2,000 to 4,000 (Merican and Yon 2002: 20)

The government plays a dominant role in the provision of preventive and promotive programmes such as immunization, control of communicable diseases, environmental sanitation, nutrition, health education, occupational health and safety, family health and anti-drug programmes. The environmental sanitation programme covers both rural and urban squatter areas with a high prevalence of communicable diseases where waste disposal and a potable water supply are not available. In 2000, 92.9% of the rural population were served by a safe water supply. Even in rural areas, 96.5% had sanitary latrines (Wong 2006: 390). The preventive dental services programme includes dental health education, clinical treatment and fluoridation of public water supplies. In maternal and child health, immunization coverage for infants is extensive: over 90% for BCG, DPT (diphtheria, pertussis and tetanus) and poliomyelitis and 80% for measles. Hepatitis B immunization coverage for infants is about 90% and immunization for rubella has been available since 1987 for all women aged 15–44 years (Malaysia 1996: 534).

The private sector is concentrated in urban areas. The working population, especially those who work for multinational companies and large establishments, receive medical benefits. Private providers are paid indirectly by employers through medical insurance or are directly reimbursed by the companies. Most of the private providers serve on the companies' panel of doctors or in managed care organizations (MCO). Other providers are the traditional practitioners who are still popular among rural people and with non-governmental organizations that provide health care free or for a nominal charge.

Health care is funded mainly through general taxation and out-of-pocket payments (Kananatu 2002: 23). Private health-care insurance is rapidly gaining popularity as health care becomes more costly. There are also the third-party payment methods for health services provided by MCOs and through community or charitable sponsorship, especially for very expensive procedures. From the trends in health-care expenditure, the percentage of health expenditure in relation to the

Table 9.2 Annual budget allocation for Ministry of Health 1970–2000 in Malaysian ringgit

Year	Total MOH budget	National budget	% National budget	GNP in millions	% GNP	Per capita allocation
1970	183,033,101		5.64	12,155	1.51	17.39
1975	405,011,250		5.78	16,916	2.39	33.97
1980	895,579,857		5.27	25,402	3.53	66.65
1985	1,256,322,300	29,191,069,194	4.30	563.37	2.23	80.13
1990	1,840,321,780	33,405,637,300	5.51	109,543	1.68	103.60
1995	2,793,731,000	48,797,932,300	5.73	208,118	1.34	135.03
2000	4,931,315,300	78,025,291,600	6.32	191,136	2.58	212.00

Source: Ministry of Health Annual Reports (1970, 1975, 1980, 1985, 1990, 1995, 2000).

national budget or Gross National Product (GNP) appears not to have increased much (Wong 2006: 225) (see Table 9.2).

The improvements in health indices are not due to the health services or health expenditure alone. Many other factors such as improved nutrition, education, higher income and better lifestyle also contributed. Above all, they were due to socio-economic development because economic growth enabled the government and individuals to invest in health-related measures including better environmental sanitation, water supplies and housing in addition to health programmes as such.

The state of health

Malaysia has been experiencing a gradual improvement in health status. In 1957, life expectancy at birth for males and females was 55.8 and 58.2 years respectively. By 1970, it was 63.5 and 68.2 years and in 1999, 69.9 and 74.9 years. The crude death rate, infant mortality rate, toddler mortality rate and maternal mortality rate have improved gradually since independence (see Table 9.3). But there are still some areas which have mortality and morbidity rates much higher than the national figures. The variation can also be seen between the urban and rural populations and different states and ethnic groups (Low et al. n.d.: 200–203).

The disease pattern has changed over the last 50 years: the primacy of communicable and nutrition-related diseases has given way to that of chronic degenerative diseases such as cardiovascular diseases and neoplasms. Motor vehicle and industrial accidents have increased consistent with rapid industrialization and urbanization. In the 1980s, accidents increased by as much as 40% and accounted for about half of admissions to public hospitals. The leading cause of death since the 1980s has been cardiovascular diseases. Out of the total of medically certified deaths, 50% are principally caused by heart disease. Lung cancer is the commonest form of neoplasm among men, with breast cancer and

Table 9.3 Vital statistics of Malaysia 1957–2000

	1957	1960	1970	1980	1990	1999
Crude birth rate	46.2	40.9	33.9	30.9	28.4	24.4
Crude death rate	12.4	9.5	6.9	5.3	4.7	4.4
Neonatal mortality rate	29.6	30.0	22.9	14.8	8.4	5.2
Infant mortality rate	75.5	69.0	40.8	24.0	13.0	7.9
Toddler mortality rate	10.6	8.0	4.2	2.0	0.9	0.1
Maternal mortality rate	2.8	2.4	1.5	0.6	0.2	0.2
Expectancy of life at birth						
Male	55.8	NA	63.5	66.7	68.9	69.9
Female	58.2	NA	68.2	71.6	73.5	74.9

Source: Vital Statistics, Department of Statistics, States of Malaya; Ministry of Health Annual Report, (1970–2000).

cervical cancer among women. Diabetes is also on the rise, with a prevalence twice as much for the urban as for the rural population (Abu Bakar et al. 1995: S3–S10) (see Table 9.4).

Future trends and challenges

Chronic degenerative diseases, related to changes in behaviour as well as population ageing, will be challenges. Cardiovascular and cerebrovascular disease and cancer rates will continue to increase with the rise of associated risk factors such as obesity, stress and smoking and other harmful lifestyle factors. Moreover, by 2010 some 2.1 million (or 7.3%) Malaysians will be 60 years or older and the number is expected to increase to almost 3.2 million by 2020 (Department of Statistics 2001: 20–46). The increase will translate into a greater demand for health-care.

Communicable and vector-borne diseases such as tuberculosis, malaria, cholera and dengue persist. The increase in incidence of HIV/AIDS is associated with the resurgence of tuberculosis and there is a problem of emerging drug-resistant pathogens. The 1997–1998 outbreak of Japanese encephalitis, the 1999 outbreak of Nipah virus cases plus the looming threat of new viruses such as SARS and H5N1 avian influenza all pose new challenges. These diseases will require more sophisticated surveillance and more advanced treatments.

Rapid industrialization, socio-economic changes and rural-to-urban migration have resulted in a segment of the population becoming marginalized: the urban poor, the *orang asli* (aboriginal people) and foreign workers. These marginalized groups are more vulnerable to illness and lack access to health care. It is estimated that about 5% of the population or nearly 1 million people consist of foreign workers, some of whom are illegal. The number of non-Malaysians has grown from 805,376 in 1991 to 1,384,774 in 2000. There is concern that the large influx of immigrant workers may contribute to the spread of communicable diseases carried from their country of origin (Merican and Yon 2002: 19).

Table 9.4 Population annual growth and vital rates, Malaysia 1970–2000

Year	Average annual growth rate	Crude rate of natural increase	Crude birth rate	Crude death rate	Perinatal mortality rate	Neonatal mortality rate	Infant mortality rate	Toddler mortality rate	Maternal mortality rate	Still birth	Life expectancy at birth (male)	Life expectancy at birth (female)
1970	3.6	25.7	32.4	6.7		21.4	39.4		1.4	19.5		
1971	2.5	26.3	32.8	6.6		20.8	37.2		1.1	19.3		
1972	2.5	25.9	32.2	6.3		21.0	36.1		1.0	18.2		
1973	2.4	24.8	31.1	6.3		21.4	36.8		1.0	17.3		
1974	2.4	25.3	31.3	6.0		20.5	33.8		0.9	16.8		
1975	2.5	24.8	30.7	6.0		19.3	32.2		0.8	15.1		
1976	2.3	25.3	30.9	5.7		16.9	28.8		0.7	14.9		
1977	2.5	24.5	30.3	5.8		16.7	29.3		0.7	14.6		
1978	2.3	24.3	29.7	5.4		15.5	26.1		0.8	13.9		
1979	2.4	25.0	30.4	5.4		14.9	25.1		0.6	13.1		
1980	2.6	25.4	30.6	5.3		14.2	23.8	2.1	0.6	13.6	66.5	71.0
1981	2.7	26.3	31.2	4.9		12.3	19.9	1.7	0.5	12.2	67.5	71.8
1982	2.7	26.0	31.0	5.0		12.1	19.5	1.7	0.5	11.6	67.3	71.7

Year											
1983	2.7	25.1	30.2	5.1		12.3	20.2	1.7	0.4	11.4	67.4	71.6
1984	2.6	25.9	31.0	5.0	19.1	11.4	17.5	1.5	0.4	9.9	67.8	72.5
1985	2.8	26.6	31.5	5.0	17.9	10.4	16.4	1.4	0.3	9.6	68.4	73.1
1986	2.8	25.8	30.6	4.7	16.8	9.9	15.5	1.2	0.3	9.0	69.1	73.4
1987	2.7	24.7	29.3	4.5	15.6	9.3	14.5	1.1	0.2	8.2	68.9	73.4
1988	2.6	25.0	29.7	4.6	15.2	9.1	14.1	1.1	0.2	8.1	69.0	73.6
1989	2.5	22.2	26.8	4.6	14.6	8.6	13.4	1.0	0.2	8.0	69.2	73.7
1990	2.5	23.3	27.9	4.6	13.2	8.5	13.1	0.9	0.2	6.7	69.2	73.4
1991	2.3	23.3	27.9	4.6	12.1	8.1	12.5	0.9	0.2	5.8	69.4	73.6
1992	2.3	23.6	28.2	4.6	12.0	7.9	12.1	0.9	0.2	5.9	69.4	73.8
1993	2.3	23.6	28.2	4.6	11.7	7.5	11.3	0.9	0.2	5.8	69.4	74.0
1994	2.3	22.8	27.3	4.6	10.8	7.1	10.9	0.9	0.2	5.2	69.4	74.2
1995	2.3	22.1	26.8	4.7	9.7	6.8	10.3	0.8	0.2	4.5	69.3	74.3
1996	2.2	21.8	26.5	4.7	9.1	6.0	9.0	0.7	0.2	4.3	69.6	74.6
1997	2.1	21.1	25.7	4.6	9.0	6.0	9.4	0.7	0.2	4.4	69.7	74.7
1998	2.3	19.9	24.2	4.6	7.9	5.2	8.5	0.7	0.3	3.9	69.9	74.9
1999	2.4	20.0	24.4	4.4			7.9	0.6	0.2		69.9	74.9
2000	2.4	20.1	24.5	4.4			7.9	0.6	0.2		70.2	75.0

Sources: Vital Statistics Time Series Malaysia (1963–1998), Department of Statistic, Malaysia (2001); Social Statistics Bulletin Malaysia (2001), Department of Statistics, Malaysia (2002).

Changes in disease patterns, improved standards of living, increased demand for high-tech medical care and a growing aged population all impact on health-care costs. The future role of the government in the light of the concentration of private health-care facilities and the rising costs of services will be a more regulatory one. Any new financing mechanism that the government adopts will have to be accompanied by measures to ensure access, affordability, quality and sustainability.

Conclusion

The development of the Malaysian public health-care system has been shaped by its colonial past. The colonial government had established medical and health services which initially were to serve the needs of the colonial economy. The postcolonial government inherited a strong state-controlled health system which laid the foundation for the development of a welfare-oriented health-care system (Phua 1989: 315–323). There was disparity in services provision between rural and urban areas and between the west coast and east coast states of Peninsular Malaysia and the states of Sabah and Sarawak in East Malaysia. The disparity had reached its peak by the time of the race riots in 1969. These led the government to address the inequity between rich and poor and its expression in racial terms. Much emphasis was placed on the objectives of the New Economic Policy to eradicate poverty and to redistribute resources to Malays.

Plans for the public health sector have followed these national development objectives. Since improved health is considered an indirect means of reducing poverty, extending access to health services is seen as an equity goal. The government has taken vigorous steps to extend health services in rural areas. Rural coverage is almost synonymous with the public health-care system. However, the relentless pursuit of narrowly defined equity goals without greater efficiency has resulted in growing imbalances between the public and private sectors. This situation has been aggravated by recent reforms in privatization and health-care financing. Thus, further development of the health services will continue to be contentious and debated in terms of cost, quality and access. To meet the challenges of an ageing population and an increasing burden of chronic conditions, future health policy should encourage cost-effective systems of disease prevention and health promotion in Malaysia.

References

Abu Bakar, S. (1995) 'The New Public Health–Meeting the Challenges of the 21st Century', paper presented at the National Public Health Conference, Ministry of Health, Kuala Lumpur, 24–26 January.

—— (2001) *Issues for the Future Health System: Vision 2020, Vision for Health, Mission for MOH, Corporate Culture and Goals of the Health System of the Future*, Kuala Lumpur: Ministry of Health, Malaysia.

Abu Bakar, S. and Jegathesan, M. (eds) (n.d.) *Health in Malaysia: Achievements and Challenges*, Kuala Lumpur: Planning and Development Division, Ministry of Health, Malaysia.

Abu Bakar, S., Lye, M. S., Mathews, A. and Ravindran, J. (1995) 'Advances in Health in Malaysia', *Medical Journal of Malaysia*, 50: S3–S10.

Ali Abul Hassan, S. (1992) 'The National Health Plan. Health Master Planning and Financing Towards 2020', paper presented at the 1992 National Health Care Conference: Health Care and Vision 2020, Ming Court Hotel, Kuala Lumpur, 2–3 November.

Aljunid, S. M. and Mohsein, N. A. A. (eds) (2002) *Health Economics Issues in Malaysia*, Kuala Lumpur: University of Malaya Press.

Barraclough, S. (1997) 'The Growth of Corporate Private Hospitals in Malaysia: Contradictions in Health System Pluralism', *International Journal of Health Services*, 27(4): 643–659.

—— (1999) 'Constraints on the Retreat from a Welfare-oriented Approach to Public Health Care in Malaysia', *Health Policy*, 47(1): 53–67.

—— (2000) 'The Politics of Privatization in the Malaysian Health Care System', *Contemporary Southeast Asia*, 22(2): 340–359.

Bin Juni, M. H. (1996) 'Public Health Care Provisions: Access and Equity', *Social Science and Medicine*, 43(5): 759–768.

Chee, H. L. (1982) 'Health Status and the Development of Health Services in a Colonial State: The Case of British Malaya', *International Journal of Health Services*, 12(3): 397–417.

—— (1990) 'Changing Patterns of Physical Health in Malaysia: Implications for the Health Care Sector', in Cho Kah Sin and Ismail Muhd Salleh (eds) *Caring Society: Emerging Issues and Future Directions. Selected Papers from the First National Conference on the Caring Society*, Kuala Lumpur: Institute of Strategic and International Studies, 197–231.

—— (1995) *Amidst Affluence: A Study of an Urban Squatter Settlement and its Access to Health Care Services*, Kuala Lumpur: Institute of Advanced Studies, University of Malaya.

Department of Statistics (2000) *Vital Statistics Malaysia (Special Edition) 2000*, Kuala Lumpur: Department of Statistics.

—— (2001) *Population and Housing Census of Malaysia 2000, Population Distribution and Basic Demographic Characteristics*, Kuala Lumpur: Department of Statistics.

—— (2001) *Vital Statistics Time Series Malaysia 1963–1998*, Putrajaya: Department of Statistics.

—— (2002) *Social Statistics Bulletin Malaysia 2001*, Putrajaya: Department of Statistics.

Economic Planning Unit (1996) *Policies and Objectives under the Seventh Malaysia Plan*, paper prepared for the 1996 National Healthcare Conference, Kuala Lumpur, 13–14 June.

Fong, C. O. (1989) *The Malaysian Economic Challenge in the 1990s: Transformation for Growth*, Singapore: Longman.

Gullick, J. (1981) *Malaysia: Economic Expansion and National Unity*, London: Ernest Benn.

Heller, P. S. (1982) 'A Model of the Demand for Medical and Health Services in Peninsular Malaysia', *Social Science and Medicine*, 18: 391–393.

Kananatu, K. (2002) 'Healthcare Financing in Malaysia', *Asia-Pacific Journal of Public Health*, 14(1): 23–28.

Lee, S. A. (1974) *Economic Growth and the Public Sector in Malaya and Singapore 1948–1960*, Singapore: Oxford University Press.

Low, W. Y., Zulkifli, S. N., Wong, S. L. and Yusof, K. (n.d.) 'Dawn of a New Millenium: Issues and Challenges of Public Health in Malaysia', in Yusof, K., Low, W. Y., Zulkifli, S. N. and Wong, S. L. (eds) *Issues and Challenges of Public Health in the 21st Century*, Kuala Lumpur: University of Malaya Press, 191–232.

Malaya (1953) *Progress Report on the Development Plan of the Federation of Malaya 1950–1952*, Kuala Lumpur: Government Press.

—— (1956) *The Development Plan and a Capital Expenditure Programme for 1956/1960*, Kuala Lumpur: Economic Secretariat.

—— (1957) *Report on Economic Planning in the Federation of Malaya in 1956*, Kuala Lumpur: Government Press.

—— (1961) *The Second Five Year Plan 1961–1965*, Kuala Lumpur: Government Press.

—— (1963) *Interim Report of the Development in Malaya under the Second Five Year Plan*, Kuala Lumpur: Government Press.

Malaysia (1966) *First Malaysia Plan 1966–1970*, Kuala Lumpur: Economic Planning Unit.

—— (1971) *Second Malaysia Plan 1971–1975*, Kuala Lumpur: Economic Planning Unit.

—— (1974) *Midterm Review of the Second Malaysia Plan*, Kuala Lumpur: Economic Planning Unit.

—— (1976) *Third Malaysia Plan 1976–1980*, Kuala Lumpur: Economic Planning Unit.

—— (1979) *Midterm Review of the Third Malaysia Plan*, Kuala Lumpur: Economic Planning Unit.

—— (1981) *Fourth Malaysia Plan 1981–1985*, Kuala Lumpur: Economic Planning Unit.

—— (1984) *Midterm Review of the Fourth Malaysia Plan*, Kuala Lumpur: Economic Planning Unit.

—— (1985) *Fifth Malaysia Plan 1986–1990*, Kuala Lumpur: Economic Planning Unit.

—— (1989) *Midterm Review of the Fifth Malaysia Plan*, Kuala Lumpur: Economic Planning Unit.

—— (1991) *The Second Outline Perspective Plan 1991–2000*, Kuala Lumpur: National Printing Department.

—— (1991) *Sixth Malaysia Plan 1991–1995*, Kuala Lumpur: Economic Planning Unit.

—— (1994) *Midterm Review of the Sixth Malaysia Plan*, Kuala Lumpur: Economic Planning Unit.

—— (1996) *Seventh Malaysia Plan 1996–2000*, Kuala Lumpur: Economic Planning Unit.

—— (1999) *Midterm Review of the Seventh Malaysia Plan*, Kuala Lumpur: Economic Planning Unit.

—— (2001) *Eighth Malaysia Plan 2000–2005*, Kuala Lumpur: Economic Planning Unit.

Merican, I. and Yon, R. (2002) 'Health Care Reform and Changes: The Malaysian Experience', *Asia-Pacific Journal of Public Health*, 14(1): 17–22.

Mills, L. A. (1942) *British Rule in Eastern Asia: A Study of Contemporary Government and Economical Development in British Malaya and Hong Kong*, London: Humphrey Milford and Oxford University Press.

Ministry of Health (1970–2000) *Annual Reports*, Kuala Lumpur: Ministry of Health.

—— (1985–2000) *Indicators for Monitoring and Evaluation of Strategy for Health for All by Year 2000 (1985–2000)*, Kuala Lumpur: Information and Documentation Unit, Ministry of Health.

—— (1999) *Policies in Health*, Kuala Lumpur: Planning and Development Division, Ministry of Health.

Ness, G. D. (1967) *Bureaucracy and Rural Development in Malaysia: A Study of Complex Organisations in Stimulating Economic Development in New States*, Berkeley: University of California Press.

Phua, K. H. (1987) *The Development of Health Services in Malaya and Singapore 1867–1960*, unpublished thesis, London School of Economics and Political Science.

—— (1989) 'The Development of Health Services in the Colonies: A Study of British Malaya and Singapore', *Asia-Pacific Journal of Public Health*, 3(4): 315–323.

Roemer, M. I. (1991) *National Health Systems of the World*, Oxford: Oxford University Press.

Wong, M. L. L. (2006) *The Development of the Health Care System in Malaysia, with Special Reference to Government Health Services 1970–2000*, unpublished thesis, National University of Singapore.

10 From colony to global city

Public health strategies and the control of disease in Singapore

Brenda S. A. Yeoh, Kai Hong Phua and Kelly Fu

The nineteenth century: the absence of systematic health care

When Stamford Raffles, an agent of the British East India Company, signed a treaty with the Temengong of Johor in January 1819 to establish a British trading post in Singapore, the island was mainly composed of *orang laut* (sea nomads) communities who were dependent for a living on fishing, the collection of jungle produce and small-scale trading and piracy (Turnbull 1977: 1, 5). At that time, Malay traditional medicine, which showed the influence of Ayurvedic medicine and the Arab pharmacopoeia, was the main form of medical treatment on this sparsely populated island (Field 1951: 19).

Not only did the establishment of British colonial rule lead to an exponential increase in the population of Singapore,[1] it was to also markedly transform the island's public health regime, although the effects were not obvious until many decades later. At first, early colonial health provision catered exclusively to the needs of the colonial administrators and the military (Tan 1991: 339). There was little or no health-care provision for the natives and immigrant lower classes other than a pauper hospital which was established around 1830 to 1833 at Bras Basah Road (Tan 1991: 340). While a number of municipal acts including the Conservancy Act were passed in 1856, directing municipal commissioners to 'administer the funds applicable to the purposes of conservancy and improvement' and 'make, cleanse, light and water streets, to remove filth...to pull down ruinous houses,...to drain the town', every report on the sanitary conditions of the town during the nineteenth century (and beyond) lamented the eminently unsatisfactory state of affairs, as exemplified in this 1872 account:

> The town was 'a nursery of disease' for 'not only [were] the drains choked with every description of filth, but the ordinary streets and thoroughfares [were] considered the proper receptacles for all kinds of accumulated impurities, and the atmosphere [was] filled with unwholesome emanations, in the highest degree dangerous to health'.
>
> (Yeoh 1996: 34)

During the second half of the nineteenth century, the health-care needs of the large number of male migrants who had come from various parts of Asia in search of work at the ports and plantations in Singapore became increasingly stark. The long and arduous journey to Singapore by sea weakened many a new arrival. The pauper hospital soon found itself overwhelmed by the large number of sick immigrants. Unable to work because of ill-health, many ended up destitute and homeless. The colonial exploitation of workers who were fed subsistence diets and made to work long hours also contributed to high death and disease rates. Indeed, 'many died, while the majority survived in poor health' (Chee 1982: 400). Mortality rates in turn-of-the-century Singapore consequently were very high in both immigrant and indigenous communities. Between 1893 and 1910, crude death rates ranged between 32.9 and 51.1 per 1,000, with an average of 42.2 per 1,000. Epidemics of infectious disease such as smallpox and cholera were also common throughout the 1800s, with particularly severe outbreaks of smallpox occurring in 1849–1850 and again in 1858–1860 (Tan 1991: 341).

The health problems of the nineteenth century were ignored by the colonial administration because sick workers were easily replaced by immigration or were repatriated. The exchange between Resident Councillor Thomas Church and the Governor of Bengal was reflective of such a mindset. Troubled by the sight of vagrants, Church commented in a 1840 letter to the Governor of Bengal that 'many a valuable life has become a victim to disease and death which might have been saved had a public Asylum been available for the reception of seamen and prompt and proper medical aid offered' (Mudeliar *et al.* 1979: 8). The Governor of Bengal was indifferent to these problems and stated in no uncertain terms that the health care of locals was neither the concern nor responsibility of the colonial authorities. In the absence of a municipal system of medical care and poor relief, native and immigrant groups developed their own networks of health care. The Chinese medical delivery system, comprising medical institutions, pharmacies, clan-based recuperation centres and *chung-i* (freelance physicians), filled a much-felt void in the lives of the Chinese labouring classes (Yeoh 1996: 112–116). Similarly, the Malay population had a well-established network of traditional medical practitioners who were able to attend to minor aliments such as indigestion, cuts and sprains (National Archives of Singapore, Oral History Interview Accession Number 1275). The main form of Western biomedical care for the local population was to be found in the Tan Tock Seng Hospital. Built in 1844, it was the brainchild of Tan Tock Seng, a rich businessman and philanthropist. The hospital was supported by funds from the local Chinese community (Mudeliar *et al.* 1979: 10).

Municipal sanitary reform and colonial health provision: 1900s–1940s

The turn-of-the-century saw a significant change in attitudes by the colonial establishment towards the provision of health and medical care for the people.

At the height of Empire-building, increasing numbers of British administrators, merchants, traders and soldiers spent large parts of their lives in the colonies exposed to the ravages produced by tropical conditions. The medical profession and colonial office in the United Kingdom were anxious to safeguard the health of expatriates and saw it as imperative to bring what were perceived to be climatic or environmental hazards under control. The setting up of Schools of Tropical Medicine in Liverpool and London in 1898 and 1899, respectively, to investigate tropical diseases on systematic and scientific lines was, according to Sir William MacGregor, 'but one of the many means devised or fostered by the Rt. Hon. Joseph Chamberlain, then Secretary of State for the Colonies, for curtailing the toll of our fellow citizens in those insalubrious, over-sea territories of the empire' (MacGregor 1900: 63).

In Singapore, it had become increasingly clear to the colonial authorities that exposure to disease was no longer a problem that confined itself to the vulnerable working classes. With the European minority living in constant interaction with the Asian masses, it was feared that the comparative immunity enjoyed by Europeans because of nutrition and living conditions would be nullified by the outbreak of virulent infectious diseases. Hence, it became imperative to reduce the incidences of these outbreaks.

In port cities like Singapore, where prosperity was largely dependent on entrepôt trade and the energies of a continuous stream of Asian immigrants, the colonial state had also to address the more intractable problems of Asian morbidity and mortality. Rampant spread of infectious diseases and high mortality rates would cripple the colony's trade. That this was the colonial government's preoccupation is clear from the colonial secretary's communication with the municipal commissioners:

> The prosperity of Singapore so entirely depends upon its use as a commercial emporium, and that use is so gravely jeopardised by the occurrence here of dangerous infectious disease which provokes other places to impose quarantine regulations against Singapore, that His Excellency [the Governor] cannot too earnestly recommend the Commissioners so to strengthen their Health Department so as to enable them to grapple with cases of disease.
> (ARSM 1895: 140)

As one of the local dailies pointedly observed: 'an epidemic mean[t] a great commercial loss to the place, apart from any more humane considerations' (*The Straits Times* 21 February 1896).

Pressure to improve sanitary conditions during the last quarter of the nineteenth century culminated in the passing of municipal ordinances to promote sanitary reform, town improvement and public health investigations into the probable causes of disease (Yeoh 1996: 85–135). Municipal investigations into public health such as the 1907 report by Professor W. J. Simpson on the 'Sanitary Conditions in Singapore' and the statistics collated by municipal health officers attributed the propagation of disease to 'Asiatic' or Chinese working class practices such as 'huddling together', and 'promiscuous spitting' (ARSM 1909: 38; Galloway 1907: 3). Recommendations for the improvement of health thus emphasized the surveillance and transformation of local practices through legislation and slum clearance. Professor Simpson's report, for example, advised the massive reconstruction of congested parts of the city. He also suggested that a housing commission be set up, a recommendation that eventually led to the establishment of the Singapore Improvement Trust in 1927 (Teo and Savage 1991: 327).

The progress of town improvements was, however, held in check by several factors, the most immediate being the lack of financial resources to fund the most basic of improvement schemes. As a result, the strategy of surveillance eventually adopted to improve the sanitary conditions of the city involved legal penalties intended to force the local population to reform their daily management of the environment. Substantive sections of the Municipal Ordinance of 1887 and 1896, and subsequent amendments, were also devoted to the policing of various aspects of Asian domestic practices including scavenging, the removal of night soil and household filth, the organization of space and the proportion of people to space within buildings, the maintenance of premises, privies and drains in a sanitary state, the proper use of water and the prevention of the spread of infectious diseases. A proliferating array of municipal bylaws conferred power on sanitary officers to carry out inspections of premises, post notices, serve court summons on transgressors and remove persons suspected to be suffering from infectious diseases. Surveillance went hand in hand with a meticulous system of penalties but this enjoyed little success.

Such strategies were little appreciated by the labouring classes. While living conditions in parts of the city were indeed congested, immigrants had few alternatives. At the very least, these houses served as cheap shelter where they could seek kin's help in case of illness or financial difficulties. Hence, when owners were served with summons, they engaged in the perfunctory cleansing of premises and minor repairs rather than more permanent improvements. Once municipal vigilance was focused elsewhere, '[c]ubicles pulled down by order of the Sanitary Department [were] frequently put up again at the earliest opportunity, improvements effected to drains and latrines [were] not properly maintained and soon [in a state of] disrepair' (Proceedings of the Legislative Council Straits Settlements 1910: 200). Fines were unlikely to deter principal tenants as their gains from increased rents were more than adequate to offset occasional fines. The Singapore Improvement Trust also failed to make much headway. Hence, the problems of overcrowding persisted throughout the colonial era and well into the 1960s.

The decades between 1900 and the 1940s coincided with an official interest in the development of tropical medicine. The establishment of the first medical school (Straits and Federated Malay States Medical School) in 1905 demonstrated this trend, as did the expansion of hospital units. In 1908, a new building for the Maternity Hospital was erected near the General Hospital. The next year, new buildings for the Tan Tock Seng Hospital were completed.

Malaria control

In 1910, a separate Health Branch of the Medical Department was established to oversee public health on the estates and mines. Health officers became responsible for antimalarial measures, enforcement of sanitary regulations, licensing of premises and examination of foodstuff. In 1911, a Malaria Advisory Board was formed that was given wide powers not only to advise, but also to execute control measures (Reid and Mohamed Din bin Ahmad 1958: 570). The setting up of the board brought about great improvements in malaria control that had previously been hindered by the use of unsuitable methods or the lack of coordination amongst agencies. In Singapore, the Anti-Malaria Committee carried out an experimental programme of drain filling, public education and the free distribution of quinine in 1912. This programme proved to be highly successful, but was unfortunately put on hold during World War I. However, the development of malaria control measures such as drainage and spraying of insecticide was accelerated after the war and it was very successful.

Maternal and child health provision

Maternal and child health in the earlier nineteenth century was not a major concern of the colonial government as the migrant population was mainly male while the native Malay population had a well-established set of birthing customs and techniques. The first eight-bed maternity hospital was only set up in 1888 (Tan 2003: 38). The health of women and children received more attention only after political events in Britain created an interest in child health. General Frederick Maurice's article in the *Contemporary Review* detailing the low standard of health of recruits for the 1899–1902 Boer War (Oakley 1984: 35) provoked a fervent discussion about health during adulthood and its implications for the maintenance and future of the empire. These ideas filtered down to the colonies and encouraged schemes to police and improve maternal and infant health. By 1907, the need for a new maternity hospital was debated in the local Legislative Council (Lee 2003: 55). In that same year, Professor Simpson made recommendations for the setting up of dispensaries where local women could be educated on 'proper' infant feeding methods; the lack of which, he commented, was responsible for the high rates of infant mortality. In 1910, investigations into the causes of infant mortality by the Municipal Health Nurse supported Simpson's views that poor infant feeding was the main contributor to infant mortality (Lim 1966: 29). As a result, a European nurse was engaged to instruct non-European mothers in childcare and a plan was approved for the training of local women as midwives. Legal provisions were also made for the recognition of different levels of midwifery training. The Midwives Ordinance introduced in the Legislative Council in 1915 has been hailed as one of 'the most important events in the history of maternity services' (Lee 2003: 58). When read for a second time, it provoked considerable debate on the effects of imposing the ordinance on local birth practitioners (particularly the *bidan*). It was eventually agreed that some provision be made for the recognition of 'untrained' Malay midwives through the award of midwifery training certificates at four levels ranging from the staff nurses with one year midwifery training to the 'untrained' customary midwife.

In 1923, the first maternal and child health clinic was started at a vaccination depot in Prinsep Street followed by many other clinics in the city (Lim 1966: 29).

By 1924, obstetric services in the colony had expanded significantly with the conversion of Kandang Kerbau Hospital into a maternity hospital (Lee 2003: 55). Rural home visiting by a public health nurse in 1927 'brought to light many cases of post-natal beriberi and numerous debilitating diseases in children, chiefly worm infestations and anaemia, severe skin diseases, cough, fever and malnutrition' (Lim 1966: 30). The government provided a travelling dispensary which had a doctor and dresser to bring medical aid to the rural population in Singapore. This service proved to be extremely popular and was one of most effective means of transforming rural attitudes towards Western biomedicine.

The role of traditional medicine

Despite these developments, traditional medicine was still the primary means of health care for non-Europeans in the colony. Hospitals, clinics and doctors of the colonial medical service mainly served those who lived in the urban areas or near important commercial districts. The services of general practitioners were out of reach of most rural folk (Field 1951: 34). It was for these reasons rather than 'ignorance' and 'superstition' that there was little use of biomedical facilities, particularly amongst rural folk living furthest from these institutions of allopathic care.

Asian migrant and native populations were also suspicious of Western biomedical care. Few understood the theories upon which it was based and many were living too far away from the city to have any contact with doctors. Inferior facilities were also a deterrent, and hospitals were seen as places of death rather than cure. The local population also rejected the derogatory labels attached to traditional practitioners. For example, although the *bidan* (Malay traditional midwife) was 'untrained' in the eyes of the colonial authorities, they were the most popular birth attendants during the early twentieth century (Lee 2003: 58). Similarly, whilst Western sanitary science advocated the removal of filth, the disinfection and ventilation of houses, and the isolation of the sick as essential preventive measures, Chinese medical theory did not necessarily give them such significance. Non-compliance followed because such measures appeared to have little direct impact on the health of the residents, but they were interpreted as a means by which the colonial government could tax and persecute the local population.

The Japanese occupation and post-war health provision: 1942–1945

During the Occupation, the General Hospital was used exclusively for Japanese military and navy personnel. Kandang Kerbau Hospital, the main maternity hospital, was converted into an emergency general hospital for the local population. This burden of care was shared with the Tan Tock Seng Hospital but these hospitals were overwhelmed with acute cases and faced a shortage of basic equipment and food. Death and disease rates were extremely high because of the lack of food and the stress of wartime conditions.

By the end of the occupation in 1945, the civil population was exceedingly malnourished. Diseases such as beriberi, pneumonia and tuberculosis affected a considerable number (Annual Medical Report of the Medical Department 1946: 2). No accurate figures exist for infant mortality rates as there are no records of live births, but estimated increases indicate a marked increase (Tan 1991: 345). Hospitals were ill-equipped and overcrowded owing to the influx of military personnel, refugees and others who sought security in Singapore. The population suffered even further when the General Hospital and the Mental Hospital were requisitioned for Allied military patients (Hone 1946: 91).

Nevertheless, public health measures were quickly reinstituted under the British Military Administration. Makeshift hospitals were opened: the Victoria Hospital, which was converted from a government school, the Katong Convent School which was converted into a tuberculosis hospital, another small hospital in Mandalay Road and a Chinese temple in Kim Keat Road that was used to accommodate the old, the destitute and the mentally ill so as to relieve congestion in major hospitals (Hone 1946: 92). Mobile clinics and welfare centres were also rapidly established: 7 in the urban areas and 15 in the rural areas and outlying islands of Singapore. Middle Road Hospital and two clinics in Kreta Ayer and Joo Chiat were used for treatment of venereal disease, while child health clinics and welfare centres carried out the bulk of the work of health maintenance. Teams were sent to investigate the nutritional state of the population and to recommend suitable diets. Milk and other foods were made available to children through welfare centres and to the general public through 'People's Restaurants'.

Water purity which had deteriorated to such an extent as to pose serious dangers to public health was improved by March 1946. A vigorous campaign was started to reinstitute antimalarial activities. During the six months of military administration, the number of malaria cases treated in the rural areas of Singapore decreased from 314 to 75 per week in spite of the expected seasonal increase (Hone 1946: 92). Throughout Singapore, there were also campaigns to inoculate against smallpox and typhoid fever. These measures proved very successful for by 1948, the health of the population had returned to pre-war levels.

Medical plan

In 1946, the Director of Medical Services, Dr W. J. Vickers, convened a committee to discuss a plan to guide medical development in Singapore. The shortcomings of the hospital system justified such a plan and included lack of funding, too few staff, inadequate medical facilities and unmet demand for medical care for the local poor (Proceedings of the Legislative Council Straits Settlement 1948: 27). The Medical Plan proposed expansion and modernization of all hospitals. The General Hospital was to be enlarged to a 1,000-bed hospital centre, Kandang Kerbau Hospital to a 500-bed maternity and gynaecological hospital, the Venereal Disease Hospital to a 200-bed facility and the Tan Tock Seng Hospital to an 800-bed, secondary hospital, all during the first stage in 1948. In the second stage, 1950–1952, a second General Hospital of 1,000 beds was to be built, the facilities of the Mental Hospital were to be improved and the Leper Hospital expanded to 300 beds. Other developments were a new infectious disease centre of 50 beds, expansion of the Orthopaedic Hospital to 120 beds and a tuberculosis hospital of 300 beds (Proceedings of the Legislative Council Straits Settlement 1948: 30–31). Finally, a chain of child and maternity clinics was to be established around the island (Choy 1954: 20).

A Select Committee, convened in May 1948 to discuss the Medical Plan, unanimously agreed that it was necessary. Although there was only limited progress before the 1950s, the plan established a sense of consciousness that the medical services could no longer simply cater for the elite. This question of equity was acknowledged by Dr Vickers who felt that 'handsome dividends' would follow if 'the most strenuous efforts [were] concentrated on giving as many as possible as much help as possible, instead of concentrating, on a lesser number and more perfect service' (Vickers 1954: 10). New attitudes towards Western biomedicine developed. No longer did the population avoid hospitals and clinics; they even demanded Western biomedical treatment as a right. This was especially clear in maternal health where the demand for hospital delivery became so great that Dr Vickers had to encourage women with uncomplicated pregnancies to seek home birth (*The Straits Times* 24 September 1953). Demand for outpatient services also stretched the resources of the hospitals: in the General Hospital, outpatient attendances in 1950 and 1955 increased from 234,593 to 433,119 (Singapore General Hospital 1976: 21). Overcrowding and long waiting times for treatment became the norm (*The Straits Times* 6 July 1958).

A fundamental reorientation of British government policy forced both politicians and bureaucrats to introduce a programme of balanced social, political and economic development. Progressive health policies, aimed at improving the welfare of all, reduced the incidence of infectious outbreaks and the percentage suffering from nutrition-related diseases. There was an expansion of preventive outpatient services, maternal and child health services and school health services with their emphasis on health education, all aimed at comprehensive coverage at the primary care level. However, a major weakness in planning in the 1950s was the failure to anticipate the growing demand for Western biomedicine. Demand continued to outstrip supply well into the 1970s.

The post-independence health-care regime: 1960s–1970s

Public health in the post-colonial era was closely related to the government's industrialization plans and the need for a healthy workforce. As the ruling People's Action Party (PAP) leader, Lee Kuan Yew, noted, the aim was to 'create the necessary social conditions for higher economic growth in industry and tourism' (Lee 1968: 6).

Ambitious plans for the expansion of health care were implemented. The most important of these was the formation of the Ministry of Health in 1959 that united the Government Health Department (responsible for rural and school health services as well as malaria control) and the Municipality Department (responsible for all municipal health matters). By 1968, the number of hospitals had doubled from 8 to 16 (Seow and Lee 1994: 149). In 1963, there was a major expansion of personal health services. Between 1964 and 1967, 21 dental health clinics were opened (Tan 1991: 347). By 1964, there were a total of 26 outpatient and 46 maternal and child health clinics across the island.

Training of medical doctors

Under the colonial regime, local medical graduates faced tremendous difficulties in obtaining further training and accreditation. Even though the British became more liberal in sending local graduates to the United Kingdom for further study after 1945, few scholarships were available (Wong 1980: 7). Local medical staff were not accorded equal status with European doctors and it was only in the mid- to late-1950s that Asian heads of department became more common. Although the colonial government attempted to increase the supply of local medical doctors in the 1950s, it was unable to meet the unprecedented demand for Western biomedicine in the 1960s (Muir and Wong 1965: 12).

Under the new government, the number of graduates produced by the Medical Faculty of the National University of Singapore increased from an annual average of 47 during 1953–1959 to 77 during 1960–1965 (Lim 1965: 13). From the 1960s, local medical doctors were able to obtain postgraduate medical training through Australian medical institutions such as the Royal Australasian College of Physicians and the Royal Australasian College of Surgeons (Wong 1980: 8). In 1965, the foundation stone was laid for the Institute of Medical Specializations that was 'conceived as a joint government project ... based on the proposition that as medical sciences advance, specialization becomes essential' (Singapore General Hospital 1976: 70). In 1970, a high-level Committee on Medical Specialization was formed to select specializations for development (Lee 1987: 23). The expansion of postgraduate training both locally and overseas also widened the scope of treatment that doctors were able to offer. In the 1960s, open heart surgery and implant surgery were inaugurated and perinatology was established as a medical discipline (Lee 1987: 23; Wong 1994: 111).

Family planning

Growth of the population was viewed as an obstacle in the way of raising the standard of living (Purcal 1989: 126). Shortly after the PAP came into power, it launched a three-month Family Planning Campaign. In 1966, a five-year plan promised every 'eligible' married woman the latest techniques in family planning (Yong 1966: 37). Maternal and child health clinics and the Kandang Kerbau Hospital were the main sites for family planning services (Maternal and Child Health Services Annual Report 1974: 17). After giving birth to her first or second child, a woman would be encouraged to go for sterilization or to use the contraceptive pill or an intra-uterine device. If she was not willing to pursue either path, she would be visited at home by the family planning staff. If all else failed, she would also bear the brunt of higher charges for hospital delivery as well as a reduced chance of housing and a school place for her child. Abortion laws were also enacted in 1974, making it legal for abortions to be performed up to the twenty-fourth week of the pregnancy (Singh 2003: 280).

These draconian measures were accompanied by a policy that encouraged fertility reduction through the promotion of infant health. When infant mortality rates were high, large family size was a means to ensure the survival of at least one child. By the 1970s, the leading causes of infant death such as prematurity were greatly reduced by nutritional supplementation and vaccination programmes as well as better access to health care (Wong 1990: 21). Better infant health and other factors such as the better education of women saw fertility rates rapidly decline from 42.7 per 1,000 in 1957 to 20 in 1970 (Singh 2003: 280–281).

Health campaigns

Intended to raise awareness of health issues through public participation, government-led campaigns were a major strand of health policies in the 1960s and 1970s. Some of these include the X-ray campaign for tuberculosis (1959), Anti-Rabies (1963), Anti-Leprosy (1963), School Cleanliness (1964) and the Keep Singapore Clean Campaign (1968) (Lim and Lee 1997: 24). The main focus of the campaign was usually an exhibition on the theme. Auxiliary projects were then used to sustain public interest such as awards for the best-kept building, school or workplace; talks and lectures; and the distribution of posters, pamphlets and other materials (Yarrall 1972: 42). Members of the government were expected to demonstrate their support and knowledge of these health issues at public appearances. In an era where modes of communication were far more limited, these campaigns were a useful method of disseminating information.

The housing and development board and health improvement

When the PAP assumed power in the 1960s, it was faced with a serious housing problem. Congestion had become so great in Chinatown that shop houses were known to accommodate as many as 100 residents (Teo and Savage 1991: 325). Slums and squatters' dwellings had mushroomed all over Singapore. In these areas, the lack of safe drinking water and waste disposal facilities and overcrowding provided fertile ground for the spread of diseases such as cholera. It was not only a serious health issue but these places were also widely perceived to be strongholds of crime. One study of squatter settlements, for example, claimed that they were hotbeds of political opposition and criminal activities in the city (Economic Research Centre n.d.: 2).

These housing and health problems were addressed through a massive public housing and resettlement scheme spearheaded by the setting up of the Housing and Development Board (HDB) in 1960. By 1965, 51,000 units of flats had been constructed by the HDB, with 23% of the island's population living in high-rise apartments (HDB 1965: 3).[2] Living conditions of the population improved as they gained easy access to clean drinking water and waste disposal facilities. Resettlement into flats also had the unintended outcome of bringing the population closer to medical facilities such as hospitals and clinics, as transportation in these urban housing estates was better developed than in the rural areas. Population planning had also reduced family sizes, thus relieving pressure on domestic living space.

Health provision in a globalizing city: 1980s and beyond

By the end of the 1970s, basic hospital and clinic infrastructure was fully set up. There was also a rising demand for private and specialized care which made health spending a major concern for the government. Patterns of disease also changed. Cancer and coronary heart disease rather than infectious diseases are now the leading causes of death.[3] According to a study of non-communicable diseases, 'lifestyles of physical inactivity, obesity, cigarette smoking, excessive alcohol intake, the consumption of rich and fatty foods... have predisposed Singaporeans to rising levels of chronic diseases' (Emmanuel *et al.* 2002: 475).

Patterns of disease and national programmes

Public education programmes that promote a healthy lifestyle through regular exercise, a healthy diet and the reduction of smoking have been one of the key areas of the government's health policies as chronic, non-communicable diseases replaced infectious diseases as the leading causes of death in the 1980s and 1990s. In the 1980s, the first Singapore Healthy Living Programme was launched. In the 1990s, similar programmes were run: for example, the National Healthy Lifestyle Campaign that featured a different theme and slogan for each year. The 'Great Singapore Workout' was introduced in 1993 to encourage physical exercise through a choreographed mass aerobic and stretching exercise. The year before, the Trim and Fit (TAF) programme was launched to reduce obesity and improve physical fitness among school children and youth. In 1998, the National Workplace Promotion encouraged companies to provide a healthy lifestyle by offering healthier options at the staff canteen and allowing workers to leave earlier to participate in sports and games. Awards were given to companies that implemented such programmes successfully (Toh *et al.* 2002: 335).

Efforts to promote a smoke-free Singapore started in the 1970s with the introduction of laws restricting smoking in public places and the prohibition of tobacco advertisements (Health Promotion Board 2005). In 1986, a National Smoking Control Programme was launched with the theme 'Towards a nation of non-smokers'. It highlighted all the ill effects of smoking and educated non-smokers on their rights in places where smoking is prohibited (Emmanuel *et al.* 2002: 477). Since then, smoking control has taken the form of public education, legislation and taxation. Legislative measures such as the Smoking (Control of

Advertisements and Sale of Tobacco) Act and the Prohibition of Smoking (Prohibition in Certain Places) Act prohibit smoking in public by under-eighteens and require that cigarette packets be labelled with health warnings. In addition, there are legal restrictions on smoking in public places and the sale of tobacco products (Toh et al. 2002: 334). Tobacco taxation has also been increasing over the years, with the current tax being SGD 210 per kg of tobacco (Health Promotion Board 2005). These measures are said to have contributed to the reduction of the overall smoking rates from 18% in 1992 to 15% in 1998 (Epidemiology and Disease Control Department 1999: 22).

Other campaigns in the last decade have focused on cancer prevention, particularly in the area of breast cancer where the most active campaigning has been carried out. Plans are also afoot to implement a National Cervical Cancer Screening Programme and to also battle colorectal cancer to reduce the morbidity rates from these increasingly common diseases (Emmanuel et al. 2002: 478).

Towards privatization: Medisave, MediShield and MediFund

In the early 1980s, the government became concerned about the rising expenditure on health and the limitations of state-subsidized health schemes such as the National Health Service in the United Kingdom. Medisave was a health savings plan that was part of the larger state-enforced saving plan, the Central Provident Fund (CPF). Under the CPF scheme, salaried Singaporeans contribute an average of 20% of their total salary to this savings fund and this is matched by an equivalent sum from their employers.[4] Medisave allocates 6–10% of this sum for potential medical and hospitalization costs, and places the onus of health consumption on the individual. Medisave also keeps tabs on individual income levels and access to medical benefits. Those who have higher levels of Medisave are given smaller subsidies and those with lower levels of Medisave are given priority in the allocation of cheaper wards. This ensures that those from the higher income groups do not lower their costs by opting for cheaper wards and absorbing the subsidies meant for the poor. Medisave is complemented by Medishield, a low-cost insurance scheme, introduced in 1990 that covers hospitalization for major or prolonged illness. It funds claims of between SGD 20,000 and SGD 70,000 a year. State-led Medifund provides for those who do not have the means to cover their medical costs, or have exceeded, or are not covered by either of the aforementioned two schemes. In this way, public subsidies are more targeted with greater cost sharing and the state is relieved of high levels of healthcare spending without totally absolving its responsibility for health care (Phua 2005: 296).

Evaluating the post-independence health-care regime

On the whole, health provision in the post-independence era has been a success. The doctor-to-population ratio has increased from 1 : 2,053 in 1965 to 1 : 757 in 1990 (Seow and Lee 1994: 150). The number of hospitals has increased from

8 in 1957 to 21 in 1990. There are also an estimated 40 nursing homes providing care for the elderly. National health outcomes have improved since the 1960s. The national childhood immunization programmes have eliminated or reduced many diseases such as poliomyelitis and tuberculosis. Maternal mortality is almost unheard of today. It would also appear that the plethora of health-related programmes and campaigns in the last decade have borne some fruit. According to the results of a 2005 study conducted by the Ministry of Health, several crucial predictors of health have improved, some notably, between 1998 and 2005: the proportion of people with high cholesterol levels fell from 25.4% to 18.7%; diabetes among adults from 9.0% to 8.2%; high blood pressure from 21.5% to 20.1%: the number of smokers from 15.2% to 12.6%: while the percentage of people taking up regular exercise improved from 16.8% to 24.9% (*The Straits Times* 25 April 2005).[5]

The main failings of health provision in the 1960s and 1970s were not so much inadequate care or poor health outcomes, but rather discriminatory tendencies arising from modernization agendas. For example: the social and physical costs of family planning measures such as abortion and the use of contraception were largely ignored. It was primarily women who were expected to adhere to family planning advice and consequently it was women who had to bear the trauma of side effects related to use of contraceptives such as bleeding and dislodged intrauterine devices (IUDs) (Lim 1979: 81).

Historically, the emphasis on specialization and high technology in the 1960s also resulted in situations where basic needs were ignored while money was spent on expensive machines that few needed. Thus, mobile coronary units were available for those suffering from a cardiac arrest (usually from the wealthier classes) whereas a mobile 'flying squad' unit for dealing with emergencies during deliveries in the rural areas was not developed (*The Straits Times* 14 September 1972). Similarly, while expensive ultrasound machines and foetal heart monitors were being purchased by the Kandang Kerbau Hospital, it took a Scottish medical specialist to comment on the shocking conditions in C class wards (less expensive wards) where 40 patients were crammed into a single ward and there was little privacy (*The Straits Times* 8 November 1978). In another incident, family of patients in the Singapore General Hospital were shocked to discover the lack of buzzers in C class wards whilst the more expensive A and B class wards had a call bell next to every bed (*The Straits Times* 5 July 1976). Such public complaints, unfortunately, did not produce much corrective action. Patients who could not afford the more expensive wards accepted these conditions. The government also denied that there were inequalities in the actual treatment provided to the rich and poor in government hospitals (*The Straits Times* 7 November 1971).

Manpower allocation in the health sector was distorted due to the focus on doctors at the expense of the development of other health professionals and traditional practitioners. Nursing and midwifery had been among the few options available to women with an O-level education. Hence, many women entered these professions. In the 1970s, the government reduced the number of nurses, a policy change which did not anticipate the changing social and economic conditions in the 1980s leading to a wider variety of jobs for women. Women today holding the same qualifications have a choice of jobs and prefer those which are less physically and emotionally demanding than nursing. As a result, there has been a shortage of nurses since the 1990s.

Finally, Medisave assumes that one's health is one's own responsibility. In long term chronic, degenerative diseases, the transfer of the burden to the individual from the state weighs heavily on the poor, especially in cases where the person does not have Medisave cover. Although last-resort measures like Medifund are available, the poor may delay seeking care until it is too late because they fear being unable to pay for hospitalization. Without the cheaper option of highly subsidized medical services provided by the State, this may seriously reduce the health-care choices available to the poor in a globalizing city. This social cost has to be balanced against the policy of cost containment in health and welfare in order to maintain the international competitiveness of the Singapore economy.

Return to infectious diseases in the new millennium?

With economic growth and a well-developed medical infrastructure, it was believed the infectious diseases which plagued the population throughout the 1960s and 1970s would cease to be public health problems. But at the beginning of the new millennium there was a series of infectious disease outbreaks that defied the conventional logic of control through improvements in sanitation and immunization. They were particularly worrying to the state as they disrupted trade, tourism and food supplies.

One of first such outbreaks was the transmission of the Nipah virus to Singapore via infected pork from Malaysia in 1998. This triggered fears about the consumption of pork and other meat products. In 2000, there was the emergence of hand, foot, and mouth disease amongst young children.[6] When this occurred, the government ordered a ten-day closure of all kindergartens and childcare centres. Parents of the 140,000 children involved were forced to find alternative childcare or take leave from work (*Asiaweek* 13 October 2000). The outbreak of severe acute respiratory syndrome (SARS) in 2003 effectively demolished the tourism industry, leaving airports, restaurants and places of interest empty. The Ministry of Health also found itself struggling to manage the outbreak as long forgotten methods of infection control had to be revived or reinvented. Paranoia also ran high in the society as people began to avoid physical contact with medical staff made identifiable by their uniforms. Many also started avoiding public places such as shopping centres. Local businesses – from food centres to malls – suffered greatly as a result. As such outbreaks triggered regional and, indeed, international concern, the government has (particularly after SARS) reassessed controls on infectious diseases. A SARS Ministerial Committee was formed to provide policy guidance and implement tough public health control measures. The search for a SARS vaccine is being pursued in research centres. In 2004 and 2005, attention switched to 'recurrent' infectious diseases such as HIV, sparked by the remarks of senior minister of State for Health, Dr Balaji Sadasivan, concerning the association between a homosexual lifestyle and the increase in HIV (Channel News Asia 9 March 2005). All pregnant women were strongly encouraged to take HIV tests to ensure that they did not transmit the disease to their children, and this measure may in time become mandatory.

Finally, the ongoing avian influenza outbreak has the potential to cause severe socio-economic damage within the Asian region and a possible global human influenza pandemic continues to create fear about the potential effects on a global business centre like Singapore. The impact of diseases is also made more significant because of the interconnectivity of regional economies where the effect within one country could send shocks which affect other countries. The effects on critical services such as health care are also important because a pandemic can be expected to result in an enormous number of hospitalizations which will overwhelm the current health-care capacity of a small country such as Singapore. Policymakers in Singapore have thus drawn up various plans for dealing with emerging and re-emerging infectious diseases including disaster plans for influenza pandemics and bioterrorism. These plans have included not only the stockpiling of therapeutic agents but also establishing surveillance networks, barriers to entry, infection control and other public health measures.

Conclusion

In the long run, the overall health of the population has improved by changing social habits and lifestyles through public health promotion and preventive programmes rather than spending on expensive, high-technology care after disease and disability have developed (Phua 1989: 322). It is hoped that public health policies will continue to reflect the basic philosophy of the past in which priority was given to easily accessible and affordable care and where public health campaigns focused on community and personal responsibility. That balance is needed to achieve an equitable, cost-effective and sustainable health-care system for Singapore.

Notes

1 Singapore was part of the Straits Settlements (which included Penang and Malacca) formed in 1826 and under control from India until 1867 after which it was ruled directly as a crown colony. Under British colonial rule, Singapore's rapidly expanding economy, coupled with a liberal open-door policy on immigration, drew ever-increasing numbers of immigrants. The population on the island grew from a few hundred at the time of Raffles to 228,555 at the 1901 census count (Innes 1901: 13). During the late nineteenth and early twentieth centuries, British Malaya expanded beyond the Straits Settlements to include the Federated Malay States of Perak, Pahang, Negri Sembilan and Selangor as well as the Unfederated Malay States of Kedah, Perlis, Trengganu, Kelantan and Johore. In 1946, Singapore became a separate colony while Penang and Malacca joined the Malayan Union, which eventually became Malaysia.
2 Within another two decades, over 85% of the population were housed in HDB flats.

3 Cancer is the principal cause of death, accounting for more than a quarter of total deaths (25.9%) in 2003, followed by heart disease (19.3%) and pneumonia (14.6%) (Ministry of Health 2004: n.p.).
4 The employer's contribution varies from year to year. During times of recession such figures have been reduced.
5 Obesity, however, inched up marginally from 6% to 6.9%.
6 The two pathogens in HFMD are EV 71 and coxsackievirus A16.

References

Administrative Report of the Singapore Municipality (ARSM).
—— (1895) *Appendix Q: Registration of Deaths*.
—— (1909) *Health Officers Report*.
Annual Medical Report of the Medical Department (1946) Kuala Lumpur: F.M.S. Government Press.
Asiaweek (now defunct magazine) *In the Grip of a Virus* (13 October 2000). Online. Available <http://www.asiaweek.com/asiaweek/magazine/2000/1013/as.health.html> (accessed 1 December 2004).
Channel News Asia, *Ministry of Health warns of Aids Spread, 311 new cases in 2004* (9 March 2005). Online. Available <http://www.channelnewsasia.com/stories/singaporelocanews/view/136436/1/.html> (accessed 5 April 2005).
Chee, Heng Leng (1982) 'Health Status and the Development of Health Services in a Colonial State: the Case of British Malaya', *International Journal of Health Services*, 12(3): 397–417.
Choy, Elizabeth (1954) *Keeping a City Healthy One Degree from the Equator: Lecture Tour of U.S.A. & Canada on Behalf of Foreign Office – London*. Singapore: Elizabeth Choy.
Economic Research Centre (1987) *Squatter Resettlement in Singapore*, Singapore: University of Singapore.
Emmanuel, S. C., Lam, S. L., Chew, S. K. and Tan, B. Y. (2002) 'A Countrywide Approach to the Control of Non-Communicable Diseases – Singapore Experience', *Annals of Academy of Medicine*, 31(4): 475–478.
Epidemiology and Disease Control Department (1999) *National Health Survey 1998*, Singapore: Ministry of Health.
Field, John William (1951) 'The Historical, Racial and Cultural Background of Western Medicine in Malaya', in J. W. Field, R. Green and F. E. Byron (eds), *The Institute of Medical Research: Fifty Years of Medical Research in Malaya*, Kuala Lumpur: Government Press.
Galloway, David (1907) 'Observations on the Death Rate', *Journal of the Malayan Branch of the British Medical Association*, January: 1–4.
HDB (1965) *50,000 up: Homes for the people*, Singapore: Housing and Development Board.
Health Promotion Board 'National Smoking Control Programme', Online. Available <http://www.hpb.gov.sg/hpb/default.asp?pg_id=979> (accessed 1 May 2005).
Hone, H. R. (1946) *Report on the British Military Administration of Malaya: September 1945 to March 1946*, Kuala Lumpur: Malayan Union Government Press.
Innes, J. R. (1901) *Report on the Census of the Straits Settlements Taken on 1st March 1901*, Singapore: Singapore Government Printers.
Lee, Kuan Yew (1968) Speech by the Prime Minister at the Inauguration of the 'Keep Singapore Clean' Campaign at the Singapore Conference Hall on Tuesday 1 October 1968. *The Singapore Public Health Bulletin*: Keep Singapore Clean Issue, 1969(5): 5–6.

Lee, Yong Kiat (1987) 'Brief History of Medical Services and Education in Singapore', in *To Commemorate the Re-opening of the College of Medicine Building, August 1987*, Singapore: Ministry of Health, 6–90.

—— (2003) 'A Short History of the Kandang Kerbau Hospital and the Maternity Services of Singapore', in Tan Kok Hian and Tay Eng Hseon (eds), *The History of Obstetrics & Gynaecology in Singapore*, Singapore: Obstetrical & Gynaecological Society of Singapore and National Heritage Board, 53–73.

Lim, Kay Tong and Mary Lee (1997) *Fighting TB: The SATA Story (1947–1997)*, Singapore: Singapore Anti-Tuberculosis Association.

Lim, Maggie (1966) 'Maternal and Child Health Services in Singapore', *Singapore Paediatric Society Journal*, 8(1): 29–41.

Lim, Tay Boh (1965) 'The Role of the University in Medical Education', in C. S. Muir and Wong Poi Kwong (eds), *Sixty Years of Medical Education 1905–1965*, Singapore: University of Singapore Medical Society, 12–14.

Lim, Veronica (1979) *History of Family Planning in Singapore, 1945–1970*, Singapore: Department of History, Faculty of Arts and Social Sciences, National University of Singapore.

MacGregor, William (1900) 'An Address on Some Problems of Tropical Medicine', *Journal of Tropical Medicine*, 3, October: 63–71.

Maternal and Child Health Services (1974) *Maternal and Child Health Services Annual Report*, Singapore: Maternal and Child Health Services.

Ministry of Health. *Health Facts Singapore 2004*. Online. Available <http://www.moh.gov.sg/corp/publications/statistics/principal.do> (accessed 25 April 2005).

Mudeliar, Viji, Nair, C. R. S. and Norris, R. P. (eds) (1979) *Development of Hospital Care and Nursing in Singapore*, Singapore: Ministry of Health.

Muir, C. S. and Wong Poi Kwong (eds) (1965) *Sixty Years of Medical Education 1905–1965*, Singapore: University of Singapore Medical Society.

Oakley, Ann (1984) *The Captured Womb: A History of the Medical Care of Pregnant Women*, Oxford: Basil Blackwell.

Phua, Kai Hong (1989) 'The Development of Health Services in the Colonies: A Study of British Malaya and Singapore', *Asia-Pacific Journal of Public Health*, 3(4): 315–323.

—— (2005) 'Singapore in World Health Organization', *Social Health Insurance: Selected Case Studies from Asia and the Pacific*, Manila: Western Pacific Region and New Delhi: South East Asia Region.

Proceedings of the Legislative Council Straits Settlements.

—— (1910) *Report of the Municipal Enquiry Commission*.

—— (1948) *Council Paper No. 4 Annexure A – The Medical Plan for Singapore*.

Purcal, John (1989) 'Some Aspects of the Political Economy of Health and Development in Singapore', in Paul Cohen and John Purcal (eds), *Political Economy of Primary Health Care in Southeast Asia*, Canberra: Australian Development Studies Network, 124–139.

Reid, J. A. and Mohamed Din bin Ahmad (1958) 'Malaria Control in the Federation of Malaya', *The Medical Journal of Malaya*, 12(4): 569–584.

Seow, Adeline and Lee Hin Peng (1994) 'From Colony to City State: Changes in Health Needs in Singapore: 1950 to 1990', *Journal of Public Medicine*, 16(2): 149–158.

Singapore General Hospital (1976) *Singapore General Hospital: 50th Anniversary Publication 1926-76*, Singapore: The Hospital.

Singh, Kuldip (2003) 'Fertility Trends in Singapore since Independence', in Tan Kok Hian and Tay Eng Hseon (eds), *The History of Obstetrics & Gynaecology in Singapore*,

Singapore: Obstetrical & Gynaecological Society of Singapore and National Heritage Board, 280–283.
Tan, Kok Hian (2003) 'The Singapore O+G Timeline', in Tan Kok Hian and Tay Eng Hseon (eds), *The History of Obstetrics & Gynaecology in Singapore*, Singapore: Obstetrical & Gynaecological Society of Singapore and National Heritage Board, 37–47.
Tan, Nalla (1991), 'Health and Welfare', in Ernest C. T. Chew and Edwin Lee (eds), *The History of Singapore*, Singapore: Oxford University Press, 339–356.
Teo, Siew Eng and Victor Savage (1991) 'Singapore Landscape: A Historical Overview of Housing Image', in Ernest C. T. Chew and Edwin Lee (eds), *The History of Singapore*, Singapore: Oxford University Press, 312–338.
Toh, C. M., Chew, S. K. and Tan, C. C. (2002) 'Prevention and Control Of Non-Communicable Diseases In Singapore: A Review Of National Health Promotion Programmes', *Singapore Medical Journal*, 43(7): 333–338.
Turnbull, C. M. (1977) *A History of Singapore, 1819–1975*, Kuala Lumpur: Oxford University Press.
Vickers, W. *Medical Progress in Singapore* (a talk given to undergraduates and graduates of the Faculty of Medicine, University of Malaya on 19 February 1954).
Wong, Hock Boon (1980) 'Postgraduate Medical Education in Singapore', in Wong Wai Chow (ed.), *75 years of Medical Education in Singapore 1905–1980*, Singapore: Faculty of Medicine, National University of Singapore, 7–11.
—— (1990) 'Neonatology in Kandang Kerbau Hospital', in Tham Kum Yang (ed), *Kandang Kerbau Hospital 1924–1990*, Singapore: The Hospital, 21.
—— (1994) 'The History of Perinatology in Singapore', in S. Srulkumaran and R. O. Daniel (eds), *A Short History of the Obstetrical and Gynaecological Society of Singapore: 1972–1993*, Singapore: The Society, 107–131.
Yarrall, Mabel C. (1972) 'Methodology on Health Campaigns', *The Singapore Public Health Bulletin*, 9(January): 42–44.
Yeoh, Brenda S. A. (1996) *Contesting Space: Power Relations and the Built Environment in Colonial Singapore*, Kuala Lumpur: Oxford University Press.
Yong, Nyuk Lin (1966) Speech in *Family Planning in Singapore*, Singapore: Government Printers.

11 Public health and the clash of cultures

The Philippine cholera epidemics

Willie T. Ong

'Hundreds of deaths daily for two weeks', blared the *Manila Times*. 'In twenty-four hours 5,094 cases and 2,724 deaths are recorded' (*Manila Times* 1 October 1902). By the end of 1903, there were 200,222 persons dead from Asiatic cholera. Such was the enormity of the 1902–1904 cholera epidemic, arguably the worst recorded epidemic of Philippine history.

Different views of the 1902–1904 cholera epidemic have been advanced by contemporary historians. Warwick Anderson uses this epidemic to illustrate the public health methods employed by the colonial government. In contrast to Anderson's non-judgmental account, two other historians give a more critical account. Reynaldo Ileto asserts that previously, historians have seen in this epidemic 'American heroism and medico-sanitary skill'. And yet, Ileto cites instances of controversial American tactics such as the burning of native houses and an ineffective quarantine (Ileto 1995: 53, 62). Ken De Bevoise goes even further to argue that the Americans disrupted the Islands' ecological equilibrium and were themselves 'agents of apocalypse'. Furthermore, De Bevoise posits that the Americans, with boundless self-righteousness, increased mortality in certain areas with their hard-handed tactics. By contrast with the less interventionist Spanish public health system, Americans with 'the power to intervene in the epidemic turned out to be only a power to make it worse' (De Bevoise 1995: 176).

Understandably, the American officials at the time thought differently. Dean C. Worcester, Philippine Secretary of the Interior, 1901–1913, insisted that the Americans were more effective in this epidemic than the Spaniards had been in the 1882 epidemic. The U.S. Bureau of Census in 1921 showed that the American-led, 1902–1904 campaign ended with approximately 200,000 deaths or 3% of total mortality, while incomplete statistics on the Spanish-led, 1882 campaign showed 76,884 provincial deaths (Worcester 1909: 21). Reviewing the documents, I suggest America and Spain ended up just about equal.

But numbers do not tell the whole story. In this paper, I will argue that rigorous American sanitary measures collided with the Filipinos' cultural and religious beliefs. Second, I will contend that this clash of cultures had both detrimental and transforming effects on American health officials; detrimental in that the Americans suffered physically and emotionally under the strain of the epidemic; and in a way, a positive transformation because it led open-minded, American health commissioners like Dr E. C. Carter to analyse what went wrong with their sanitary campaign and adopt a more culturally sensitive stand. In reshaping the customs of the colony, some colonizers were themselves transformed.

Historian of medicine, David Arnold notes that earlier historians saw medicine as one of the 'nobler and redeeming features' of Western colonialism, while more recent historians have seen it as an instrument for social control. Furthermore, historians are now more inclined to see colonial medicine from the colonized's point of view (Arnold 1997: 1393–1394). My chapter is a step in that direction.

Cholera in Spanish times

During the Spanish occupation, the major epidemics were cholera, smallpox and beriberi. Filipino historian Jose Bantug believes the 1628 epidemic had features suggestive of cholera. Historical records show 'cholera' outbreaks during the following years: 1812, 1817, 1820, 1843, 1879, 1882 and 1888–1889 (Bantug 1953: 28–31). Several of these epidemics coincide with the time of worldwide migration of cholera from India. The scanty records that exist show that in the 1820 epidemic, thousands had died in Manila.

The classic index epidemic during the Spanish era was the 1882 cholera epidemic. According to Dr D. R. Alba y Martin, the Director of Health for the port of Zamboanga, the first case in Zamboanga occurred on 7 July 1882. When the patient died, Alba had the victim's clothing and other personal effects burned. Cholera ran its brutal course in 1882 and Spanish authorities were helpless to stop it. Local boards of health were appointed in various towns but according to De Bevoise, they did not make a great difference. Dr Rebelo, who led the local board in Capiz City, could not hide his frustration as people quickly lost faith in the orthodox medicine: 'they handed themselves over to traditional healers, stupid and uncivilized people who are devoted to giving poultices and sticking plaster for all sorts of ailments' (De Bevoise 1995: 173).

According to American sources, under the Spanish, sanitation and the water and sewer systems were inadequate. Dr Victor Heiser, Director of Health in 1905–1915, wrote: 'With the exception of an antiquated and polluted Spanish water system in the capital, there was not a reservoir, not a pipeline, and not an artesian well in the islands' (Heiser 1936: 39). This adverse view of the Spanish was a recurring theme in the writings of American health officials after the United States took over the Philippines in 1898. In the first decade of American rule, Dean C. Worcester, a zoology graduate of the University of Michigan, was the key person in health administration. As Secretary of the Interior, Worcester controlled the appointments of health commissioners and approved the Board of Health's actions (Worcester 1909: 28). He was instrumental in establishing three medical institutions: the Bureau of Science (1901); the University of the Philippines Medical School (1905); and the Philippine General Hospital (1907). Indeed, according to Lewis Gleeck, Worcester was the most influential man in the Philippines in 1901–1912. Despite his contributions, many Filipinos disliked him, finding him disagreeable, tactless and belligerent (Gleeck 1976: 190).

Although showing a degree of humanitarianism, some Americans discriminated against Filipinos. In 1900, Dr Louis Atlee delivered a speech before the College of Physicians in Philadelphia. He said that 'our troops look like giants among a lot of monkeys when mixed in a crowd of Filipinos' (Atlee 1900: 12). Equally arrogantly, Colonel Arthur L. Wagner reported that the natives had 'scarcely more power of intelligent initiative than the same number of cattle' (De Bevoise 1995: 179).

In 1902, the Philippine Islands had a population of more than 7.5 million, with over 90% native Filipinos. In Manila, the population was around 300,000, including most of the 8,315 Americans and 3,888 Spaniards in the Islands. The hot and humid climate had only two seasons, dry and wet, with cholera flourishing in the rainy months of June to October. Despite the inadequacies of the Spanish health system, the death rate in Manila was fairly low at 28 per 1,000 in non-epidemic years in contrast to India with a high 76 per 1,000 and New York with a low 19 per 1,000 (U.S. Bureau of the Census 1905: 74).

The political climate in 1902 was intense because of the Filipino-American War of Resistance. This had started on 4 February 1899 and, on paper at least, had ended on 4 July 1902. The Americans suffered 4,234 casualties with 2,818 wounded. The Filipinos, on the other hand, suffered 20,000 deaths. The war had cost the Americans USD 600 million, or USD 4 billion in current value (Karnow 1989: 194). De Bevoise claims that some American generals were guilty of war crimes, including the wholesale burning of villages to stamp out resistance (De Bevoise 1995: 243). Reynaldo Ileto writes that in 1902, it was difficult to differentiate the war against disease and the pacification of Filipinos when public health measures were seen as continuing acts of war (Ileto 1995: 53).

The 1902–1904 cholera epidemic

As cholera had done in the past, it migrated from India. In successive order, the following countries and cities reported cholera outbreaks from January 1900 to October 1901: India, the Straits Settlements, Singapore, Buenos Aires, Batavia (Jakarta), Yokohama, Formosa, Borneo and Sumatra (*Manila Times* 7 May 1902). On 3 March 1902, cholera was reported in Canton; it arrived in Hong Kong six days later. As cholera crept closer to the Philippines, everyone was apprehensive. Worcester confessed: 'No one in the islands had any experience with cholera... and we had to get this [experience] as we went along' (Worcester 1921: 413). Victor Heiser described how cholera supposedly migrated from Hong Kong to Manila

> Under the terms of this embargo, a large shipment of cabbages from Canton, was refused, and the angry shipmaster thereupon dumped the cargo into Manila Bay and sailed off, leaving the surface of the water literally covered with the bobbing heads. From the nipa huts of Farola, Tondo, and Meisic, the Filipinos swarmed to the waterfront, launched their praos and bancas, and went fishing for cabbages. They welcomed the succulent vegetables as manna.
>
> (Heiser 1936: 104)

On 20 March 1902 at 2:30 PM, two cases resembling Asiatic cholera were admitted to San Juan de Dios Hospital for treatment. Hospital physicians immediately notified the Board of Health. Within one hour, Health Commissioner L. M. Maus, Chief Inspector Meacham and Bureau of Laboratory officers Paul Freer and Richard Strong arrived. After twenty-four hours, Strong demonstrated the deadly comma bacillus in hanging drop slides (U.S. Philippine Commission 1903: 267). The Islands proved to be a fertile ground for cholera. In the first three days, 37 cases were confirmed (*Manila Times* 23 March 1902). In ten days, the number ballooned to 102 with a case fatality rate of 90% (U.S. Philippine Commission 1903: 267). Most of the cases were traced to the Farola district in Tondo, an area where the poorest classes lived in unsanitary shanties.

Worcester immediately ordered American soldiers to quarantine the entire district. In fear and confusion, the natives tried to escape. By the third day of quarantine, a cholera-stricken native had escaped, spreading the disease to the nearby province of Rizal. With the mortality in the quarantined district rising, Worcester thought it best to transfer the natives into the San Lazaro detention camp. With Worcester's approval, the Board of Health carried out Government Order 66, which called for the burning of infected nipa huts and the disinfection of houses made of wood (Ileto 1995: 64). On 27 March, the infected Farola district was burned to the ground. The Americans, led by Worcester and Heiser, and a hundred natives watched this event (*Manila Times* 30 March 1902). Heiser wrote

> Under a blazing sky, the terrified and resentful owners watched the shooting sparks as shack after shack crackled and collapsed. The report spread about the homes of the poor were being burned to make room for future dwellings and warehouses of rich Americans. Further rumors that the foreign doctors had poisoned the wells were also widely credited; it was even said the American aim was to annihilate the Filipino race.
>
> (Heiser 1936: 105)

If the Americans saw the burning of the Farola district as the extermination of the cholera germs, to the natives it was American oppression. The burning of this Tondo district, publicized by the media, proved to be a turning point in the increasing conflict between the colonizers and the colonized. Filipino resistance took the form of non-reporting of cases and secret burial of the dead. Just six days after the destruction of Farola, reports came out of concealment of bodies in outlandish ways. Under the cover of night, cholera-stricken corpses were disposed of in the Pasig River, further polluting the already polluted waters (*Manila Times* 4 April 1902). In one case, a mother hastily buried her seven-month old infant in a shallow grave (*Manila Times* 16 May 1902). The American health officials were incensed by the natives' defiance. This prompted them to employ more stringent measures, which only provoked the natives more. The vicious cycle contributed to the discord between Filipinos and Americans.

Concurrent with the failed quarantine of the Farola district, Worcester ordered a quarantine along the Mariquina river, which rose in the mountains above Montalban. For 16 miles it flowed through picturesque canyons and 14 miles through a thickly populated valley where natives had built shanties beside it (*Manila Times* 28 February 1903). Heavily used, the river was polluted. Health officials found the bacterial content of the river water to be as high as 613,703 per cc. This contrasted with the New York Croton water supply, which had a count of 75 per cc (U.S. Philippine Commission 1903: 329).

Like the Farola quarantine, the river quarantine had undesirable effects for it prohibited the use of the river for trade, travel or drinking (Worcester 1909: 24). In addition, one native was killed in an attempt to breach the quarantine line. As one American soldier said : 'Why is this senseless guard kept on the Mariquina river? It is of no use; it gives the soldiers extra duty and by preventing the people from sending their sugar and lumber to market, it creates hard times and adds every month to the present discontent and the number of ladrones [bandits] in the mountains' (*Manila Times* 22 October 1902).

Worcester also ordered the quarantine of all exits from Manila, further hampering trade. When it became obvious that this land quarantine would not prevent the spread of cholera to the provinces, he had no choice but to remove it. He later confessed that the worst mistake was to establish the land quarantine (Worcester 1909: 28). The Americans vacillated between discipline and leniency in handling the epidemic. Dr C. F. De Mey, captain and assistant surgeon of the U.S. volunteers, recounted his experience

> [In front of my] quarters there was a small house in which lived a man, a woman and their little son. One day I noticed the little one picking a chicken, and was interested in the deftness with which he picked it. The next morning the child was dead. I went immediately into the house and told the father and mother to throw all food away. The mother told me that she had [no food] left but a piece of chicken which the little one had been eating... I made the serious mistake of not throwing it away myself. And the next day the mother died of cholera. I went immediately to the water-closet, and sure enough, there were chickens feasting [on the feces].
> (U.S. Philippine Commission 1903: 413)

In the face of such behaviour, it would be difficult to find fault in De Mey's resolve that the health officer must 'rule with a rod of steel'. He also advocated burning of contact houses to stamp out the infection (U.S. Philippine Commission 1903: 412).

Rigorous inspections were pursued. Within the first three weeks of the epidemic, Board Inspector Meyer Herman had employed over 1,500 native men as sanitary inspectors. But the colonial officials claimed that around 300 were 'mentally and morally unfit' for their work and they were subsequently discharged (*Manila Times* 30 May 1902). Hence, American teachers were put to work as sanitary inspectors. With such a large number of inspectors, no one was exempt. The house-to-house inspections continued both day and night. This was done to counteract the natives' tendency to conceal cases (*Manila Times* 3 September 1902). In the town of Santa Cruz alone, almost 18,000 houses were inspected and reinspected a month later. This epidemic had the longer-term effect of acting as catalyst to the Board of Health's development, thus illustrating John Duffy's contention that dramatic outbreaks of disease may increase the powers of public health institutions (Duffy 1997: 424).

Cholera cases and contacts were transferred to detention hospitals. There were nine such hospitals and two detention camps but these proved inadequate for the burgeoning number of cases. The larger San Lazaro detention camp could accommodate 2,000 patients. However, it was poorly equipped and barely completed (Worcester 1909: 29). For the period of March to May 1902, the Americans enforced the policy that all cholera cases and contacts be isolated in hospitals or camps (U.S. Philippine Commission 1903: 269). Heiser himself later admitted the error of pursuing this measure because of the panic that ensued. In four out of five cases, the patients died and relatives never saw their loved ones again (Heiser 1936: 106).

Treatment of cholera in 1902 was mostly ineffective and even harmful. It consisted of cleansing the bowels with an enema, application of a hot-water bottle and use of a new drug called Benzozone. This drug, however, proved inefficacious and case fatality rates remained high. For patients close to dying, injections of strychnia were given to stimulate the heart's contraction. But these heroic treatments only further ingrained the natives' belief that being taken to a hospital meant certain death (Ileto 1995: 61).

For several months, cholera spread geographically, reaching the farthest province of Mindanao by October (*Manila Times* 9 October 1902). Iloilo was the province hardest hit, reporting over 100 deaths a day for two weeks at the height of the epidemic (*Manila Times* 26 September 1902). The situation got so out of hand that long lines waited at churches for burials to take place.

The destruction of infected nipa huts continued in the provinces. In one incident in Batangas, the burning of a house led to the destruction of 81 neighbouring huts (De Bevoise 1995: 181). Some American teachers refused to implement Government Order 66. As compensation, the Philippine Commission paid USD 4,692.39 for the houses burned in Lumbang which worked out at USD 15 per house. Compensation took six months to be paid and people had nothing to live on in the meantime (Ileto 1995: 64–65). Filipino opposition swelled. In San Pablo, Laguna, the mayor exchanged words with an American army surgeon who had reprimanded the mayor for being slow. The mayor retorted that the surgeon was insulting and impatient (Ileto 1995: 68).

The cultural conflict

There was some inconsistency in American policy. Lewis Gleeck notes that 'it was a common anticipation that there would be an immediate revolution of custom and condition from the American presence' (Gleeck 1976: 274). Though

President McKinley said that America would not interfere with Filipino habits and customs, the Bureau of Health had no choice but to do this (Heiser 1936: 64).

The American health officials believed at least four customs encouraged the spread of infectious diseases. First, there was the custom of eating with the fingers, oftentimes, with inadequately washed hands. Second, there were the religious fiestas. Food was brought from cholera-infested districts and distributed to all who would partake (Heiser 1936: 114). A third problem lay in the habit of visiting the sick. Following the Biblical admonition to comfort the sick, Filipinos dutifully visited neighbours who fell ill (Heiser 1936: 109). Cholera could also spread because Filipinos refused cremation (U.S. Bureau of the Census 1921: 1060). It was easy to understand the Americans' horror at seeing crowded interments with Filipinos eating beside a cholera-stricken corpse.

Gossip is said to be the Filipinos' favourite pastime. As noted earlier, a rumour spread that the houses of the poor were being burned to make room for the future residence of Americans. Another rumour was that once Filipinos were isolated in a detention camp, they were abused and murdered (U.S. Philippine Commission 1903: 271). It was also believed that hospitals patients were poisoned with 'vino', a strong alcoholic drink (Worcester 1921: 416). One persistent but baseless rumour was that the Americans were poisoning the wells to revenge themselves on the insurgents.

Another important cultural difference was in the approach to illness. While Americans struggled to overcome the disease, Filipinos would generally accept their fate with resignation. American Dr Siever of the Santiago Hospital said that Filipinos, despite extreme thirst, rarely asked for water. Americans on the other hand fought the disease and sought every measure available to survive (*Manila Times* 25 September 1902).

Religious beliefs also appeared to have hampered the drive against cholera. Spain's four hundred years of rule had brought Catholicism to the land and by the time of the American occupation, more than 90% of the Filipinos were devout Catholics. Epidemics were seen as punishment from God and they approached them with fatalism. Bert Emerson, an American businessman, was disgusted with the local peoples' ignorance and superstition. Emerson described continuous prayers and daily religious processions instead of boiling water and cooking food thoroughly. He noted that in place of carbolic acid as disinfectant, people relied on holy water (*Manila Times* 19 October 1902).

Another American eyewitness claimed that Filipinos from all classes, including Catholic priests and professionals, opposed American rule. The priests perpetuated the belief that cholera was part of God's will. The priest would paint the door with a red cross analogous to the marking of the door by the Jews during the Passover (Banister 1906: 151). Priest Gregorio Tabar was particularly opposed to the Americans' heavy-handed tactics. He claimed that cholera did not exist except in the minds of Americans. Having sheltered cholera patients in his home, he was promptly quarantined (*Manila Times* 4 April 1902).

In Vigan, Ilocos, a priest claimed he had seen Patron Saint San Roque emerging from a well, which he interpreted as a sign of a miraculous cure. As many as 6,000 natives flocked to the well, which turned out to be infected with cholera. After much hesitation, the provincial governor decided to disperse the crowds (*Manila Times* 17 November 1902b). Thus, Americans faced the constant problem of protecting public health while not trampling on Filipino beliefs.

The brunt of the responsibility for curtailing the epidemic lay with Commissioner L. M. Maus. By May 1902, the Board of Health had backed down on its tactics of burning and cremation (Ileto 1995: 65–66). Maus called a meeting with Filipino physicians on 13 July 1902, which was also attended by two Filipino members of the Philippine Commission. Maus could not hide his exasperation with local customs (*Manila Times* 13 July 1902).

To their surprise, the Filipino physicians' recommendations were unanimously approved by the Board. Four crucial issues were debated: (1) removal of land quarantine; (2) withdrawal of compulsory isolation and treatment; (3) free distribution of cholera medicines; and (4) removal of sanitary inspectors without medical training (*Manila Times* 13 July 1902). Speaking for the Filipino physicians, an unnamed doctor also insisted on domiciliary care. He reasoned that since the Americans were not able to provide facilities for the mounting number of cases, there should be no forced isolation of patients, thus avoiding separation of families. The Filipinos also lobbied for treatment to be carried out by their countrymen to ease the problem of cultural barriers. Throughout the long meeting, the Filipino physicians attacked and the Americans defended. Maus eventually agreed to carry out the physicians' wishes, and there was some softening of American policy with the establishment of auxiliary boards composed of native physicians. The quarantine around towns was also lifted, but later on Worcester, reacting to a rise in cases, resumed the quarantine.

Shortly after the meeting, Maus quit his post. It appears that he was close to breaking point when he called the meeting for he was willing to accede to the Filipino physician's wishes. Worcester had no choice but to accept his resignation and appoint Frank Bourns as replacement. Apparently, Maus was close to a nervous breakdown. Worcester wrote

> Throughout the early months of the epidemic Major Maus had labored unceasingly to check it, displaying an energy and indifference to fatigue and personal discomfort which were highly commendable. The long-continued strain ultimately began to tell on him severely and it became evident that while he was quick to throw an organization into the field he easily became discouraged and then wanted to smash his machine and build a new one to take its place.
> (Worcester 1909: 23)

The complex relationship of American doctors with the elite Filipino and Spanish doctors involved political considerations. Having lost their positions of power with the coming of the new colonial government, these elite doctors were obviously jealous of the Americans. Worcester complained that although these local doctors had verbally agreed to assist the board, they gave no tangible assistance. They failed to report cases or even falsely reported cases.

The conflict escalated. Philippine Commissioner T. H. Pardo de Tavera wrote to Governor Taft concerning the abuses and barbarities of American sanitary inspectors (Anderson 1992: 91, 105–106). The Americans also had their complaints. Special sanitary inspector, Frank Dubois, claimed that most Filipino doctors were ignorant of disinfection measures and also lacked the capacity to do sanitary work (U.S. Philippine Commission 1904: 225). However, some local physicians did help in the epidemic. Worcester acknowledged the good work of Dr Ariston Baustista Lin and Dr Manuel Gomez, the board secretary. There must have been other instances wherein Filipinos had helped their countrymen, but here the historical evidence is lacking.

Undoubtedly, the effects of the epidemic on the Americans were substantial. As early as April 1902, many Americans, including a judge, had succumbed to cholera. Moreover, bandits continued to kill Americans. Sadly, a diligent police inspector named Kiely was killed by two men while visiting cholera victims in Panay, Iloilo (*Manila Times* 17 November 1902a). Stress would also take its toll. Major Franklin Meacham, the Board's chief health inspector, succumbed to the stress. He had been expecting his wife and two young daughters to arrive from New York. However, his existing heart and liver ailments were exacerbated and he died before his family arrived.

Unlike Maus, Bourns, a major in the Army Medical Corps, understood the Filipino culture. For one, Bourns could speak the Filipino and Spanish languages fluently (U.S. Philippine Commission 1902: 272). His approach evoked less antagonism and may have led to a decrease in cases in August and September. But Bourns too would quit and cholera deaths increased by November. Worcester believed Bourns' tactics had produced this decline and was reluctant to let him go.

In September 1902, Major E. C. Carter took over as Health Commissioner. Fresh from the United States, Carter started with the typical no-nonsense approach. Worcester proudly proclaimed that Carter was efficient and fair (U.S. Philippine Commission 1904: 4).

But after two years of the epidemic, he too had changed. We see this in the tone of his annual reports from 1902 to 1904. Carter had started with an abhorrence of native culture saying: 'Undoubtedly the greatest obstacle to improving the conditions of the native is the native himself' (U.S. Philippine Commission 1903: 65). Later, writing on the lessons from the epidemic, Carter showed he understood that science must take into account other variables: 'The change [must be done] through lines of least resistance rather than scientific accuracy. Changes are doomed to failure unless it understands the susceptibility of the population'. In his last report to the President of the United States, he admitted that he felt compelled (but stopped himself after some thought) to write over his signature his belief that 'nothing could be done except to relieve the suffering of the sick and the destitute, and the epidemic would cease only when the vulnerable material was exhausted' (U.S. Philippine Commission 1906: 69). In the end a total of 200,222 people including 66,000 children had perished (U.S. Bureau of the Census 1905: 47–56).

In April 1904, the Board of Health declared that the Philippines was cholera free. But this declaration was premature. For by 1905, new cases were reported.

With the possibility of another epidemic looming, Carter submitted his resignation (Worcester 1921: 419). The 1902–1904 cholera epidemic had been the collision of the irresistible force of the disease against the immovable object of American science.

Subsequent cholera outbreaks under American rule

On 20 August 1905, cholera reappeared in Taytay, Jalajala and other towns in Laguna de Bay. Three days later, it was reported in the Bilibid prison. At the end of two weeks, 137 cases had appeared but the increase in cases did not continue. As before, cholera affected the poorer natives first before spreading to the upper classes. However, newly appointed Director of Health Victor Heiser could not see any epidemiological connection with the 1902–1904 epidemic. This led physicians to theorize that cholera was endemic in Manila and simply resurfaced during the rainy seasons (Heiser 1908: 93).

Heiser proved to be the most resilient health chief not because of his intellectual superiority but because he understood Filipino culture. As a former federal agent of the U.S. Public Health Service, Heiser no doubt benefited from his previous experiences with American immigrant populations. Heiser also sought to increase the Director of Health's power, and he lobbied for more funds since money was an 'ever-present and pressing problem in the Bureau of Health' (Heiser 1936: 61).

From 1905, there was a generally decreasing cholera mortality trend. Learning from his predecessors, Heiser tried to circumvent the Filipino's cultural and religious beliefs. Moreover, the conditions in the San Lazaro detention hospital and other hospitals were being improved. Heiser also tried to avoid the controversial sanitary tactics used in the 1902–1904 epidemic.

By February 1906, the epidemic had subsided, leaving 6,067 dead, just 6% of 1902 mortality levels. Worcester praised Heiser for practically terminating the epidemic in Manila on 21 February 1906. Fewer cases occurred in 1907 and there were 745 deaths. But in 1908, cholera surged back, claiming 17,770 lives before decreasing again in subsequent years (Worcester 1909: 32). Until the end of Heiser's term in 1915, mortality rates from cholera and other infectious diseases declined. One major factor was the construction of modern water and sewer systems, which started in 1907. The water system cost USD 1.5 million and the sewer system cost USD 2 million (Worcester 1921: 431–432). Undoubtedly, declining cultural conflict and the greater scientific understanding of cholera also played a role.

One major public health strategy against cholera was health education. Hygiene rules were published in newspapers and printed on handbills in various native languages. They were circulated to teachers who taught them to schoolchildren (U.S. Philippine Commission 1905: 7). Glaring red posters were posted on public buildings. In addition, Heiser formed the 'knife and fork society' for children hoping that they would persuade their parents to use utensils instead of their hands in eating (Heiser 1936: 117–118).

Religion would also be used to promote education on disease prevention. Heiser visited two rival church leaders. First, he convinced Catholic Archbishop

Harty to have the priests distribute cholera pamphlets to the people. Afterwards, Heiser went to Father Aglipay, head of the Philippine Independent Church, and said: 'The Roman Catholics are sending out cholera circulars. Don't you want to save the lives of your people also?' (Heiser 1936: 118).

In 1908, scientific research played a pivotal role in reducing cholera mortality. Henry Nichols and Vernon Andrews made a comparative study showing the efficacy of intravenous saline injections in decreasing by 80% mortality from circulatory collapse, and preventing kidney failure due to dehydration (Nichols 1909: 83, 91). In another landmark study, Assistant Director of Health McLaughlin proposed four areas of action to suppress cholera: (1) a good water supply; (2) safe disposal of excreta; (3) early discovery of cases, suspects and carriers; and (4) habits of cleanliness (McLaughlin 1909a: 54). In a related article, Mclaughlin said that the teaching of sanitary habits was best done by school teachers and local priests (McLaughlin 1909b: 107–109).

Many modern health strategies had their inception in the 1910s. The first 'Clean-up Week' was started by Victor Heiser in 1914. The Bureau of Health led this one-week activity of street sweeping, garbage collection and the simple cleaning of houses and immediate surroundings. In the same year, the Pure Foods and Drugs Act was enforced to ensure the quality of food products and medicines being sold to the public.

In the 1920s, the country was spared any serious cholera outbreak. Continuing efforts were made to improve general sanitation and keep the food and water supplies safe. Health education activities persisted, with an average of 22,000 lectures given in schools and town plazas every year. Cholera re-emerged in March to May 1930, eventually causing 3,000 deaths out of the 5,000 reported cases. Although it was much smaller than the previous epidemics, the Philippine Health Service embarked on an extensive health education campaign, even participating in the 1932 Manila Carnival with health streamers, slogans and a display booth. The Philippine Health Service also continued to distribute its official publication, *The Health Messenger*, increasing print distribution to 30,000 copies nationwide.

By the early 1940s, deaths from cholera and smallpox had waned. But even as the Americans prepared to leave, they expressed disappointment at not being able to rid the Philippines of two other infectious diseases: tuberculosis and malaria. Then came the Japanese occupation from 7 December 1941 to 26 February 1945 when Philippine health-care activities came to a standstill. Health institutions, libraries and key documents were destroyed. Anecdotal reports show that although no cholera epidemics were reported, health parameters took a turn for the worse. The incidence of tuberculosis, malaria and severe malnutrition increased, especially among the lower classes. Over 5,000 segregated lepers escaped in search of food. But most striking of all was the number of venereal disease cases, which according to Health Secretary Antonio C. Villarama grew by leaps and bounds.

After the Liberation, the Philippines underwent a decade of unprecedented growth and medical progress. In the 1950s, a multitude of international agencies poured in funds and other assistance. The World Health Organization (WHO) chose Manila as the site of their Western Pacific Regional Headquarters, further enhancing the country's image. The prototype rural health units, which the Americans instituted, were also a great success. The goal was to bring health services closer to the people. Widespread reduction in infant mortality, maternal mortality and the general death rate was attributed to the spread of the rural health units. This led Undersecretary of Health Dr Regino Padua to label the 1950s as a golden era of public health.

The El Tor epidemic of 1961–1965

In the 1960s, with continuing aid from foreign donors like the USAID, WHO and UNICEF, the Department of Health pursued programmes on infectious diseases control, nutrition and family planning. Gastroenteritis, including cholera, ranked third in the list of major killer diseases. Pneumonia and tuberculosis were the first two. Amidst the high hopes for the decade, cholera returned stronger and deadlier in 1961 as the dangerous strain, El Tor. During the 1961–1965 El Tor epidemic, public anxiety increased to fever pitch. Media frenzy was heightened by the number of deaths worldwide. Because of the tense situation, the WHO in 1962 called for an interregional meeting on cholera control to be held in Manila. The meeting sought to exchange information on the epidemiology, prevention and control of El Tor. A follow-up meeting was held there in 1964, with delegates coming from all over the world.

El Tor started on 22 September 1961, producing as many as 2,000 cases per month and 182 deaths for the year. In 1962, there were an astonishing 17,000 cases with 272 deaths and in 1963, 3,000 cases with 300 deaths. El Tor would rise again in the rainy month of August 1964. In one month, 1,479 cases and 11 deaths were reported in Pampanga, and in the cities of Pasay, Quezon, Caloocan, Cavite, Cabanatuan, San Pablo and Lipa. As in previous epidemics, the slum area of Tondo would yield the largest number of cholera victims. At the San Lazaro Hospital cholera ward, an average of 40 cases were admitted daily.

There are chilling similarities between the El Tor epidemic of the 1960s and the Asiatic cholera of the early 1900s. First, the El Tor vibrio is so similar to the Asiatic cholera strain that it takes detailed serological tests to differentiate them. Second, public health measures invoked by the Health Department were similar to those of the early 1900s. Manila Mayor, Antonio Villegas, wanted to follow the American example by lobbying to lift the injunctions against the demolition of squatter shacks, especially those in Tondo. Unless this was done, the Mayor said, cholera would strike again and again. The notorious area of Tondo has been labelled by health authorities as a reservoir of infection. The slum dwellers were castigated for their hostility and complacency (Nollido 1964: 5, 92–93).

The stress on the health authorities was reminiscent of that produced by the 1902–1904 epidemic. Although Health Secretary Rodolfo Canos issued numerous health bulletins and the Philippine government released PHP 1,022,000 in funds, this epidemic could not be controlled. Like the American health authorities before him, a frustrated Secretary Canos said

> We have many skilled doctors in our hospitals to combat El Tor...the Department of Health is doing its job in health-educating the masses...(but) the people, especially there living in the slum areas, must cooperate. They must rise out of their apathy...apathy, that is the monster of any national crisis...The trouble is the general attitude of the people.
> (Nollido 1964: 5, 92–93)

The problems were identified as culture and attitude. The health authorities felt discouraged in their health education campaign as there was not enough 'social consciousness' to go around. The El Tor epidemic ended in 1965 but the basic conditions for its re-emergence remained present.

On 21 September 1972, the country was stunned when President Ferdinand Marcos announced that, under Proclamation Order No. 1081, martial law was in effect throughout the country. Although the *Times Journal* headline on 3 January 1974 read 'State of health of nation better. Less deaths', some health professionals questioned the accuracy of that data. Some quarters accused the government of deliberately promoting a positive outlook when the health picture was in fact bleak. For example: health workers believed that cholera was listed under gastroenteritis to avoid international scrutiny. However, this claim cannot be verified, especially because of the paucity of records. In 1986, the Marcos administration was overthrown by the People Power Revolution and President Corazon Aquino quickly restored democracy. Clearly prioritizing health, Aquino increased the health budget from PHP 4 billion to PHP 11 billion. The proportion of Gross National Product (GNP) going to health rose from an average of 2.8% during the Marcos years to an average of 4.2% under Aquino.

Then, in the 1990s, lifestyle diseases overtook infectious diseases as the leading causes of deaths. Although cholera had all but disappeared from the mortality list, diarrhoea still ranked first in terms of morbidity statistics in 1997. Diseases of the heart ranked first in terms of mortality while the scourge of tuberculosis remained the number five killer.

Cholera outbreak in 2003

One century after the 1902–1904 cholera epidemic, could history repeat itself? In September 2003, an outbreak of diarrhoea cases baffled not only the health department but the country as well. By 31 October 2003, there were 242 reported cases of diarrhoea with 4 deaths from at least 8 streets in Tondo, including Capulong, Velasquez, Varona, Raxabago streets and Dagupan extension (Felipe and Crisostomo 2003). Confirmed cholera cases numbered 29. According to the Department of Health Press Release on 5 November 2003, rectal swabs from patients showed that many were positive for the cholera vibrio. Others were positive for *Salmonella typhi* (the cause of typhoid fever) and *E. coli*, indicating sewage contamination. 'It is an outbreak most probably due to sewage contamination of the water lines', said Health Secretary Manuel Dayrit. Old, leaking water pipelines, illegal connections and low water pressure were all blamed.

According to the latest statistics, 23.7% of the Philippine population have no access to a safe water supply and 30.7% have no sanitary toilets. The worst sanitation data can be found in the Autonomous Region of Muslim Mindanao where 38.4% have no access to safe water and 57.2% have no toilets. This is hardly surprising as the water pipes date back to the American era. Environmentalist Allen Padua says, 'After the war, the Americans established the Balara water facility to supply their military installations. Quezon City, Pasig and Fort Bonifacio were former American military facilities' (Chin 2004). The lack of safe water, toilets and sewer systems explains why diarrhoea is persistently the number one cause of morbidity in the country.

The Alliance of Progressive Labor, a non-governmental organization, made a public statement blaming the Maynilad Water Services Inc. (MWSI) for this public health disaster. The Tondo water pipes are old but the company said they did not have the funds to repair them (Alliance 2003). MWSI has employed stopgap measures such as adding chlorine to the water, increasing the water pressure and repairing faulty lines.

The Manila Health Department, led by Mayor Lito Atienza, also started rationing safe water but many residents refuse to use it. Dr Rachel Garcia, director of the National Capital Region, is frustrated by the residents' refusal to use these safe water outlets. Unaware of the dangers of tainted water, residents still use tap water because it is more convenient. Boiling water entails too much time and too many additional costs. Moreover, the Filipino culture of eating with poorly washed hands continues to this day. It is no wonder that cholera has struck again.

Politics and economics, as well as cultural factors, play a part in disease outbreaks. Not surprisingly, the government downplayed the latest disaster by calling it a 'cluster of cases' instead of an outbreak. The term cholera was rarely mentioned in newspapers as the terms gastroenteritis, diarrhoea or 'gastro' disease dominated the headlines. It is hard to blame government officials for this ploy because of the economic implications of having a cholera outbreak in modern times. In a country where 40% of the people are below the poverty line, the often frustrating tasks of teaching sanitary practices and providing safe water need to continue to be carried out.

References

Alliance of Progressive Labor (2003) 'Maynilad to Blame for Tondo Deaths Due to Water Contamination', Online. Available <http://www.apl.org.ph/ps/20031029waterdeaths.htm> (accessed 30 October 2004).

Anderson, W. (1992) 'Colonial Pathologies: American Medicine in the Philippines 1898–1920', unpublished doctoral dissertation, University of Pennsylvania.

Arnold, D. (1997) 'Medicine and Colonialism', in W. F. Bynum and R. Porter (eds) *Companion Encyclopedia of the History of Medicine*, Vol. 2, New York: Routledge, 1393–1416.

Atlee, L. F. (1900) 'Some Observations by a Naval Surgeon in the Philippines', *International Clinics*, 1: 10–16.

Banister, J. M. (1906) 'Medical and Surgical Observations During a Three Years Tour of Duty in the Philippines', *Journal of the Association of Military Surgeons*, 18(3): 149–169, 259–334.

Bantug, J. P. (1953) *A Short History of Medicine in the Philippines*, Quezon City, Philippines: University of the Philippines Press, Inc.

Chin, L. (11 January 2004) 'The Water Crisis in Our Midst', *The Sunday Times*, Online. Available <http:www.manilatimes.net/national/2004/jan/11/yehey/weekend/20040111wek1.html> (accessed 30 October 2004).

De Bevoise, K. (1995) *Agents of Apocalypse: Epidemic Disease in the Colonial Philippines*, Princeton: Princeton University Press.

Department of Health (5 November 2003) 'Press Release: DOH Commends Atienza, Says Outbreak is Lessening', Department of Health, Online. Available <http://www.doh.gov.ph/press/November052003.htm> (accessed 30 October 2004).

Duffy, J. (1997) 'Social Impact of Disease in the Late 19th century', in J. W. Leavitt and R. L. Numbers (eds), *Sickness & Health in America*, Wisconsin: University of Wisconsin Press, 418–425.

Felipe, C. S. and Crisostomo, S. (30 October 2003) 'Manila Government Contains Disease Outbreak', *The Philippine Star*, Online. Available <http://www.newsflash.org/2003/05/ht/ht003847.htm> (accessed 30 October 2004).

Gleeck, L. E. Jr (1976) *American Institutions in the Philippines*, Manila: Carmelo and Bauermann.

Heiser, V. G. (1908) 'Some Considerations with Regard to the Cause of the Frequent Reappearances of Cholera in the Philippine Islands', *The Philippine Journal of Science*, 3(2): 89–106.

—— (1936) *An American Doctor's Odyssey: Adventures in Forty-Five Countries*, New York: W.W. Norton and Co.

Ileto, R. (1995) 'Cholera and the Origins of the American Sanitary Order in the Philippines', in V. L. Rafael (ed.), *Discrepant Histories*, Philadelphia: Temple University Press, 51–82.

Karnow, S. (1989) *In Our Image: America's Empire in the Philippines*, New York: Random House.

McLaughlin, A. (1909a) 'The Suppression of a Cholera Epidemic in Manila', *The Philippine Journal of Science*, 4(1): 43–67.

—— (1909b) 'The Suppression of a Cholera Outbreak in the Provinces', *The Philippine Journal of Science*, 4(2): 107–119.

Manila Times (23 March 1902) 'Dreaded Cholera is Now with Us', 1.

—— (30 March 1902) 'The Burning of Farola', 8.

—— (4 April 1902) 'Secreting of Cholera Cases', 1.

—— (7 May 1902) 'Asiatic Cholera', 5.

—— (16 May 1902) 'Buried Under House', 1.

—— (30 May 1902) 'Health Report for March', 5.

—— (13 July 1902) 'Discussed Situation', 4.

—— (3 September 1902) 'Report of Cholera Scare in Manila', 3.

—— (25 September 1902) 'Cholera Mocks Efforts of Science', 4–5.

—— (26 September 1902) 'And Still Those Forced Fingers Rule', 4.

—— (1 October 1902) 'Awful Ravages of Cholera in Panay', 1.

—— (9 October 1902) 'Cholera Invades Mindanao', 1.

—— (19 October 1902) 'Cholera Swept Province of Iloilo, in Beautiful Panay, is a Charnel House', 1.

—— (22 October 1902) 'The Mariquina River Quarantine', 4.

—— (17 November 1902a) 'Murder of Inspector Kiely', 1.
—— (17 November 1902b) 'Saint Roque Descends Into a Well', 1.
—— (28 February 1903) 'Sanitation in Manila', 2.
Nichols, H. J. and Andrews, V. L. (1909) 'The Treatment of Asiatic Cholera During the Recent Epidemic', *The Philippine Journal of Science*, 4(2): 81–98, 141–146.
Nollido, W. D. (19 September 1964) 'The Return of El Tor', *Philippines Free Press*, 5: 92–93.
U.S. Bureau of the Census (1905) *Census of the Philippine Islands 1903*, Washington: U.S. Bureau of the Census.
—— (1921) *Census of the Philippine Islands 1918*, Manila: Census Office of the Philippine Islands.
U.S. Philippine Commission (1903) *Third Annual Report of the U.S. Philippine Commission to the President 1902*, Washington: Government Printing Office.
—— (1904) *Fourth Annual Report of the U.S. Philippine Commission to the President 1903*, Washington: Government Printing Office.
—— (1905) *Fifth Annual Report of the U.S. Philippine Commission 1904*, Washington: Government Printing Office.
Worcester, D. C. (1909) *A History of Asiatic Cholera in the Philippine Islands*, Manila: Bureau of Printing.
—— (1921) *The Philippines Past and Present*, New York: The Macmillan Company.

12 Public health in Australia from the nineteenth to the twenty-first century

Milton J. Lewis

Introduction

From the late eighteenth century, Europeans were an increasing presence in the Pacific, first as explorers, then as beachcombers, traders and missionaries and finally as representatives of their governments. Two models of colonialism emerged in the Pacific. The first was settler colonialism. In the course of the nineteenth century, there was extensive emigration from Europe to Australia and New Zealand (as well as to other parts of Europe overseas such as North America and Latin America). In these Australasian settler colonies, transplanted European cultural, political, economic and social institutions became dominant, largely sweeping away indigenous, tribal ones; and the indigenes lost their land. The second model, that applying in Polynesia, Micronesia and Melanesia, saw the islanders very largely retain the land but political control pass to a European colonial elite who also introduced the market economy and as part of this process brought in Asian migrant labourers. Europeans brought to Asia and the Pacific the concepts of the nation state and of modern capitalism, both of which survived the passing of their empires after World War II (Denoon *et al.* 1997: 185–186; Basch 1999: 25, 32).

The modern mortality decline

Australian age-standardized mortality rates declined from the 1860s. Life expectancy at birth increased from 47 years for males and 50 years for females in 1875 to 74 and 76, respectively, in 1990. In fact, Australia enjoyed a distinct advantage in life expectancy over the 'Mother Country' (England and Wales) up to 1945. In the case of cause-specific mortality decline in England and Wales in the period 1875–1950, 40% to 43% of the decline was due to reduction in infectious disease mortality, 13% to 16% to reduction in bronchitis, pneumonia and influenza, and 7% to 11% to reduction in diarrhoea and enteritis. The Australian picture is similar (Taylor *et al.* 1998a: 29–30; Taylor *et al.* 1998b: 41). Indeed, the mortality decline in Australia, and the timing in the change in the leading causes of mortality from communicable to non-communicable diseases, resemble those in England and Western Europe rather than in Asia.

Even in Japan (the first Asian nation to modernize) in 1900, life expectancy at birth was only 44 years for males and 45 for females, and in 1940, 50 and 54; whereas in the United Kingdom it was already 51 and 55 by 1910. Japan made great gains after World War II. By 1985 it was leading the world with 75 years for males and 80 for females; in comparison, China (1981) returned 66 and 69; India (1975–1980), 51 and 50; and Indonesia (1980–1985), 51 and 53, while England and Wales (1981–1983) returned 71 and 77. By the 1980s, in Japan, in cause-specific mortality, the dominant place of infectious diseases had been taken by heart disease, cancer and cerebrovascular disease (Powell and Anesaki 1990: 63–64). In China, life expectancy was 33 years in 1840–1899, and still only 35 in 1949, but it had risen to 70 by 1992. Before 1949, infectious diseases including tuberculosis were the dominant causes of death. By the 1980s, non-communicable diseases were to the fore, and the cause-specific mortality pattern was approaching that of economically advanced nations (Bray 2000: 720–721; Caldwell 2001: 8). In India in the five decades from 1870, famines, plague and influenza produced large, intermittent increases in mortality like those found in the crisis mortality pattern of seventeenth-century Europe. Only from 1921 is there a sustained rise in life expectancy: in 1921–1931, 28 years for males and females; in 1961–1970, 46 and 45 respectively, and in 1975–1980, 51 and 50 respectively (McAlpin 1983: 351–354; Powell and Anesaki 1990: 63). In the early nineteenth century, the life expectancy of Southeast Asians was about 25 to 30 years. By the late 1980s, it ranged from about 55 in Burma to over 70 years in Singapore (Elson 1992: 180; Owen 1992: 495).

Urbanization and health

By the late nineteenth century, Australia was one of the most urbanized countries in the world. The two largest cities, Sydney and Melbourne, were, by the turn of the century, noteworthy even by international standards. Sydney had grown from 96,000 in 1861 to 496,000 in 1901; Melbourne from 125,000 to 478,000. The three decades from 1860 were the period of the 'long boom' in the Australian economy. Per capita income was at least as high as in Britain and the United States. However, detailed inquiry into urban working class life suggests that a good proportion of the working class did not enjoy the benefits of this economic growth (Lee and Fahey 1986: 1–2). The more populous Australian cities had much substandard housing. Thus, compared with large European and American cities, Melbourne may have had small-scale, 'clean' industries and low population densities, but its hectic growth created a stock of poor-quality, 'jerry-built' dwellings. As in other cities, typhoid had become endemic by the 1870s and was a more lethal threat then than the automobile in the mid-twentieth century (Sinclair 1975: 154).

Infant mortality

Sydney, Melbourne and London had the same order of infant death rates until the early 1890s, after which those of Sydney and Melbourne fell below those of London but the gap was not great. High infant mortality from diarrhoeal disease was as common in Australia as in Europe. In Sydney, 1875–1900, mortality from diarrhoea was usually around 32 per 1,000 births. During the 1880s and 1890s, London's infant diarrhoeal death rate averaged about 23 per 1,000 live births. But mortality returned under diarrhoea was only the most obvious aspect. In contemporary Third World countries, diarrhoea and malnutrition interact to decimate infant life. A similar problem of weanling diarrhoea existed in nineteenth-century Sydney (and other western cities), although it was perhaps not as great as in poor countries today (Armstrong 1905: 395; Central Board of Health 1885: 17; Meyer 1921: 19; Newsholme 1935: 351; Scrimshaw *et al.* 1968: 253).

Public health legislation

The first Public Health Act passed was modelled on the famous 1848 English Act. Passed in Victoria in 1854, it created a Central Board of Health. Smallpox in New Zealand, Victoria and New South Wales (NSW) persuaded Queensland in 1872 to provide for a temporary board if a 'formidable' epidemic threatened. The next year South Australia passed an Act providing for a range of measures to prevent the spread of 'epidemic, endemic or contagious disease'. However, it was the example of the English Public Health Act (1875) and the spur of smallpox epidemics that gave rise to a plethora of legislation: in NSW, the Infectious Diseases Supervision Act (1881), the Dairies Supervision Act (1886) and a comprehensive Public Health Act (1896). In Victoria, the existing Act was amended in 1883 to provide for notification of 'malignant, infectious or contagious disease', while the long-standing problem of excessive illness and deaths from typhoid prompted legislators to enact the Public Health Act (1889). In South Australia, an Act was passed in 1884 providing for notification and isolation of cases of smallpox, cholera, plague and yellow fever. Queensland also passed new legislation in 1884. Western Australia passed a new Act in 1886 as a result of an official inquiry into the appalling sanitary condition of Perth. Tasmania enacted the main legislation of this era in 1885 (Lewis 1989: 6).

One clear difference from the English administrative system was the supervision exercised from the centre because of the comparative weakness of local government. Lacking funds and administrative skills, and, often, the resolve to act against local interests, local government in Australia had to be controlled by the colonial/state health authorities.

Did the building of sewerage systems markedly influence the course of typhoid mortality? The typhoid death rate began to decline more than seven years before houses were first connected in Melbourne in 1897. Moreover, the Victorian decline from about 1890 was occurring in extra-metropolitan areas as well. The construction of sewerage systems in Sydney in the 1880s, and in Perth in the 1900s, coincided with the beginning of the downward trend in each city. Adelaide obtained sewers in the early 1880s but the typhoid death rate is not available until the 1890s so little can be said about this city. In Hobart the decline began a few years before a sewerage system was constructed in the second decade of the twentieth century. Progress in sanitation, better drainage and safer water supplies would seem to be the most likely causes of the decline from about 1890. But sewerage reinforced the existing downward trend (Cumpston 1989: 234–237).

Professionalization of public health

The first modern public health professional was John Ashburton Thompson. In 1896, as NSW chief medical officer, he embarked upon the construction of an up-to-date public health service.[1] He won international recognition for his epidemiological publications on leprosy and bubonic plague. The coming of bubonic plague to Sydney in 1900 enabled Thompson to contribute significantly to aetiological understanding of plague which was still unclear about the role of the rat flea. His war on rats contained the epidemic. From Hong Kong in 1894, bubonic plague had spread to Bombay in 1896 and in the 1900s was in Europe, and, for the first time, in Japan, the Americas, South Africa and Australia.

Thompson insisted medical staff possess a postgraduate diploma of public health or equivalent. W. G. Armstrong and Robert Dick, the new medical officers of health for Sydney and Newcastle respectively, conducted courses for sanitary inspectors from 1898. The first Royal Sanitary Institute examination was held in 1900. Impressed by the NSW initiative, other Australian states and New Zealand instituted such examinations ('Public Health' 1897: 359; Report of Medical Officer of Health to Metropolitan Combined Districts 1900: 9; Armstrong 1925: 97–100; Rosen 1977: 60–61). The University of Melbourne offered a diploma of public health from 1906. The University of Sydney also offered a diploma of public health, awarding it occasionally from 1910 (Russell 1977: 103; Young et al. 1984: 401).

Public health development to World War I

In 1914, the NSW Labor government raised the status of public health by appointing the first Minister for Public Health and creating the post of Director General of Public Health. Between 1898 and 1914, the central administration increased its inspectorial and professional staff from 15 to 86. Like NSW, Queensland was affected by plague. Although plague died out in 1909, that state's Health Department maintained its examination of rats until 1916, after which it became the duty of local authorities. The Health Act (1900) provided for a full-time commissioner of public health. As elsewhere in the Western world, Victoria set up machinery to apply bacteriological knowledge to control of infectious diseases. The authorities established a public health laboratory in the University of Melbourne's Department of Bacteriology in mid-1897. The Pasteur Institute in Paris had only been established in 1887. A Microbiological Laboratory was established in NSW in 1897, and a Bacteriological Institute set up in Queensland in 1899. Similar facilities were created in the other Australian states early in the new century (Cummins 1979: 189; 'Health Administration in Victoria' 1935: 1190; Woodgyer and Forsyth 1997: iii).

Food surveillance

Health authorities in Australia sought to make the urban milk supply safer by attention to the hygiene of dairies and retailers and the health of dairy cattle. Where in 1901, 12% of Sydney diaries were classified as in bad condition, in 1910, about 1% were so classified. From 1903, the use of chemical preservatives to control growth of bacteria in milk was regulated. Declining numbers of tuberculous animals from metropolitan herds destroyed between 1901 and 1913 *prima facie* indicate a declining incidence of diseased beasts.

Victoria's Meat Supervision Act (1900), Milk and Dairy Supervision Act (1905) and Pure Food Act (1905) reflected a shift in thinking about control from focusing on adulteration (with water and excessive amounts of chemicals) in public health legislation to specific legislation on food purity. The first Act introduced expert inspection of the whole beast at slaughter. The second transferred regulation of dairies from local councils to the more reliable hands of the State Agriculture Department. One indicator of improvement is that the proportion of udder tuberculosis to total tuberculosis fell from almost 72% in 1906–1907 to just over 6% in 1913–1914. The Pure Food Act provided for a Food Standards Committee to advise on the standards required for commonly used foods and drugs. The NSW Pure Food Act (1908) strengthened the Board of Health's capacity to eliminate adulteration. South Australia's Food and Drugs Act came into operation in 1909, while Tasmania followed with a Food and Drugs Act in 1910. Western Australia's Health Act (1911) created an advisory committee. Similarly, Queensland relied on provisions in its general Health Act (1911) to control the quality and purity of food (Cumpston 1989: 400–403; Lewis 1976: 61).

The interventionist state

In 1901, the six colonies came together as the Commonwealth of Australia. In the first decade of the new nation's life, the Liberals pursued a national policy of protection of the European nature of the population, manufacturing industries and the standard of living. For six decades, all political parties supported an immigration policy involving exclusion of Asians and Pacific Islanders (the 'White Australia' policy) because of concern about race and fear of competition from cheap labour. Industry received protection in return for providing reasonable wages for European workers. A third pillar of policy was compulsory arbitration in industrial disputes. When in government, Labour extended the Liberals' nation-building and industrial measures (Crowley 1974: 274–307).

Ideological influences on public health

Liberal and Labor alike were influenced by larger ideological currents. Although Labor simply sought a greater share of the product of a capitalist economy, not fundamental social change, British Fabian ideas of state socialism had some influence. Michael Roe has suggested American Progressivism best exemplifies the dominant ideology of this era in Australia as in the rest of the 'Anglo-Saxon' world. A meritocracy pursuing the common good would civilize capitalism and apply scientific solutions to social and economic problems. The successful use of bacteriology to prevent disease was a marvellous justification for the Progressives' faith in applied science. With their belief in the superiority of the Anglo-Saxon race, they were deeply concerned with 'racial health'. A key issue in 'the health of the race' was the decline in the birth rate. The quantity and quality of population came to be seen as a vital aspect of power in the competition between nations and empires. Infant and maternal health became a primary concern in part because of this larger issue (Goodwin 1966: 370–371; McBriar 1966: 74–75; Roe 1984: 7–14).

The event which heightened public awareness of infant health was the NSW Royal Commission on the Birth Rate of 1903–1904, which linked Australia's future as a 'white' power in the Pacific to population growth. Indeed, W. G. Armstrong began the first organized infant health work in Australia while the Commission was in progress. The core message for the mother was to breastfeed. Other public health doctors and lay enthusiasts in the other capital cities initiated infant health work. Isabel Younger Ross and Constance Ellis led the movement to create infant clinics in working-class Melbourne from 1917. In Queensland, the preferred approach initially was distribution of clean milk to poor mothers. While Western Australia lacked an infant health centre until the 1920s, it shared in the national decline in infant mortality in the early 1900s (Mein Smith 1990: 117–121; Raftery 1995: 71–72). This major turning point occurred in the early 1900s just when the first public health interventions (in Sydney) were beginning so they cannot account for the sudden nationwide decline, although the subsequent clinic and educational interventions undoubtedly reinforced the downward trend in mortality due to other factors.

School health services

In 1907, medical inspections of Sydney and Newcastle schoolchildren were carried out. By 1919, the staff consisted of 11 medical officers, 12 dental officers, 6 dental assistants and 7 nurses. The medical inspection schemes in the various states unearthed a great deal of chronic, if usually minor, disease. However, the services were restricted by poor funding and a focus on diagnosis. Treatment was normally to be provided by the child's own doctor (a provision which disadvantaged children from poorer families). The medical profession guarded the preserves of private practice. Thus, in 1914, the NSW Education Department created a small travelling clinic for children in remote areas. In 1916 special meetings of doctors decided to oppose appointments to the clinic. Provision of treatment ceased. As late as 1931, the NSW Director of Maternal and Baby Welfare said he would prevent infant clinic nurses from providing therapeutic advice (as opposed to health education). The clinics' work was similarly constrained in other States (Cumpston 1989: 122–125; 'Baby Clinics' 1931: 792; 'Public Health in Victoria' 1954: 20; Thame 1974: 233).

The Commonwealth and health

The Commonwealth's powers in health were limited to quarantine. But with World War I over, enthusiast for preventive medicine J. H. L. Cumpston, federal director of quarantine, pressed the Commonwealth to take complete control of public health. The states would not transfer powers. Establishment of a Federal Health Department was finally secured by the 1921 visit to Australia of V. G. Heiser, representative in the Far East of the Rockefeller Foundation's International Health Board, whom Cumpston had met while visiting the Philippines in 1905. Heiser offered to finance training of Australians in public health to fill the leading posts. Cumpston became foundation Commonwealth Director General of Health.

Tropical medicine had from the late 1870s in European countries and their empires been developing to serve the economic and political interests of imperial governments, and only secondarily the health of indigenes. As early as 1902, the Australasian Medical Congress had called for a School of Tropical Medicine to tackle health problems faced by Europeans developing the tropical north. The focus on the tropics continued to be significant until the late 1920s when research showed whites could safely work in the north and when J. S. C. Elkington, a great proponent of tropical medicine, left the Federal Health Department. He had strongly supported the idea of his colleague R. W. Cilento of a Tropical Medical Service covering Queensland, the Northern Territory, Papua and New Guinea, the British Solomon Islands and the New Hebrides. The service was to be a forward defence against importation of communicable diseases from the Pacific. The second defence was exclusion from 'Fortress Australia' of non-European immigrants under the 'White Australia' policy. But the main focus of the Commonwealth's interests had shifted to the temperate southern part of the continent where the vast majority of European Australians lived, and the service was not established. The Federal Health Department acted as an epidemiological intelligence centre in the Austral-Pacific area for the League of Nations Health Organization, Geneva and the Office International d'Hygiene Publique, Paris (Cumpston 1989: 417; Hone 1920: 273–275; Lewis 1989: 11–12, 25).

The Royal Commission on Health

After strong lobbying by Cumpston and his allies, in 1925 a federal royal commission on Health was set up. Its two most important recommendations were the creation of a federal health council to facilitate Commonwealth-state administrative cooperation and a national public health scheme to be directed by the Commonwealth. The grand plan for a national public health scheme was not implemented. All that resulted from the Royal Commission was the rather anaemic Federal Health Council which held its first meeting in 1927. The basic problem was that the states too often rejected Commonwealth proposals, seeing them as threats to their sovereignty in health matters (Gillespie 1991: 43–45; Lewis 1989: 12–13).

A National School of Public Health

The Commonwealth and states approved a Royal Commission proposal for a school to train medical officers of health which opened at Sydney University in 1930. The plans for the School of Public Health were much influenced by the example of the London School of Hygiene and Tropical Medicine. In this sense it was indirectly the product of the Rockefeller Foundation's policy of funding public health schools across the world. Entomological and parasitological surveys of diseases like malaria in North Queensland, Papua, and New Guinea became established aspects of the research programme. During World War II, the school's staff provided invaluable assistance to the Allied military forces concerning disease control (Lee 1980: 13–18).

A National Health Research Council

The Royal Commission on Health had called for a health research council. The National Health and Medical Research Council (NHMRC) emerged in 1936 as a compromise between the objectives of the medical profession and those of Cumpston and his allies. Cumpston believed research and its applications should be closely related so public health practice and administration were made central to the work of the Council ('A Medical Research Council' 1928: 529; 'A Medical Research Council for Australia' 1935: 497; Gillespie 1991: 51; Lewis 1989: 15–16).

Infant and maternal health

The infant death rate declined slowly from almost 31 per 1,000 live births in 1906–1910 to just over 26 per 1,000 in 1936–1940. It fell to just above 19 in 1946–1950. From the 1920s, reduction of neonatal mortality had been the focus of public health concern and it was linked by experts to wider access to antenatal care and safer obstetrics. While there was a historic shift from home to hospital delivery in the interwar period, antenatal care for most mothers remained inadequate. There were some public clinics for the poorer woman or outpatient services for those booked into a public hospitals in urban areas. Only with the appointment of professors of obstetrics did medical graduates emerge in the 1930s with the capacity to give this care properly (Mein Smith 1990: 302–307).

The maternal mortality rate showed no inclination to fall. The point of transition came in the later 1930s when the sulfonamides dramatically reduced deaths from puerperal sepsis. In Australian cities, the same technical factors bringing down mortality across the Western world in the 1940s were present – penicillin, blood transfusion services and specialist care for patients otherwise unable to afford it (Lewis 1992: 42; Loudon 1992: 23–28).

Control of tuberculosis and venereal disease

In the period up to about 1880, colonial governments did not concern themselves with TB control. Inadequate financial support for working class sufferers was the weakest part of early control schemes. It was not adequately addressed until after World War II. Institutional facilities were also quite inadequate. Public health doctors and medical specialists had spearheaded the development of control facilities in the 1920s but they had failed to promote much growth in the 1930s (Thame 1974: 23, 89–109; Walker 1983: 440–453).

A powerful stimulus to official action concerning VD was the threat of high infection rates among Australian troops returning from overseas in World War I presented to the civilian population. In 1915, the Commonwealth urged the states to introduce compulsory notification. Western Australia introduced legislation establishing compulsory notification; treatment defaulters (treatments were prolonged and unpleasant) could be compelled to resume treatment; free care was provided; knowingly communicating VD and the provision of treatment by persons not medically qualified were made illegal; and anyone suspected of being infected could be detained for examination. The Commonwealth offered 15,000 pounds on a matching basis to the states to help establish a clinic system. Between 1916 and 1920, other states passed legislation like that of Western Australia (Lewis 1998a: 232–233; Thame 1974: 135–152, 163–168, 211). But Robert Dick, a senior NSW public health doctor, pointed out that in larger cities like Sydney, 'compulsory notification was a hopeless procedure' (quoted in Lewis 1998a: 229) because doctors were reluctant to report such stigmatizing infections and patients too often gave false names and addresses.

Mass immunisation

With the introduction of an effective toxoid in the 1920s, diphtheria control became possible. At first only administered to case contacts, from the early 1930s, it was employed in school immunization programmes. But substantial control only came with the widespread immunization of infants in the 1940s and 1950s. While immunization campaigns were a significant cause of the decline in mortality and morbidity from diphtheria, non-specific factors that contributed to the fall were improved nutrition and the advent of the small family contributed (Feery 1981: 174; Thame 1974: 74–83).

A national health service

In 1941, the NHMRC endorsed a report on a national health service by a subcommittee consisting of Cumpston, Cilento, J. N. Morris (the British Medical Association in Australia) and Harold Dew (the Royal Australasian College of Surgeons) calling for: a national system of hospitals and clinics staffed by salaried doctors; official supervision of the preventive work of private practitioners; and taxes, not national insurance, to fund the service.

The Federal Labor Government began in 1943 to address post-war planning. The centre of health planning moved from the NHMRC (and the Joint Parliamentary Committee on Social Security) to the Treasury as the objective changed from 'socialization' to payment of cash benefits to citizens who would purchase services from private practitioners. This also meant the end of the ambitions of Cumpston and colleagues to shift the balance of the health system from the curative to the preventive side. The Liberal attorney-general of Victoria in 1945 pursued an action in the High Court concerning the Commonwealth's Pharmaceutical Benefits Act (1944), claiming it was beyond the powers of the Commonwealth (a claim the court accepted); and the Commonwealth's expenditure power only concerned matters falling within its legislative, executive and judicial capacity. The government felt obliged to seek by referendum in 1946 constitutional power over social and health services. The referendum conferred power to provide medical and dental services (but not so as to authorize any form of civil conscription). The restriction on its power over medical services was accepted by the Labor government because it wanted to demonstrate it would not exercise compulsion. The restriction was used by the profession to prevent implementation of the second Pharmaceutical Benefits Act (1947).

The claim of the opposition parties and business interests that the government's policy of bank and airline nationalization was socialism by stealth was easily extended to socialized medicine. The NHMRC plan for a salaried service bringing together preventive and curative medicine disappeared in the struggle between a now united profession and the government over doctors' autonomy. Labor's National Health Service Act (1948–1949) provided for regional clinics to do preventive work, but only remote areas would have a salaried service and the great bulk of the population would continue to be served by fee-for-service, private practitioners. The opposition and the profession rejected the legislation. The Liberal-Country Party government came to power in 1949 and introduced its own national health service which involved federal subsidization of citizens who took out private insurance with which to pay for fees for services (Gillespie 1991: 131–154, 185–193, 224–249; Lewis 1989: 18–22).

Public health problems in the 1950s and 1960s

In the six decades from 1945, it is possible to identify three main public health strategies: the medical; the lifestyle; and the 'new public health' approach. Two examples of the medical approach are the campaigns against tuberculosis and poliomyelitis. A national campaign against tuberculosis using mass radiography was initiated under the Commonwealth Tuberculosis Act (1945–1948). Mortality declined from 24.8 per 100,000 population in 1949 to 2.7 in 1966, although a secular decline had been occurring since the late nineteenth century. By 1976, when the Commonwealth announced it would cease to fund the states, Australia had moved to a position of international best practice in control of TB (Boag 1976: 8–12; 'Compulsory Mass X-Ray Surveys: The Future' 1971: 61–62; Palmer and Short 1994: 206–215; 'The Control of Tuberculosis in Australia' 1960: 225; 'Tuberculosis and Complacency' 1967: 459–460).

The first reported epidemic of poliomyelitis took place in South Australia in 1895. The last great epidemic occurred in 1949–1956 during which time a total of 16,000 cases nationwide were reported. The Commonwealth supplied, free of charge, Salk vaccine to the states, and mass immunization began in mid-1956.

From 1967, the oral Sabin replaced the injected Salk vaccine. No case of polio due to a wild virus was reported from 1986 (Buxton 1977: 18–22, 62–64; Cleland and Ferguson 1913: 262–264; Cumpston 1989: 326; Herceg and Hall 1995: 399–400; Patrick 1987: 239–240).

The second epidemiological transition

In Australia, public health began to respond to chronic, non-communicable diseases in the 1950s and 1960s. As the wealth of Western countries increased, so the incidence of coronary heart disease rose. Mortality rose markedly after World War II. But from the 1970s it declined sharply in West European and North American countries, and in Australia. By 1993, heart disease mortality had declined by 66%, and stroke mortality by over 70%. Both prevention and treatment contributed to the decline, although the precise contribution of each is unclear (Magnus 1996: 517–518; Marmot and Mustard 1994: 189–200).

Cancer and smoking

Male cancer mortality increased slowly from the 1900s to 1950, from when a sustained linear increase occurred to the mid-1980s. The increase was almost wholly due to expanding lung cancer mortality. From the late 1980s, it began to fall. Since the 1960s, female lung cancer mortality has continued to rise (NHMRC 1997: 2; Taylor *et al*. 1998b: 42).

In 1962, the Australian Medical Association, the Royal Australasian College of Physicians, the Royal Australasian College of Surgeons, the Australian College of General Practitioners and the Anti-Cancer Council of Victoria expressed support for the report of the Royal College of Physicians on smoking and health. They urged the Federal Government to introduce an education programme and restrict advertising. In 1969, the NHMRC proposed warnings on cigarette packets, control of advertising and a campaign about the dangers of smoking. In 1980, the Liberal-National Party Government decided to implement some of the recommendations of a Senate inquiry including having the tar and nicotine content stated on packets.

In 1979, the Movement Opposed to the Promotion of Unhealthy Products was established. It called for prohibition of all advertising and sports promotion by tobacco companies. Billboard Utilizing Graffitists Against Unhealthy Promotions was started in 1979, and members frequently defaced poster advertisements for cigarettes. In 1972, some Liberal members of Federal Parliament had had legislation passed requiring television and radio advertisements to carry a warning that smoking is a health hazard.

In 1987, the Victorian Labor government imposed a tax on tobacco products to fund the Victorian Health Promotion Foundation. Governments in some other jurisdictions followed suit: Foundation SA in 1988, the Australian Capital Territory Health Promotion Fund in 1989 and Healthway in Western Australia in 1991. These bodies provided funds for sponsorship of sports and cultural activities, replacing tobacco companies' funding (NHMRC 1997: 4–9; Walker 1984: 97–112).

Tobacco use fell steadily in the 1980s and early 1990s, but with the decline stalling in the mid-1990s, public health workers called for new initiatives. In 1996, new Federal Health Minister Dr Michael Wooldridge promised to introduce fresh measures to reduce smoking prevalence. Recognizing the gains to be had from pooling the expertise in different jurisdictions, the federal government funded a National Tobacco Campaign (NTC). Coordinated by the Federal Health Department, the NTC commenced in mid-1997. It proved to be the longest-running, Australian, anti-tobacco campaign, with the states and territories meeting the costs of the greater demand for local smoking-cessation services generated by the federal government's mass media advertising (Hill and Carroll 2003: ii 9).

Traffic accidents

In 1971 Victoria introduced legislation on compulsory use of seat belts in vehicles, and within a year all states and territories had done the same thing. In 1976 random breathalyser testing (RBT) of drivers was introduced. RBT was introduced in the 1980s in the other jurisdictions. The mandatory use of bicycle helmets was brought in between 1990 and 1992. The success of anti-drink driving measures is shown by the fact that, nationally, the percentage of fatally injured drivers and motor cyclists with a blood alcohol concentration of 0.05 or over fell from 44 in 1981 to 30 in 1995. A multi-pronged approach to road safety has, historically, been the key to reduction of mortality and morbidity. A combination of legislation, education and strict enforcement has worked well (NHMRC 1997: 15–21; Report of Royal Commission into Sale, Supply, Disposal or Consumption of Liquor in State of Victoria 1964–1965: 949–994; Room 1988: 430).

Alcohol and other drugs

As early as 1872, Victoria enacted legislation providing for medical treatment of inebriates. But it was the 1890s and early 1900s which saw considerable legislative action across Australia. In the first flush of official enthusiasm, some effort was made to make available specialist treatment facilities. Enthusiasm had waned by the 1920s in part because 'cures' were notoriously difficult to obtain (Garton 1987: 43–44; McCarthy 1888: 9–12; 'The Treatment of Inebriates' 1906: 481).

In 1961, the *Medical Journal of Australia* noted Australia had an estimated 300,000 'problem' drinkers. Doctors themselves were showing renewed concern. New services were being set up in hospitals like the Royal Brisbane Hospital, St Vincent's Hospital, Sydney, and the Alfred and the Royal Melbourne Hospitals. Specialist centres were opened: Langton Clinic in Sydney in 1959, Wacol Clinic in Brisbane in 1965 and St Anthony's Hospital in Adelaide in 1968. There was a spate of new legislation, and the central proposition was alcohol abuse was a disease to be cured.

By the 1970s, a preventive approach was being advocated as an alternative to a curative one. The Western Australia Honorary Royal Commission on alcohol and drug dependence observed in 1973 that one of the key factors blocking progress was the fact that there was no clearly successful treatment. By the late 1980s, a consensus was established that fiscal measures and reduction of availability, supplemented by mass education campaigns, was the royal road to victory ('Alcoholism' 1961: 55; Paton 1985: 1; Report of Honorary Royal Commission to Inquire into Treatment of Alcohol and Drug Dependants in Western Australia 1973: 52; Stoltz 1978: 227–243; Wodak 1986: 1–2).

The federal government became concerned in the 1950s about Australia's high per capita consumption of heroin, which was due mainly to medical use for pain control. It banned importation in mid-1953. In the course of the 1960s, illegal drug use increased markedly. Cannabis became a prohibited drug in 1966. All states now punished trafficking as a separate offence.

Between 1969 and 1980, five official inquiries took place into the non-medical use of drugs. Only one, the Senate Standing Committee on Social Welfare inquiry 1974–1977, looked at alcohol and tobacco. But all were concerned with illegal use. The federal government announced in 1980 support for the committee's recommendation that a national strategy concerning the dangers of alcohol, tobacco, analgesics and illegal drugs be developed. In alcohol policy, the government supported overall reduction of consumption, but remained vague about how it would intervene. In the middle of the 1984 federal election campaign, the Labor Prime Minister, R. J. L. Hawke, promised to initiate a National Campaign against Drug Abuse (NCADA).

A draft national alcohol policy had already been put together in 1984. After NCADA came into existence in 1985, the objective of harm minimization was widely accepted. But the alcohol industry argued health education alone was enough, ignoring environmental determinants like price and availability.

In early 1988, South Australia, the leading wine-producing state, expressed reservations about those areas dealing with availability, pricing and advertising. In 1989 the Ministerial Council on Drug Strategy accepted a modified version of the draft policy. South Australia had had two offending sections of the draft removed. But at least governments had committed themselves to harm minimization; accepted harm arose from normal as well as heavy drinking; and acknowledged advertising, availability and pricing were as important as education and treatment in control of alcohol abuse.

The second evaluation of NCADA, in 1992, recommended it continue as the National Drug Strategy (NDS). The Ministerial Council on Drug Strategy in 1992 agreed to raise the share of funding for law enforcement to 10%. The NDS Plan (1993–1997) identified three goals: minimization of the level of disease and death; of drug-related crime and violence; and of the level of personal and social disruption, and economic losses.

Between 1985 and 1995, the prevalence of smoking by males fell from 40% to 30% while female prevalence fell from 30% to 26%. The prevalence in males had been falling since 1945 so too much cannot be made of the impact of the national campaigns. Probably too much cannot be made of the effect of the national campaigns on the downward trend in alcohol consumption from the early 1980s because the trend began before they commenced. The campaigns appear to have had no moderating effect on cannabis consumption.

Two international experts, Eric Single and Timothy Rohl, who reviewed the NDS at the end of the 1990s believed it should support development of new treatments rather than established services; harm minimization had proved influential in bringing about a more consistent national approach to drug problems; but inadequate coordination of planning between Commonwealth and states had led to a situation where at least 50% of funds eventually went to support established treatment facilities (Drug Problems in Australia: An Intoxicated Society? 1977: 12; Hawks 1989: 9–16; Manderson 1993: 117–159, 170–172; National Health Policy on Alcohol 1989: 6–8; Single and Rohl 1997: vii–viii, 3–66).

The community health centre concept

Dr Sidney Sax, who had been impressed by Sidney Kark's experiments with community health services in South Africa, was made chairman of a NSW committee on the care of the aged. Sax in 1965 proposed development of community services at two levels – at local level, personal services like home aides and at regional level, general practitioner and other services.

In 1971, the first community health centre was opened. In mid-1972, the second centre was opened in Blacktown, a socially disadvantaged, outer suburb of Sydney. At the end of 1972, a community centre was opened to provide services for an inner city population – the Glebe Community Care Centre. It functioned in close association with the Community Care Teaching Unit of Royal Prince Alfred Hospital, a teaching hospital of the University of Sydney. There are other examples of community-based centres which predate the national programme. In mid-1971, members of Sydney's Aboriginal community set up the Aboriginal Medical Service in Redfern, an inner city, low-income suburb (Crouch and Coulton 1983: 17–20; Fagan 1984: 20; Raftery 1995: 22–23; Sax 1984: 103).

A National Community Health Program

Soon after the Whitlam Labor Government assumed office in 1972 (this government ended all discrimination on grounds of race, colour or nationality in immigration, burying the White Australia policy, although restrictions had been easing since the 1960s), two bodies were established to carry out health policy: the Health Insurance Commission to introduce the universal insurance scheme, Medibank; and the Hospitals and Health Services Commission (HHSC), charged with increasing the supply of services. Yet, the government's financial support for community services was minor compared with its support for universal health insurance, although it needs to be said while Medibank underwrote 'sickness' care and reinforced the predominant, fee-for-service, private practice system, the clear constitutional (and probably political) barriers to 'nationalization' of the medical profession (discussed above) meant greater equity had to be pursued within the existing private practice system. Also, with the luxury of hindsight, we can see the HHSC was unclear about how to advance health status. Although reference was made to the effect of the social environment on health, the HHSC appears to have intended to use mainly the individualistic patient–doctor relationship to promote prevention. The Australian Medical Association (AMA) saw the community centres having only a supportive role in relation to the general practitioner and was opposed to salaried medical practice in centres. The socially progressive Doctors' Reform Society warmly supported the programme whereas the conservative General Practitioners Society opposed it (*Review of the Community Health Program* 1976: 29–45; Sax 1984: 101–103, 141–142).

Community medicine

The 1973 report of the interim committee of the HHSC had called for courses in community medicine. In 1976, Ian Webster was appointed foundation professor of community medicine at the University of New South Wales. Webster noted community medicine had existed in medical practice for some time whether as public health, social medicine or preventive medicine. But it had been separated from mainstream medicine. In 1975, Charles Bridges-Webb had been appointed to the foundation chair of community medicine at the University of Sydney. His department was focused on the education of general practitioners (Bridges-Webb 1979: 65; Webster 1979: 38–40).

The states and the programme

The NSW Liberal government was suspicious of the Whitlam government's health policy. Yet it allowed the Health Commission to work with the Community Health Program. A major constraint was its understanding with the AMA that no general practitioner services would be provided by centres in order that the salaried doctors did not compete with private practitioners. The Victorian conservative government would not allow centres to open. Commonwealth funds were then forwarded directly to community groups. Later, the Victorian government assumed responsibility for the programme. The conservative Queensland government willingly accepted Commonwealth funding, using it mainly to develop existing health services. The conservative government in Western Australia made a similar response. In South Australia and Tasmania where Labor was in power, a range of initiatives (including centres employing salaried doctors) were introduced.

The conservative Fraser government took power at the federal level in the mid-1970s, with the national economy in recession. Although it promised to preserve the programme with its 350 health centres, it effectively ended federal funding by mid-1981 (Palmer and Short 1994: 120–121; *Review of the Community Health Program* 1976: 30–35).

Evaluation of the programme

Preventive services played a relatively small role in the overall functioning of most community centres, said Lindsay Davidson, principal of the School of Public

Health, University of Sydney, reporting on health promotion in Australia in 1979. In 1986, an Australian Community Health Association review made two major observations. First, the services had become solidly established. Second, community health had become reduced to an illness-oriented service. To a large extent, the original objectives of primary prevention and community participation had been lost to sight. However, in retrospect it is clear health education and promotion received unprecedented recognition and the ground was prepared for the coming of the 'new public health' (Cohen 1987: 11; Davidson *et al*. 1979: 101; Palmer and Short 1994: 124–126; Raftery 1995: 30–34).

Health promotion

In 1978, in an environment of rising health-care costs, the Federal Health Minister, Ralph Hunt, had announced an inquiry by Lindsay Davidson into health education, promotion and prevention. Davidson recommended national objectives for health promotion be established; a national health promotion centre be created; and the Commonwealth fund research. The only fruit of the Davidson inquiry was the Fraser government's commitment of AUD 500,000 to a media campaign encouraging individuals to change to healthier lifestyles. In 1984, the NHMRC produced *Towards a National Policy on Health Promotion*, identifying a number of areas where national goals needed to be set. The AMA had released a report on health education in 1981, basically advocating production of literature for doctors and the public (Davidson *et al*. 1979: 48–49, 93–124, 192–195, 230–236; Milio 1986: 427–430; NHMRC Community Health Promotion and Education Standing Committee 1984: 2–4). As noted above, in 1987–1991, Victoria, South Australia, the ACT and Western Australia established health promotion foundations that successfully worked to reduce tobacco industry influence on hearts and minds.

In 1985, Neal Blewett, the Federal Health Minister, established the Better Health Commission as Australia's response to the WHO's Health for All by the Year 2000 policy. In an historic report (1986), it proposed setting national goals and targets in three areas – cardiovascular disease, nutrition and injury. Among its strategies the only identifiably new public health proposal was for a national community development fund to assist local communities in health advocacy. In 1987, the Health Targets and Implementation Committee was established to devise strategies to attain these goals. It drew up Australia's first set of national goals and targets for three areas – population groups, major causes of illness and death, and risk factors. It made use of new public health terminology but the focus was on more traditional prevention. The National Better Health Program came into being to implement the goals. When it was evaluated in 1992–1993, the programme was found to have much developed health promotion infrastructure and made real progress in injury prevention, health of older people, primary prevention of lung and skin cancer and secondary prevention of breast and cervical cancer, and prevention of high blood pressure and nutrition.

Don Nutbeam and colleagues in the Department of Public Health at Sydney University were commissioned to identify goals and targets for 2000. They focused on morbidity and mortality; healthy lifestyles and risk factors; health literacy; and healthy environments. The first two built on the earlier set of goals and targets. But the last two represented a move towards a new public health approach, encouraging people to include non-health factors like transport, and not just doctors and hospitals, when thinking about health. The review did act as a catalyst for inclusion of national goals and targets in the Medicare Agreements in 1993. However, the important but politically controversial new public health issue of the social and economic determinants of health was not seriously addressed (Better Health Commission 1986: vii–xv; Nutbeam 1997: 355–358; Milio 1986: 430; Palmer and Short 1994: 216–218; Wise and Nutbeam 1994: 9–10).

Public health as a profession

The Hawke Labor government decided to commission an overseas expert to review public health research and educational requirements. American academic Kerr White's 1986 recommendations were for: an Australian Academy of Health; the Australian Institute of Health to provide policy analysis; a National Centre for Health Statistics; a National Centre for Technology and Health Services Assessment; a National Centre for Epidemiology and Population Health; funding for academic appointments in public health; NHMRC scholarships in public health disciplines; the Medical Research Committee of the NHMRC to become the Health Research Committee; a Health Development Committee; and a range of other arrangements to promote public health education and research.

Following strong but unsuccessful opposition from some members of the public health professional community, in 1987 the public health functions of the national School of Public Health were transferred to the University of Sydney Faculty of Medicine. The Australian Institute of Health became a statutory authority. The National Centre for Epidemiology and Population Health was set up at the Australian National University. Sydney, Adelaide and Monash Universities expanded existing Master of Public Health (MPH) programmes. The University of Western Australia introduced an MPH course, while Queensland University provided Master's courses in tropical health. The James Cook University of North Queensland brought into being a Tropical Health Surveillance Unit. Newcastle University increased its postgraduate training capacity in clinical epidemiology. By 1992–1993, 21 institutions ran 29 MPH or related courses (Chapman and Leeder 1991: 432–433; Reid 1994: viii–ix; White 1986: 4–14).

Senior public health figure Tony Adams said of the post-Kerr White educational development, it was 'a flowering of public health' (Adams 1992: 99). On his return from America in the 1960s, Adams had sought to establish an equivalent of the long-established and influential American Public Health Association. In 1968, he convened a meeting where it was resolved to establish the Australian Society for Epidemiology and Research in Community Health (ASERCH). It held its first meeting in 1969. In 1974 a working party proposed the organization include New Zealand in its name. Then, the Australian and New Zealand Society for

Epidemiology and Research in Community Health (ANZSERCH) and APHA (the Australian Public Health Association, formed in 1969 from five State associations) amalgamated as ANZSERCH/APHA. In 1986, a motion was carried to change the name of the organization to Public Health Association of Australia and New Zealand (PHA/ANZ). After New Zealand formed its own public health association, the PHA became the Public Health Association of Australia (PHAA). The international role of the PHAA was expanding, especially in the Asia-Pacific region: for example, it worked with the Indonesian Public Health Association to strengthen this organization and helped Vietnam develop a national public health association (ASERCH Minutes 15 June 1968: 1–3; 20 August 1969: 1–2. Report of Meeting to Discuss Future of ASERCH 1974: 1; Minutes of AGM of ANZSERCH/APHA 1981: 3; Minutes of AGM of PHA/ANZ 1986: 1–3; PHAA Annual Report 1989–1990: 3–11; 1990–1991: 3–8; 1991–1992: 4–13).

The National Public Health Partnership

From a new public health perspective, partnerships between a variety of players are integral to the advancement of population health. Creation of the National Public Health Partnership (NPHP) in 1997 presented opportunities for better coordination of policy and administration. A series of vertical national health programmes had come into being in the 1980s and 1990s. These in effect produced barriers between the Commonwealth and the states, and between each other. As health outcomes and resource-allocative efficiency became important goals of the health system, the NPHP offered a chance to remove such barriers and move towards a more strategic approach to public health ('The National Public Health Partnership and Public Health Funding Agreements' 1997: 5; 'Introducing You to the National Public Health Partnership' 1997: 1–2).

The health of Aborigines

The first modern reports on Aboriginal health were those produced in 1911 by the Northern Territory Aboriginal Department. These noted the spread of syphilis and tuberculosis among Aborigines, and the practice of abortion, encouraged by local Chinese, that was resulting in widespread female sterility. In 1919–1920, a high level of infectious diseases and infant mortality was noted as Aborigines changed from nomadic to fringe-camp lifestyles. But, government health workers were more concerned with containing diseases in Aboriginal populations that might threaten Europeans than promoting the health of Aborigines for its own sake.

The NSW Aborigines Welfare Board reports of the 1940s and 1950s reveal whooping cough, influenza, measles, mumps and scabies regularly swept through the reserves. However, some improvements were occurring. High and low estimates of infant death rates among non-metropolitan Aborigines were: in 1950–1954, 90 and 72 per 1,000 live births respectively; and in 1960–1964, 76 and 61. Even so, the Aboriginal population had rates three to four times those of Australia as a whole. Aboriginal rates declined steadily in the 1970s as did childhood mortality rates. But since the 1970s, adult mortality from chronic disease, accidents and violence has been growing.

The National Aboriginal Health Strategy in the 1980s acknowledged sexually transmitted infections were a serious health problem. The key to their control and that of HIV/AIDS was community health services. When a national indigenous Australians' sexual health strategy (1996–1997 to 1998–1999) was developed, it supported a 'horizontal' approach in a primary health-care context because indigenous involvement was critical.

Alcohol abuse is responsible for about 10% of deaths. For some time, communities have pursued various self-help schemes like alcohol-free areas. Poor living conditions have been identified by official inquiries as health hazards since the early 1970s. At the end of the 1980s many, especially remote communities throughout the country, still lacked a safe water supply, let alone other basic amenities (Federal Race Discrimination Commissioner 1994: 1–5, 17–19; Lewis 1998a: 379–405; Miller and Torzillo 1996: 3–8; Moodie 1973: 48–116; National Aboriginal Health Strategy Working Party 1989: 7; *The National Indigenous Australians' Sexual Health Strategy* 1997: 2–3; Parry 1992: 34–42).

The Aborigine-run medical services have often been at odds with state health departments which see professional expertise as vital to programmes. In contrast, the Aboriginal services have cleaved to a belief in the health-promoting involvement of community members. Each has its strengths and weaknesses: for example, horizontal programmes (concerned with social, cultural and economic factors) may be better able in the long term to respond to multifactorial 'diseases' like alcohol abuse, but may make it difficult to pursue effective interventions with individuals in the short term. A persisting problem has been the institutionalized fragmentation of policy between Commonwealth and states (Brady 1999: 34–36; Kunitz 1994: 110–114; Kunitz and Brady 1995: 552–555).

HIV/AIDS

HIV/AIDS has been one of the most significant public health challenges Australia has had to confront. Under the able leadership of Federal Health Minister Dr Neal Blewett, a bipartisan approach to national policy was established early. Indeed, Australia was at the forefront internationally of initiatives in education and prevention. From 1985, with an American test available, universal blood donor screening was introduced. Free testing sites encouraged voluntary testing when compulsory testing might have deterred people from finding out their infection status. Later, needle exchange programmes were introduced. In the absence of a vaccine or cure, the focus was on prevention. In an innovative move, the federal government began direct funding of community-based organizations for educational work, even funding education of prostitutes.

A National Task Force had been set up in 1984 to guide the work of the medical and scientific communities. A National Advisory Committee, headed by magazine editor Ita Buttrose, advocated partnerships between high-risk people and the health authorities, and effective input by the former into policy development.

The Task Force, headed by haematologist David Penington, put priority on testing of high-risk people and wanted medical leadership. The gay community opposed compulsory testing, arguing it would further stigmatize gay men. By mid-1986, agreement was reached that testing would be voluntary. However, conflict erupted again in 1987 over the 'Grim Reaper' education campaign (involving graphic television images) aimed at the general public. The spread of HIV into the heterosexual community did not happen, but the campaign had the effect of justifying greater public funding for HIV/AIDS work.

Within medical circles, compulsory testing continued to be strongly supported. Victoria, Western Australia and South Australia established cooperative relations with their respective AIDS councils. NSW was rather slow to develop community-based programmes. Conservative governments in Tasmania and Queensland refused to work with their councils in educational work aimed at gay men. With the advent of Labor governments in both states at the close of the 1980s, cooperation with gays and greater efforts to educate schoolchildren were initiated.

The first national strategy (1989–1993) laid down six areas of action – education; prevention; treatment, care and counselling; community participation; research; and international cooperation. The federal opposition expressed general support for the strategy. The second national strategy (1993–1994 to 1995–1996) continued to focus on partnerships between governments, affected groups, and health and scientific professionals. Education and prevention remained the centrepieces. Male homosexual sex and injecting drug use continued to be the primary routes of spread at the close of the 1990s. Both the second and third national strategies enjoyed great success in containing the virus. The fourth national strategy was implemented in mid-1999 (Lewis 1998b: 8–12; Palmer and Short 1994: 238–241).

Australia and HIV/AIDS in the Asia-Pacific region

Government and community organizations became more and more involved in Asia and the Pacific in education, prevention, treatment and care work. Federal Health Minister Brian Howe pointed out in mid-1990 that in addition to supporting the WHO Global AIDS Program, Australia was contributing AUD 1 million a year for assistance programmes in Southeast Asia and the Western Pacific. He announced his department would host an international conference on AIDS in Asia and the Pacific.

By the early 1990s, Australia was providing more assistance to countries in the region – for example, the Australian International Development Assistance Bureau (AIDAB) was helping to fund the South Pacific Commission's AIDS and STD Prevention Project. This provided information, technical assistance, training and small grants to member states. AIDAB also gave bilateral aid to various countries, and through funds provided to the Australian Federation of AIDS Organizations was supporting two Pacific Island, non-governmental organization training courses plus a street outreach programme in one country.

At the beginning of the new millennium, good progress was being made against HIV/AIDS in Thailand and Cambodia, and the governments of China and

India were at last responding seriously to the massive problems each faced; but crises were looming in other Asian and Pacific nations. Former Federal Senator, Chris Puplick, Chair of the Australian National Council on AIDS, hepatitis C and Related Diseases, in 2002 observed that Australian aid programmes were already in place in China and Australian expertise still had more contributions to make there, as it did in Indonesia where the situation was 'close to being out of control'; Australia would have to do more for Papua New Guinea which in any case was on the verge of becoming a failed state. HIV/AIDS had become the greatest killer of young Port Moresby males.[2] By 2006, an estimated 2% of the adult population of Papua New Guinea was infected and 75% of people living with HIV in the Pacific resided in that country. In response to the deteriorating situation in such countries, the Foreign Minister, Alexander Downer, had announced in July 2004 that Australia would provide another AUD 300 million to be spent on HIV/AIDS programmes in the Asia-Pacific region (Lewis 1997: 270; Puplick 2002: 17; *The Australian* 12 July 2004, 2–3 December 2006).

Australia and the future of public health in the Asia-Pacific region

Clearly, management of HIV/AIDS is one area of public health strength that Australia will continue to share with countries of the region. Another is tobacco control after Asia in the 1990s became a focus of the global anti-smoking movement's attention as national markets were flooded with American cigarettes and smoking rates in the region rose rapidly. Indeed, half the world's smokers now live in Asia.

As a world leader in tobacco control measures, Australia has provided, at home and in Asian venues, cutting-edge training for public health workers from Asian and Pacific countries. In addition, Australia has helped pioneer research through the Australian and Asian Tobacco Documents Project at the School of Public Health, University of Sydney, into the influence of the transnational tobacco companies on anti-smoking policy in Asian countries (Knight and Chapman 2004a: ii 22–ii 23; Knight and Chapman 2004b: ii 30–ii 31; Mackay 2004: ii 1–ii 2; Woodward and Kawachi 2003: ii 1).

Finally, Australia has a population in which more nationalities are represented than the population of almost any other country in the world. The ethnic diversity is the legacy of two considerable migration waves that ended the historical Anglo-Celtic character of the population: the first, from the late 1940s, included migrants from Western and Southern Europe and North America; the second, from the mid-1970s, from Southeast and South Asia, the Middle East and Latin America. Since the introduction of multiculturalism into official health and welfare policy in the 1970s, health professionals, health authorities and non-governmental organizations have developed considerable expertise in delivering to different ethnic groups in Australia health care and public health in culturally sensitive ways (Lewis 2003: 259–260). Recently, it has been realized that people working in multicultural health in Australia, those involved in international health

Public health in Australia 243

initiatives, and those working in the home countries of migrants to Australia should meet more formally and more frequently to share knowledge and skills. For example, a health symposium entitled 'Working across Borders: Sharing Experience in Diversity: Health in Local and Global settings' was held in Sydney in mid-2005. Such initiatives promise to open up other fruitful lines of cooperation across a range of areas in public health between Australia and other countries in the Asia-Pacific region.[3] This policy of cooperation in areas from HIV/AIDS to tobacco control is as distant from the 'Fortress Australia' policy of the early twentieth century as today's open multiracial and multicultural society is from 'White Australia'.

Notes

1 In Australia public psychiatric services developed separately from public health services so mental health is not discussed here. Readers concerned with the history of mental health services and policy might want to consult Lewis (1988).
2 By 2005, globally, 40.3 million people had HIV/AIDS, of whom 17.5 million were women and 2.3 million were children under 15 years of age. The annual report of the Joint UN Programme on HIV/AIDS and the WHO said the epidemic was almost out of control in Indonesia and Pakistan; and 10,000 of the 11,200 cases reported in 21 Pacific nations were in Papua New Guinea, although the real figure for that country could be five times greater.

   There are currently an estimated 14,800 cases in Australia. Between 1995 and 2000 there was a reduction of 25% in cases, but since 2000 the number of cases has increased each year. By 2006, 10% to 18% of Sydney's gay male population were infected with HIV; so that this group has an infection rate of the same order as poor African countries struggling with the pandemic (*The Australian* 23 November 2005, 1 December 2006). Injecting drug use is driving the HIV epidemic in Indonesia (50% to 60% of new cases are the result of injecting drug use) and there may well be 2 million infected people by 2025 if efforts at prevention are not increased; of these, 145,000 will be located in Indonesia's New Guinea province (total population, 2.3 million) and in the case of that culturally distinct subsection of the largest Muslim nation in the world sexual transmission is the driver of the epidemic.

   Australia has provided AUD 37 million over five years for the Indonesia HIV/AIDS Prevention and Care Project which will be completed in 2007. The team leader, Tim Mackay, has recently said provision of clean needles and syringes to injecting drug users (to prevent spread of the virus) is an urgent priority (*The Sydney Morning Herald* 19–20 August 2006).
3 At the Asia-Pacific Economic Cooperation meeting in South Korea in late November 2005, the prime minister of Australia, John Howard, was reported as pointing out Australia had been playing a leading role in developing a coordinated regional response to the contemporary threat of an avian influenza epidemic. Having a record of dealing well with public health crises like HIV/AIDS, Australia wanted to share its expertise with its neighbours. Rapid response teams of experts would be trained to fly in to deal with outbreaks and prevent the spread of the infection. He pledged AUD 100 million over four years (in addition to AUD 41 million already committed) to fund WHO work and train health professionals in the region. He urged countries to be honest in reporting outbreaks and not to repeat China's mistake of attempting to hide infectious episodes caused by the SARS (severe acute respiratory syndrome) virus. SARS infected about 8,500 people but fewer than 1,000 died. In stark contrast an avian influenza-derived pandemic is estimated to cause 7.4 to 150 million deaths worldwide, depending on the infectivity of the virus. The World Bank concluded the SARS

outbreak of 2003 had caused a 2% decline in GDP in one quarter alone across Southeast and East Asia. This translated into a USD 7 billion loss in production. If the avian influenza virus exchanges genetic material with a human strain and the new virus is spread by person-to-person contact, the resulting influenza pandemic would cause a global loss of production of USD 500–USD 600 billion (when the morbidity and mortality projections developed for the United States by the Centers for Disease Control are applied worldwide) (Lokuge *et al.* 2005: 1; *The Australian* 23 November 2005; *The Sun-Herald* 20 November 2005).

References

'Alcoholism' (1961) *Medical Journal of Australia*, 1: 55–56.
'A Medical Research Council' (1928) *Medical Journal of Australia*, 1: 529–530.
'A Medical Research Council for Australia' (1935) *Medical Journal of Australia*, 1: 497–498.
Armstrong, W. G. (1905) 'Some Lessons from the Statistics of Infantile Mortality in Sydney', *Transactions of Australasian Medical Congress*: 385–395.
—— (1925) 'An eminent epidemiologist', *Health*, 3(4): 97–100.
ASERCH Minutes, 15 June 1968; 20 August 1969, Noel Butlin Archives, Australian National University, Canberra.
'Baby clinics' (1931) *Medical Journal of Australia*, 2: 792.
Basch, P. F. (1999) *Textbook of International Health*, New York: Oxford University Press.
Better Health Commission (1986) *Looking to Better Health*, Vol. 1, Final Report, Canberra: Australian Government Publishing Service.
Boag, T. C. (1976) 'Australia Wins Fight to Control Tuberculosis', *Health*, 26: 8–12.
Brady, M. A. (1999) 'Difference and Indifference: Australian Policy and Practice in Indigenous Substance Abuse', unpublished thesis, Australian National University, Canberra.
Bray, F. (2000) 'The Chinese Experience', in R. Cooter and J. Pickstone (eds), *Medicine in the Twentieth Century*, Amsterdam: Harwood Academic Publishers, 719–738.
Bridges-Webb, C. (1979) 'Community Medicine: Little Sister or Big Brother?', in R. Walpole (ed.), *Community Health in Australia*, Ringwood, Victoria: Penguin Books Australia, 63–72.
Buxton, A. J. G. (1977) 'Poliomyelitis in South Australia 1937–1956', unpublished thesis, University of Adelaide.
Caldwell, J. C. (2001) 'What Do We Know about Asian Population History? Comparisons of Asian and European Research', in Ts'ui-jung Liu, J. Lee, D. S. Reher, O. Saito and Wang Feng (eds), *Asian Population History*, Oxford: Oxford University Press, 3–23.
Central Board of Health (1885), *Report of the Board for 1885*, Melbourne: Government Printer.
Chapman, S. and Leeder, S. (1991) 'Public Health Services in Australia', in W. W. Holland, R. Detels and G. Knox (eds), *Oxford Textbook of Public Health*, Vol. 1, Oxford: Oxford University Press, 423–438.
Cleland, J. B. and Ferguson, E. W. (1913) 'Acute Anterior Poliomyelitis, Including Landry's Paralysis', in *Report of Director General of Public Health, New South Wales*, Sydney: Government Printer.
Cohen, M. (1987) 'Unintended Consequences of Medicine', *New Doctor*, 43: 11–13.
'Compulsory Mass X-Ray Surveys: The Future' (1971) *Medical Journal of Australia*, 2: 61–62.

Crouch, M. and Coulton, C. (1983) *The Course of Community Health in New South Wales, 1958–1982*, Kensington, New South Wales: School of Sociology, University of New South Wales.

Crowley, F. K. (1974) '1901–14', in F. K. Crowley (ed.), *A New History of Australia*, Melbourne: William Heinemann, 260–311.

Cummins, C. J. (1979) *A History of Medical Administration in New South Wales, 1788–1973*, Sydney: Government Printer.

Cumpston, J. H. L. (1989) *Health and Disease in Australia: A History* (ed. M. J. Lewis), Canberra: AGPS Press.

Davidson, L., Chapman, S. and Hull, C. (1979) *Health Promotion in Australia 1978–1979*, Canberra: Australian Government Publishing Service.

Denoon, D., Firth, S., Linnekin, J., Meleisea, M. and Nero, K. (1997) *The Cambridge History of the Pacific Islanders*, Cambridge: Cambridge University Press.

Drug Problems in Australia: An Intoxicated Society? Senate Standing Committee on Social Welfare Report (1977) Canberra: Australian Government Publishing Service.

Elson, R. E. (1992) 'International Commerce, the State and Society: Economic and Social Change', in N. Tarling (ed.), *The Cambridge History of Southeast Asia*, Vol. 2, *The Nineteenth and Twentieth Centuries*, Cambridge: Cambridge University Press, 131–195.

Fagan, T. (1984) 'The Aboriginal Medical Service', *New Doctor*, 34: 19–20.

Federal Race Discrimination Commissioner (1994) *Water. A Report on the Provision of and Sanitation in Remote Aboriginal and Torres Strait Islander Communities*, Canberra: Australian Government Publishing Service.

Feery, B. (1981) 'Impact of Immunization on Disease Patterns in Australia', *Medical Journal of Australia*, 2: 172–176.

Garton, S. (1987) ' "Once a Drunkard always a Drunkard": Social Reform and the Problem of "Habitual Drunkenness" in Australia, 1880–1914', *Historical Studies*, 53: 38–53.

Gillespie, J. A. (1991) *The Price of Health: Australian Governments and Medical Politics 1910–1960*, Cambridge: Cambridge University Press.

Goodwin, C. D. W. (1966) *Economic Inquiry in Australia*, Durham: Duke University Press.

Hawks, D. (1989) 'The Watering Down of Australia's Health Policy on Alcohol', Keynote Address to Winter School in the Sun: Lifestyles, Culture and Drugs Conference, Brisbane, 1989.

'Health Administration in Victoria 1834–1934' (1935) *Health Bulletin*, 42: 1, 190–192.

Herceg, A. and Hall, R. (1995) 'Polio Vaccination and Polio Eradication', *Medical Journal of Australia*, 163: 399–400.

Hill, D. and Carroll, T. (2003) 'Australia's National Tobacco Campaign', *Tobacco Control*, 12(3): ii 9.

Hone, F. S. (1920) 'The Teaching of Preventive Medicine to Medical Students', *Transactions of Australasian Medical Congress:* 273–275.

'Introducing You to the National Public Health Partnership' (1997) *National Public Health Partnership News*, 1: 1–2.

Knight, J. and Chapman, S. (2004a) ' "Asian Yuppies ... are always Looking for Something New and Different": Creating a Tobacco Culture among Young Asians', *Tobacco Control*, 13(4): ii 22–ii 29.

—— (2004b) ' "Asia is Now the Priority Target for the World Anti-Smoking Movement": Attempts by the Tobacco Industry to Undermine the Asian Anti-Smoking Movement', *Tobacco Control*, 13(4): ii 30–ii 36.

Kunitz, S. J. (1994) *Disease and Social Diversity: The European Impact on the Health of Non-Europeans*, New York: Oxford University Press.

Kunitz, S. J. and Brady, M. A. (1995) 'Health Care Policy for Aboriginal Australians: The Relevance of the American Indian Experience', *Australian Journal of Public Health*, 19(6): 552–555.

Lee, D. J. (1980) *The School of Public Health and Tropical Medicine, 1930–1980*, Sydney: School of Public Health and Tropical Medicine.

Lee, J. and Fahey, C. (1986) 'A Boom for Whom? Some Developments in the Australian Labour Market, 1870–1891', *Labour History*, 50: 1–6.

Lewis, M. (1988) *Managing Madness: Psychiatry and Society in Australia, 1788–1980*, Canberra: AGPS Press.

—— (1997) 'Sexually Transmitted Diseases in Australia from the Late Eighteenth to the Late Twentieth Century', in M. Lewis, S. Bamber and M. Waugh (eds), *Sex, Disease and Society: A Comparative History of Sexually Transmitted Diseases and HIV/AIDS in Asia and the Pacific*, Westport and London: Greenwood Press, 249–276.

—— (1998a) *Thorns on the Rose: The History of Sexually Transmitted Diseases in Australia in International Perspective*, Canberra: Australian Government Publishing Service.

—— (1998b) 'Control of STDs and the History of Public Health in Twentieth Century Australia', unpublished paper, Microbiological Unit Centenary Conference, University of Melbourne.

Lewis, M. J. (1976) ' "Populate or Perish": Aspects of Infant and Maternal Health in Sydney, 1870–1939', unpublished thesis, Australian National University, Canberra.

—— (1989) 'Editor's Introduction', in J. H. L. Cumpston *Health and Disease in Australia: A History* (ed. M. J. Lewis), Canberra: AGPS Press, 1–31.

—— (1992) 'Maternity Care and the Threat of Puerperal Fever in Sydney, 1870–1939', in V. Fildes, L. Marks and H. Marland (eds), *Women and Children First: International Maternal and Infant Welfare, 1870–1945*, London: Routledge, 29–47.

—— (2003) *The People's Health. Public Health in Australia, 1950 to the Present*, Westport and London: Praeger Press.

Lokuge, B., Drahos, P. and Neville, W. (2005) 'Pandemics, Antiviral Stockpiles and Biosecurity in Australia: What about the Generic Option?' *Emja* (rapid online publication), 26 October: 1–7.

Loudon, I. (1992) 'Some International Features of Maternal Mortality, 1880–1950', in V. Fildes, L. Marks and H. Marland (eds), *Women and Children First: International Maternal and Infant Welfare, 1870–1945*, London: Routledge, 5–28.

Mackay, J. M. (2004) 'The Tobacco Industry in Asia: Revelations in the Corporate Documents', *Tobacco Control*, 13(4): ii 1–ii 3.

Magnus, P. (1996) 'The Cardiovascular State of Australia: Good or Bad News?', *Medical Journal of Australia*, 164: 517.

Manderson, D. (1993) *From Mr Sin to Mr Big: A History of Australian Drug Laws*, Melbourne: Oxford University Press.

Marmot, M. G. and Mustard, J. F. (1994) 'Coronary Heart Disease from a Population Perspective', in R. G. Evans, M. L. Barer and T. R. Marmor (eds), *Why Are Some People Healthy and Others Not? The Determinants of Health of Populations*, New York: Aldine de Gruyter, 189–214.

McAlpin, M. B. (1983) 'Famines, Epidemics, and Population Growth: The Case of India', *Journal of Interdisciplinary History*, 14(2): 351–366.

McBriar, A. M. (1966) *Fabian Socialism and English Politics 1884–1918*, Cambridge: Cambridge University Press.

McCarthy, C. (1888) *Inebriate Retreats: Their Origin, Utility, Necessity, and Management*, Melbourne: Stillwell.

Mein Smith, P. (1990) 'Reformers, Mothers and Babies. Aspects of Infant Survival, Australia, 1890–1945', unpublished thesis, Australian National University, Canberra.
Meyer, E. C. (1921) *Infant Mortality in New York City*, New York: Rockefeller Foundation International Health Board.
Milio, N. (1986) 'Promoting Health Promotion: Health or Hype?', *Community Health Studies*, 10(4): 427–437.
Miller, P. and Torzillo, P. (1996) 'Health, an Indigenous Right: A Review of Aboriginal Health in Australia', *Australian Journal of Medical Science*, 17: 3–8.
Minutes of AGM of ANZSERCH/APHA (1981) Noel Butlin Archives, Australian National University, Canberra.
Minutes of AGM of PHA/ANZ (1986) Noel Butlin Archives, Australian National University, Canberra.
Moodie, P. M. (1973) *Aboriginal Health*, Canberra: Australian National University Press.
National Aboriginal Health Strategy Working Party (1989) *A National Aboriginal Health Strategy*, Canberra: Australian Government Publishing Service.
National Health Policy on Alcohol in Australia: Presented to Ministerial Council on Drug Strategy: Adopted 23 March 1989.
Newsholme, Sir Arthur (1935) *Fifty Years in Public Health. A Personal Narrative with Comments*, London: Allen and Unwin.
NHMRC (1997) *Promoting the Health of Australians: Case Studies of Achievements in Improving the Health of the population, December 1996*, Canberra: Australian Government Publishing Service.
NHMRC Community Health Promotion and Education (Standing) Committee (1984), *Towards a National Policy on Health Promotion*, Canberra: Commonwealth Department of Health and Aged Care.
Nutbeam, D (1997) 'Creating Health–Promoting Environments: Overcoming Barriers to Action', *Australian and New Zealand Journal of Public Health*, 21(4): 355–358.
Owen, N. G. (1992) 'Economic and Social Change', in N. Tarling (ed.), *The Cambridge History of Southeast Asia*, Vol. 2, *The Nineteenth and Twentieth Centuries*, Cambridge: Cambridge University Press, 467–527.
Palmer, G. R. and Short, S. D. (1994) *Health Care and Public Policy: An Australian Analysis*, South Melbourne: Macmillan Education Australia.
Parry, S. (1992) 'Disease, Medicine and Settlement: The Role of Health and Medical Services in the Settlement of the Northern Territory, 1911–1939', unpublished thesis, University of Queensland.
Paton, A. (1985) 'The Politics of Alcohol', *British Medical Journal*, 290: 1–2.
Patrick, R. (1987) *A History of Health and Medicine in Queensland 1824–1960*, St Lucia, Queensland: University of Queensland Press.
PHAA Annual Report, 1989–1990: 3–11; 1990–1991: 3–8; 1991–1992: 4–13, Noel Butlin Archives, Australian National University, Canberra.
Powell, M. and Anesaki, M. (1990) *Health Care in Japan*, Routledge: London and New York.
'Public Health' (1897) *Australasian Medical Gazette*, 16: 359.
'Public Health in Victoria' (1954) *Health Bulletin*, 112: 16–19.
Puplick, C. (2002) 'Region in Crisis', *HIV Australia*, 2(2): 16–17.
Raftery, J. (1995) ' "Mainly a Question of Motherhood": Professional Advice-Giving and Infant Welfare', *Journal of Australian Studies*, 45: 66–78.
Reid, J. (1994) 'Public Health Education in Australia: Nobody's Child', *Social Science and Medicine*, 38(8): v–ix.
Report of Honorary Royal Commission to Inquire into Treatment of Alcohol and Drug Dependants in Western Australia (1973), *Western Australia Votes and Proceedings*, 6.

Report of Medical Officer to Metropolitan Combined Districts, 1900 (1900), Sydney: Government Printer.
Report of Meeting to Discuss Future of ASERCH, Melbourne, 23 October 1974 (1974), Noel Butlin Archives, Australian National University, Canberra.
Report of Royal Commission into Sale, Supply, Disposal or Consumption of Liquor in State of Victoria (1964–1965), *Victoria Parliamentary Papers*, 2.
Review of the Community Health Program: Report from the Hospitals and Health Services Commission, March 1976 (1976), Canberra: Australian Government Publishing Service.
Roe, M. (1984) *Nine Australian Progressives: Vitalism in Bourgeios Social Thought 1890–1960*, St Lucia, Queensland: University of Queensland Press.
Room, R. (1988) 'The Dialectic of Drinking in Australian Life: From the Rum Corps to the Wine Column', *Australian Drug and Alcohol Review*, 7: 413–437.
Rosen, B. (1977) 'Australia's Contribution to the Conquest of Plague', *Journal of Royal Australian Historical Society*, 63(1): 60–71.
Russell, K. F. (1977) *The Melbourne Medical School 1862–1962*, Carlton, Victoria: Melbourne University Press.
Sax, S. (1984) *A Strife of Interests: Politics and Policies in Australian Health Services*, Sydney: Allen and Unwin.
Scrimshaw, N. S., Taylor, C. E. and Gordon, J. E. (1968) *Interactions of Nutrition and Infection*, Geneva: World Health Organization.
Sinclair, W. A. (1975) 'Economic Growth and Well-Being: Melbourne 1870–1914', *Economic Record*, 51: 153–173.
Single, E. and Rohl, T. (1997) *The National Drug Strategy: Mapping the Future: An Evaluation of the National Drug Strategy 1993–1997*, Canberra: Australian Government Publishing service.
Stoltz, P. (1978) 'The Australian Foundation on Alcoholism and Drug Dependence: a National Perspective', in A. P. Diehm, R. F. Seaborn and G. C. Wilson (eds), *Alcohol in Australia: Problems and Programmes*, Sydney: McGraw-Hill, 227–243.
Taylor, R., Lewis, M. and Powles, J. (1998a) 'The Australian Mortality Decline: All-Cause Mortality 1788–1990', *Australian and New Zealand Journal of Public Health*, 22(1): 27–36.
—— (1998b) 'The Australian Mortality Decline: Cause-Specific Mortality 1907–1990', *Australian and New Zealand Journal of Public Health*, 22(1): 37–44.
Thame, C. (1974) 'Health and the State: The Development of Collective Responsibility for Health Care in Australia in the First Half of the Twentieth Century', unpublished thesis, Australian National University, Canberra.
'The Control of Tuberculosis in Australia' (1960) *Medical Journal of Australia*, 2: 225–226.
The National Indigenous Australians' Sexual Health Strategy 1996–1997 to 1998–1999. A Report of the ANCARD Working Party on Indigenous Australians' Sexual Health, Canberra: Commonwealth Department of Health and Family Services.
'The National Public Health Partnership and Public Health Outcome Funding Agreements: How are These Related?' (1997) *National Public Health Partnership News*, 2: 5.
'The Report of the Health Commission' (1926) *Medical Journal of Australia*, 1: 81–82.
'The Treatment of Inebriates' (1906) *Australasian Medical Gazette*, 25: 480–482.
'Tuberculosis and Complacency' (1967) *Medical Journal of Australia*, 2: 459–460.
Walker, R. (1983) 'The Struggle against Pulmonary Tuberculosis in Australia, 1788–1950', *Historical Studies*, 20(80): 439–461.

—— (1984) *Under Fire: A History of Tobacco Smoking in Australia*, Carlton, Victoria: Melbourne University Press.
Webster, I. W. (1979) 'Where the Healing Starts', in R. Walpole (ed.), *Community Health in Australia*, Ringwood, Victoria: Penguin Books Australia, 37–52.
White, K. L. (1986) *Independent Review of Research and Educational Requirements for Public Health and Tropical Health: Report to Hon. Neal Blewett M. P., Minister for Health*, Canberra: Commonwealth Department of Health and Aged Care.
Wise, M. and Nutbeam, D. (1994) 'National Health Goals and Targets: An Historical Perspective', *Health Promotion Journal of Australia*, 4(3): 9–13.
Wodak, A. (1986) 'Australian Alcohol Consumption', *Medical Journal of Australia*, 144: 1–2.
Woodgyer, A. J. and Forsyth, J. R. L. (1997) *Microbiological Diagnostic Unit 1897–1997: 100 Years of Service in Public Health Microbiology: A History*, Parkville, Victoria: Department of Microbiology and Immunology, University of Melbourne.
Woodward, A. and Kawachi, I. (2003) 'Tobacco Control in Australia', *Tobacco Control*, 12(3): ii 1–ii 2.
Young, J. A., Sefton, A. J. and Webb, N. (1984) *Centenary Book of the University of Sydney Faculty of Medicine*, Sydney: Sydney University Press.

13 Papua New Guinea

Epidemiological transition, public health and the Pacific

Vicki Luker

This chapter reviews the changing patterns of health in Papua New Guinea (PNG)[1] from 1884, when the era of colonial administration began, until the present. It also considers the role played in these changes by public health – that is, measures taken by the State to protect and cure PNG's people from disease. Today PNG, which has by far the largest population and land area among the Pacific island states and territories, also has the worst health status (see Table 13.1; PNG MOH 2000, Vol. 3: 2–5). One purpose of this review is to indicate how and why this predicament arose.[2]

But the discussion has three other objectives: First, in using Abdel Omran's classic model of the 'epidemiological transition' to offset the distinctive features of PNG's experience, I wish ultimately to reflect on this model and concepts of transition (Omran 1971). That Omran's standard periodization (an age of pandemics and famine, followed by an age of receding pandemics, and finally by one of degenerative or man-made diseases) ill-fits PNG in certain respects should come as no surprise. As Caldwell has noted, there are probably as many models of transition as there are societies (Caldwell 2001: 160). Yet it can be instructive to contemplate the discrepancies between experience and a potent model; and to ask the question: where, for PNG, is the 'epidemiological transition' heading?

Second, historians of public health are frequently pulled towards either heroism or anti-heroism, eulogy or indictment, particularly of self-interest and inflated claims in the name of public health (Porter 1994: 1–5). Historiography of colonial public health in PNG and the Pacific, particularly for the period prior to World War II, tends towards indictment.[3] But the time has perhaps come to reassess some common critiques, while addressing current potentials of public health services to do good and, at the same time, their inherent limitations.

Third, because PNG is the giant among the Pacific island states and territories, in many international surveys it figures as the token representative of this region. But how does PNG's experience of changing health and modern public health illuminate the wider experiences of the island Pacific, which, when bracketed with Asia, or with Australia and New Zealand, are so often elided? To these last three objectives my conclusion will return.

Land and people

Two adjectives routinely describe PNG: 'diverse' and 'isolated'. Comprising the eastern half of the great island of New Guinea and adjacent islands, its varied terrain encompasses high inter-montane valleys, steep forested mountainsides, immense swampy deltas and coastal lowlands.[4]

PNG's people largely descend from two waves of immigrants. The first probably moved into the region 60,000 years ago, reaching the highlands some 30,000 years later. Their descendants mostly speak one of PNG's 500 or more non-Austronesian languages as their mother tongue. Descendants of a later wave settled on the coast and islands, mingled to some extent with their predecessors, and are loosely identified with PNG's 200 Austronesian languages (Foley 1992: 139, 137). PNG's long history of human settlement in many different environments produced great cultural diversity.

While this diversity makes generalizations hazardous, some can be useful. Large, centralized polities never developed in PNG pre-colonially and, on the eve of the colonial era, three broad patterns of livelihood can be distinguished. These still figure, since about 85% of PNG's citizens continue to live rurally and engage to greater or lesser degrees with traditional modes of subsistence. First, a large proportion (perhaps, by analogy with today, roughly 40%) of the population depended on sweet potato cultivation – a pattern of production characterizing the highlands. Second, coastal and lowlands people combined some or all of the following: the harvesting of sago or the cultivation of root crops; coconuts and bananas; and fishing. Third and least advantaged were small groups on mountainsides and in other marginal environments, relying on bush foods and where possible shifting cultivation.

The epithet 'isolated' carries two shades of meaning – one referring to the internal isolation of PNG's peoples from each other, due to topographical barriers or hostilities; the other to the isolation of the area as a whole from the outside world. Though most researchers now reject a stress on 'isolation', preferring to explore the ways in which PNG's peoples participated in wider networks,[5] concepts of both isolation and connectedness assist understandings of historic changes in health.

Pre-colonial health

Nutrition was and is a crucial determinant of health. Though patterns of nutrition have changed in PNG over time and varied according to environment and livelihood, two basic points must be made. Then, and to a great extent still now, breast milk was essential for the survival of infants and small children and all PNG cultures had customs to support lengthy lactation. But even with sufficient breast milk, complementary nutrition was often inadequate, while pregnancy and prolonged breastfeeding depleted women (Gillett 1990: 54–55). Second, many of PNG's peoples, especially those who could not fish, had become accustomed to limited intakes of protein. This was especially so in the highlands, where pig meat was reserved for special occasions and hunting-prey was scant. In addition to little protein, traditional diets were also relatively low in calories (Heywood and Jenkins 1992: 260–261).

Table 13.1 Country data: Melanesia, Micronesia and Polynesia

Country	Last census	Population as counted at last census[a]	Land area km²[a]	Estimated annual population growth rate 2004–2015 %[a]	Urban population %[a]	TFR[a]	IMR[a]	LEM[a]	LEF[a]	GNI US$[b]
Melanesia										
PNG	2000	5,190,786	462,840	2.2	13	4.6 (2000)	64 (2000)	53.7 (2000)	54.8 (2000)	580 (2004)
Solomon Islands	1999	409,042	28,370	2.3	16	4.8 (1997–1999)	66 (1997–1999)	60.6 (1997–1999)	61.6 (1997–1999)	550 (2004)
Vanuatu	1999	186,678	12,190	2.7	21	4.8 (1999)	27 (1999)	65.6 (1999)	69.0 (1999)	1,340 (2004)
New Caledonia	1996	196,836	18,576	1.9	60	2.4 (2002)	6.9 (2002)	69.9 (2002)	77.6 (2002)	14,060 (2000)
Fiji	1996	775,077	18,272	0.7	46	2.7 (2000)	22 (1996)	64.5 (1996)	68.7 (1996)	2,690 (2004)
Micronesia										
FSM	2000	107,008	701	1.2	27	4.1 (2000)	40 (2000)	66.6 (2000)	67.5 (2000)	—
Guam	2000	154,805	541	1.4	38	2.9 (2001–2003)	9 (2001–2003)	74.5 (2001–2003)	80.8 (2001–2003)	—
Kiribati	2000	84,494	811	2.3	37	4.3 (2000)	44 (2000)	61.2 (2000)	66.9 (2000)	970 (2004)
Marshall Islands	1999	50,840	181	1.6	65	5.7 (1999)	37 (1999)	65.7 (1999)	69.4 (1999)	2,370 (2004)
Nauru	2002	10,065	21	1.0	100	4.0 (1997–2002)	42.3 (1997–2002)	52.5 (1997–2002)	58.2 (1997–2002)	—
NMI	2000	69,221	471	3.1	90	1.6 (2000)	5 (2000)	72.5 (2000)	77.8 (2000)	—

Country	Year	Population	Area	Growth rate	% urban	TFR	IMR	LEM	LEF	GNI per capita #
Palau	2000	19,129	488	2.0	71	2.5 (2000)	5 (2000)	66.5 (2000)	71.9 (2000)	6,870 (2001)
Polynesia										
American Samoa	2000	57,291	200	2.0	48	4.0 (2000)	8.5 (2001)	69.0 (2000)	76.0 (2000)	—
Cook Islands	2001	18,027	237	-1.3	59	2.9	21	68.0	74.3 (1996–2002)	—
French Polynesia	1996	219,521	3,521	1.8	53	2.4 (2002)	6.9 (1996–2002)	70.3	75.4	16,150 (2000)
Hawai'i [c]	—	1,211,537 (2000)	6,423.4 sq. ml	—	—	—	7.8 (2000)	75.9 (1990)	82.06 (1990)	34,946
Niue	1997	2,088	259	-3.8	35	3.0 (1997–2001)	29.4 (1997–2001)	68.8 (1997–2001)	71.2 (1997–2001)	—
Pitcairn	1999	47	39	—	0	—	—	—	—	—
Samoa	2001	174,140	2,935	0.9	21	4.6 (2001)	19.1 (2001)	71.7 (2001)	74.2 (2001)	1,860 (2004)
Tokelau	2001	1,537	12	0	0	4.9 (1997–2000)	33	68.4 (1997–2000)	71.3 (1997–2000)	—
Tonga	1996	97,784	649	-0.3	32	3.8 (1999–2001)	12 (1999–2001)	69.8 (1995–96)	71.8 (1995–1996)	1,830 (2004)
Tuvalu	1991	9,043	26	0.4	42	3.7 (2000–2003)	35 (1997–2002)	61.7 (1997–2002)	65.1 (1997–2002)	—
Wallis & Futuna	1996	14,166	255	0.5	0	3.0 (2000–2003)	7.4 (2000–2003)	70.2 (2000–2003)	74.3 (2000–2003)	—
New Zealand	2001	3,737,277[d]	268,021[e]	1.1[d] (2000–2005)	85[d]	1.95[f]	5[d] (2000–2005)	76.6[d] (2000–2005)	81.4[d] (2000–2005)	20,310 (2004)

Sources: a SPC (2005); b World Bank (2005); c Hawai'i (2001); d New Zealand (2005a); e New Zealand (2005b); f New Zealand (2005c).

Notes

— data not obtained; # per capita gross state product; TFR total fertility rate; IMR infant mortality rate; LEM male life expectancy at birth; LEF female life expectancy at birth. GNI gross national income (formerly referred to as gross national product, or GNP).

Malaria was the most important disease, widely established in the lowlands. Genetic adaptations conferring advantages against malaria testify to its antiquity among many lowland populations (Serjeantson et al. 1992: 204–216). Prehistorically, malaria helped shape population distribution and density (Riley 1983: 131). In terms of the tripartite analysis of livelihood above, the superior sources of protein enjoyed by coastal dwellers were generally compromised by malaria; in the highlands, intensive sweet potato cultivation and freedom from malaria facilitated dense population amidst, however, scarce protein; while people on mountain slopes inland from the coast often suffered both malaria and short protein supplies. Iodine deficiencies were also marked among some marginal groups (Heywood 1992: 356).

Other diseases appear to have included pneumonia (a big killer, especially in the highlands); yaws; intestinal parasites; tropical ulcers; fungal infections; some gastrointestinal diseases; and filariasis. But certain major tropical diseases – such as trypanosomiasis and schistosomiasis – were absent, while many 'crowd' and other diseases from the metropolitan world – for instance smallpox, cholera, whooping cough, measles, influenza, and the major sexually transmitted infections (STIs) – had few opportunities for importation before the nineteenth century.

How did people in PNG live and die prehistorically? Rates of infant and child mortality were perhaps five times higher than now (see Table 13.1) and life expectancy at birth was probably around 30 years. Aside from the hazards of childbirth, infancy, disease and injury (with the toll from violence, in some societies, considerable) (Knauft 1987: 462–463; Lindenbaum 1979: 65; Meggitt 1977: 100–112), many lives would have been affected, from time to time, by disasters to which PNG is prone – due to drought (although PNG is one of the wettest places on earth), flooding and, depending on location, tectonic activity, cyclones or unusual spells of frost.

'Medicine' was not, traditionally, a discrete body of theory and practice (Frankel and Lewis 1989: 3–4). Concepts of contagion were probably widespread, but sickness, particularly among young adults, was attributed mostly to sorcery or to punishment by spirits and therefore called for ritual remedies. Sophisticated midwifery seems to have been uncommon among PNG societies, but some communities had specialists in, for instance, bone-setting, trepanning, or medicinal plants (see, e.g. Kiki 1968: 17). Other responses to disease could include abandoning the sick or sites of sickness (cf. Allen 1989: 52). The likely best pre-colonial checks on disease were, however, the smallness of PNG communities (mostly ranging in populations from 10s to 100s, though some coastal communities were much larger) and their modes of isolation. These defences, as will be seen, were broken by colonialism.

The early colonial period to World War II

Colonialism's onset and the 'missing' transition

Changes to health in PNG since the beginning of the colonial era have been pronounced and complex but, as in many developing countries, gaps in data are big. Even today, most births and deaths are unregistered. Many sick people do not or cannot attend health facilities and the reliability of records provided by these varies. The first census of the entire population was not attempted until 1966 and census-taking remains difficult. Even when the arms of government were farthest reaching – probably in the decade or so before and after independence in 1975 – many groups were barely touched by the State, which since the early 1990s has arguably receded. Before the 1930s, most of the highland populations, numbering perhaps a million people, were not even known by the colonial administrations to exist. Valuable colonial records have been lost.

Omran's well-known description of the three stages of the epidemiological transition has already been mentioned: an age of pestilence and famine, characterized by high mortality, life expectancies at birth between 20–40 years, and no sustained population growth; an age of receding pandemics, when mortality progressively declines, life expectancy increases from about 30 to 50 years, and populations grow; and finally, an age of degenerative and so-called man-made diseases, when infectious disease further declines, non-communicable disease (NCD) takes its place, mortality rates reduce, life expectancy at birth extends beyond 50 years, and rates of population growth decline as fertility falls (Omran 1971: 516–517).

The first difficulty with this sequence for PNG (and all the other Pacific Island states and territories) is that it misses an early transition at the beginning of the colonial era: what could be called, to adapt historian William McNeill's image, the transition into the 'global disease pool'.[6] The peoples of PNG were among the isolated communities introduced to a range of metropolitan diseases by the expansion of European empires that, by the late nineteenth century, had knitted nearly all the world's peoples into a network of pathogenic exchange. Though the nature of this transition and its effects varied, and within Pacific scholarship contention surrounds the thesis that new diseases devastated immunologically naïve Pacific populations, there can be no doubt that many suffered demographic decline.[7]

PNG's transition into the global disease pool began comparatively late, even by Pacific standards. Malaria was an important factor in the delay, because it thwarted the establishment of a European presence and subsequently limited it, even after the management of malaria was improved through quinine prophylaxis and mosquito control. Nevertheless, from the 1880s to the late 1920s, most coastal peoples engaged somehow with administrative, economic or evangelistic activities managed by Europeans. In the 1930s, the opening-up of the highlands accelerated and, after World War II, the process of 'first contacts' continued in remote areas right into the 1980s. Despite this staggering, it can be helpful, as demonstrated by historian Alfred Crosby, to think of two phases of 'first contacts' in PNG: earlier for most lowlanders and later for highlanders (and, by extension, other inland populations) (Crosby 1997: 151–167). I discuss first the earlier phase, affecting the coastal regions of both northern PNG, which was initially under German and then Australian administration and is referred to here as New Guinea; and in southern PNG, which was first ruled as a British protectorate, then from 1906 as an Australian territory, and which I call simply Papua.[8]

The lowlands' transition into the 'global disease pool'

Diseases introduced into the lowlands from the late nineteenth century included smallpox, influenza, tuberculosis (TB), leprosy, whooping cough, gonorrhoea and new intestinal parasites.[9] They were brought to communities by visitors (Europeans, Islander missionaries, and other foreigners, including men from elsewhere in PNG); by locals returning from labour plantations and, in due course, from other new communities created under colonialism, such as mining camps, prisons, schools and ports; and by contacts with neighbours and associates who had already been exposed to new infections, for secondary and tertiary transmission carried many infections far. Dysentery, introduced to the islands region in northeastern PNG in the 1880s, spread violently, sweeping away whole communities (Cilento 1927: 78). Smallpox entered northern PNG in the 1890s and travelled much more widely than many Europeans then guessed (Allen 1989: 41–43). Oral traditions suggest that this was not, perhaps, PNG's earliest smallpox epidemic, and other introductions were possible via indigenous trading and other networks, increasing in the nineteenth century, with the Dutch East Indies (see, e.g. Williams 1933: 8–9). Gonorrhoea, first observed in labour enclaves and settlements touched by shipping routes (Turner 1905: 32), had spread so far in the lowlands that by the 1920s Raphael Cilento – speaking of New Guinea – described the infections as having 'already run all over' (Cilento 1927: 82).

The extent of such epidemics suggests that while barriers may have blocked transmission in certain directions, simultaneous patterns of, probably for the most part, short-range interaction could promote it in others, sometimes producing far-flung networks of dissemination. Under colonial conditions, the number of people on the move and their range of movement moreover increased, due to the circular migration of indentured labourers, particularly in New Guinea which was economically more advanced; the progressive extension of missions and administrations; and the reduction of hostilities between communities under their influences.

These same dynamics also spread more widely diseases that had been established in PNG pre-colonially, such as yaws, tinea imbricata and, most significantly, malaria or locally unfamiliar malarial strains. Populations on the western islands of New Guinea, for example, suffered grievously from malaria introduced in the 1880s (Black 1957: 418; Cilento 1928: 2). Thus the transition into 'the global disease pool' entailed the expansion of 'local' diseases too.

What was the effect of this pathogenic spread? In the late nineteenth and early twentieth centuries many lowland populations were observed to be declining. In 1903, one official declared that 'tribes' near Port Moresby would 'within measurable time, die out. Some communities have decreased by one-half in the past ten years; others are declining less rapidly, and the majority are at a standstill' (Barton 1904: 16). Similar concerns exercised German commentators and their Australian successors in New Guinea (Commonwealth of Australia 1923: 33–39). Such writings reflect the confused thinking about native depopulation in the Pacific. Disease was usually understood as a factor, but the weight of disease relative to other causes, and precisely which diseases, and how, were and continue to be debated.

Three points are worth stressing: First, there was no epidemiological and demographic uniformity in this lowlands transition. Though population decline was evidently common, pre-existing conditions, different dates of 'first contacts', differing kinds of interaction, the mix of new diseases (metropolitan and local), the timing of their introduction, dynamics of transmission, and their consequences varied from population to population, as surveys then and later made clear (see, e.g. Cilento 1928: 1–11; Murray 1923: 10; Scragg 1957: 122; 1977). Second, despite a common tendency in the literature to stress the impacts of epidemics (a stress found too in Omran's characterization of 'the age of pandemics'), there were other important, and sometimes less conspicuous, dynamics. These could include routine or perennially raised morbidity and mortality due to new diseases, and the role of reduced fertility – often but not only due to STIs – in limiting reproductive capacity.[10] Third, while many scholars have noted that Europeans often 'saw' native depopulation after it had ceased, or perhaps where it had never been (see, e.g. Nelson 1976: 45–46), it is easy to forget that this transition into the 'global disease pool' – even for those PNG populations that were among the first to undergo it – is relatively recent and its repercussions can still be felt. The force of the first wave of introduced diseases in PNG, as Ian Riley has observed, 'is by no means spent' (Riley 2000: 2).

Public health: inexcusable ineffectiveness?

In the first 60 years of the colonial era, new diseases plainly degraded health for much of lowlands PNG. While conditions might have been even worse without some of the administrations' measures in public health, particularly quarantine and the progressive regulation of labour recruitment, nevertheless the public health tools and resources available were unequal to the magnitude and nature of the task and essentially compromised by the underlying commitment of the administrations to activities that required the movement of people.

Throughout this period, indenture was the main engine for the dispersal of disease. By the 1930s, roughly 60,000 labourers were under contract in the territories of New Guinea and Papua at any one time (ANGAU 1944: 2). Proponents of indenture asserted its benefit to the people (Commonwealth of Australia 1923: 51–52). There was striking evidence to the contrary, dramatized by examples of high morbidity and mortality in plantations and mining camps and further accentuated by the decline of communities that had been weakened by the removal of too many able-bodied men and eroded by the diseases they brought home (Nelson 1976: 146–147, 198–210). In response to depopulation, the German administration banned recruiting from some areas (Firth 1982: 126–132). Later surveys, tracking for instance the spread of gonorrhoea, found disease following the routes of workers returning home (Cilento 1927: 81). Subsequent health measures did contribute to overall mortality declines on plantations (Shlomowitz 1988: 78), while other regulations – for instance, checking labourers as fit for discharge and locking up men and women with STIs – were intended to protect the population at large; but the rigour and comprehensiveness of these measures, and their effectiveness even in the best of circumstances, must be doubted.

Quarantine was the most effective preventive tool available and on occasion did stymie particular potential epidemics (see, e.g. Commonwealth of Australia 1923: 70). Perhaps most notably, Australian quarantine procedures protected PNG and the Solomon Islands from the first and most virulent wave of the 1918–1919 influenza pandemic that caused so much destruction to other island populations (see, e.g. Tomkins 1992: 181). But strict and total quarantine, were it possible to police, would have impeded the circulation of people that was colonialism's lifeblood.

Notwithstanding differences among the various administrations of Papua and New Guinea, Donald Denoon's study of colonial health in PNG is critical of their efforts, particularly between the wars (Denoon 1989). Though acknowledging their meagre establishments and resources, the limited medical technology of the day and PNG's challenging conditions, he stresses that, as a priority, the health of ordinary villagers in practice ranked third after Europeans and labourers; nineteenth-century lessons about sanitation as the most effective way of improving people's health *en masse* were neglected;[11] more Papua New Guineans, male and female, should have been medically trained, to a higher level, and sent back to work among their people; more European nurses should have been employed; and, instead of dispensing bootless hookworm and yaws treatments by the tens of thousands on village patrols in the 1920s and 1930s, the administrations should have focused on the health of PNG mothers. The various Christian missions, he argues, did better.[12] They put down roots in their communities; employed more European women with nursing skills; trained local helpers; and targeted babies and children (Denoon 1989: 85–86). By the late 1930s, the administrations were supporting or enlisting missions in specific projects – relating to infant and child welfare; leprosy and TB asylums; and village outreach.

Yet some criticisms of the interwar administrations warrant reconsideration. Take just the linked question of water and human waste, so central to the control of major diseases such as malaria and dysentery. The administrations were emphatically alive to the need for sanitary village conditions, but the kind of engineering that had enabled great improvements to the health of nineteenth century European populations was impossible to replicate in PNG on a wide scale – and sanitation is still an elusive goal today, with 70% of PNG's people lacking safe water (PNG MOH 2000 Vol. 2: 27). Rather, attempts to promote village latrines, to confine pigs and their excrement, or reduce malaria by introducing larva-eating fish into lakes and rivers had the same ultimate health benefits in view, but were 'do-able'. That such efforts were usually unsuccessful, sometimes even counter-productive, is another matter (Allen 1989: 55).

The history of public health in PNG before World War II highlights certain basic conditions that remain challenging even now. The population was dispersed; transport was difficult; supra-local structures and systems for the administration and delivery of services needed building; resources, including the human resources, were short; and the ideas, methodologies and values of the state's health officials and those of villagers mostly failed to synergize.

World War II to independence

War and two transitions

World War II had far-reaching effects on Papua New Guineans. From 1942 to 1945, when PNG's indigenous population may have totalled 1.5 million, nearly as many Japanese and Allied soldiers served in the country. Local men were commandeered to work for different armies, food supplies were disrupted and depleted, many villages were abandoned for the bush, malaria thrived and virulent strains of dysentery were introduced, spreading to reaches of the highlands that were otherwise little affected by the fighting (Allen 1983; Burton 1983). War-related declines of some native populations were 'alarming' (Commonwealth of Australia 1947: 10). At the end of the war, in Denoon's words, the health of Papua New Guineans was probably worse than ever (Denoon 1989: 63).

After the war, patterns of health were remarkable for two transitions. The first was the highlands' transition into the global disease pool. Between World War I and World War II, European observers noted the freedom of highlanders from, among other diseases, TB, yaws, malaria and gonorrhoea (Commonwealth of Australia 1938: 52). Thereafter, infections from the lowlands were increasingly carried into the interior. In the post-war decades, the return of highlanders from labour contracts on the coast, curtailed local warfare, the building of churches and schools, the development of coffee plantations, markets and administrative centres, the clearing of roads and the immigration of some lowlanders into the highlands all promoted a mixing of people and diffusion of infection that produced, as geographer John Connell notes, 'a rather more homogeneous pattern of diseases within the country' (Connell 1997: 276). Malaria and tuberculosis became more common, STIs spread (with an epidemic of syphilis, in the late 1960s, following the construction of the Highlands Highway) (Garner *et al.* 1972), and the scale of measles, influenza and other epidemics increased. The actual effects of new diseases and longitudinal changes in health were tracked among some groups: such as the Huli in the Tari Valley, whose contacts with the wider world increased from the 1960s (Allen 2002), and the Hagahai of the Schrader foothills, whose contacts (only formalized in the 1980s) entailed elevated infant mortality, population decline and cultural distress (Jenkins *et al.* 1989).

Yet the highlands transition into the 'global disease pool' did not apparently cause overall the pronounced population declines earlier noted among many coastal communities, and this has struck some commentators as globally exceptional: a large, late and unique departure from the classic 'fatal impact' scenario. Crosby concludes, 'Of all the isolated peoples snatched into the great world in the past half-millennium, Papua New Guinean highlanders have in all likelihood weathered the trauma best' (Crosby 1997: 162; cf. Wigley 1990: 195–197).

The second transition approximates that outlined by Omran for a population moving from 'the age of pandemics and famine' to 'the age of receding pandemics'. Average life expectancies lengthened, from roughly 30 after the war to 49.6 in 1981, due largely to declines in infant mortality from perhaps 350–450 per 1,000 births to a national average of 100 per 1,000 births in the mid-1960s, and 72 in 1981 – though this varied markedly from place to place, with predictably more babies dying in rural and isolated areas (Bell 1973a: 134). Yet with improved infant survival and little change to fertility, the population grew: from 2.1 million in the first census of 1966 to 3 million in 1981.

In the 1960s and 1970s, so often portrayed as decades of rapid modernization for PNG, the first hints of 'modern diseases' were also detected. With the growth of the cash economy, more people – rural and urban – could buy imported foods such as tinned fish, salt, flour, oil, sugar and rice; and a few did less physical work. Longitudinal studies of changes to bodyweight in the periurban village of Pari, Port Moresby, recorded early tendencies towards obesity, which in many parts of the Pacific has entailed a 'modern' syndrome of NCDs, including diabetes and heart disease (Maddocks and Maddocks 1977: 113). These latter began appearing in PNG's hospital statistics from the 1970s (Sinnett et al. 1992: 381–382) but could not compare with those of more urbanized populations in Polynesia and Micronesia where NCDs had already become heavy burdens (Zimmet and Whitehouse 1981).[13] New diets also worsened dental health (Maddocks 1973a: 73).

Other habits of consumption changed too. Smoking became more common; after the ban on alcohol for Papua New Guineans was lifted in the 1960s, men began drinking more alcohol; and the chewing of betelnut spread into the highlands (Scragg 1971: 10). New sexual behaviours also spread STIs. But with the exception of the latter, which had long been a colonial health problem, the negative health consequences of most of these new habits were not yet much felt.

Total fertility rates (TFRs) in the 1960s and 1970s approximated 5.4 in 1960, 5.8 in 1971, followed by 4.8 in 1980 (Bakker 1986: 13). Yet regional differences were great, influenced by long-standing variations in nutrition and disease as well as more recent changes – including disease introductions, improved nutrition and new customs relating to marriage and sex – all of which could variously subtract from or add to fertility. According to Omran's model, fertility declines should not be expected until further along the epidemiological transition. Yet some findings were read as possibly early signs of predicted fertility falls (see, e.g. Biddulph 1970: 26) while others seemed at odds with such expectations: the arguably least modernized part of the country, the highlands, had the lowest, not the highest TFRs; and in the late 1960s women in households where the male head earned cash tended to have more, not fewer, children (Bakker 1986: 101). Modern family planning techniques, promoted on a small scale from the first clinic opened in Port Moresby in 1962, anyway made little headway (Muirden 1973: 481–483).

For most people in PNG, life however remained very traditional and rural. When first formulating his model, Omran had drawn largely from European data and explained the health transition in terms of 'the modernization complex', thus downplaying the specific impact of public health measures. But for developing countries he proposed a variant explanation: there the epidemiological shift was propelled largely by modern medicine (Omran 1971: 527, 536). This thesis has been popularized by some historians of health in the developing world (see, e.g. Watts 1996: 353). Was it true of PNG?

Public health: making a big difference?

On balance, almost certainly yes. Public health pushed both an overall transition in PNG to lower infant mortality and higher life expectancy in the post-war era, and also reduced the pain of the highlanders' transition into the global disease pool.

After the war, several developments combined to deliver services that saved lives – particularly babies' and children's. These included an expanded repertoire of new and powerful drugs, vaccines and insecticides; a zeal owing something to the military ethos of World War II and post-war idealism; increased financial support from Canberra; a more effective centralized service from combining the separate health administrations for the territories of Papua and New Guinea; the boosted number and expertise of health workers, due to employment of former military medical orderlies, refugee doctors from Europe and Papua New Guinean health workers, now trained in greater numbers as village aid-post orderlies, health extension officers, nurses, laboratory assistants and medical doctors (Scragg 1990: 23–45); and the expansion of infrastructure to maximize geographic coverage and depth of service. Dr (later Sir) John Gunther, director of medical services in PNG from 1946 to 1957, set the momentum and direction. By the end of his term, there were 332 mission aid posts (missions also expanded post-war), 1,091 government aid posts, 69 mission hospitals and 97 government hospitals. The process of integrating both government and mission services into a single national system began in earnest in the late 1960s and was completed just prior to independence (Denoon 1989: 99–102).

Most gains in people's health during these decades could be attributed to dedicated campaigns, using new technologies, against specific diseases. Campaigns against leprosy and, in more circumscribed areas, goitre and tetanus would warrant examination in a fuller discussion, but most significant were the comprehensive efforts against yaws, TB and malaria. In 1955 a campaign was launched to inject every person in PNG with penicillin aluminium monostearate against yaws; from the late 1950s an ambitious programme against TB endeavoured simultaneously to prevent its spread into the highlands and control it in the lowlands through a three-pronged strategy of mass vaccination, mass case-finding and intensive therapy; at the same time the campaign against malaria used residual spraying with Dichloro-Diphenyl-Trichloroethane (DDT) and by 1970 nearly half the population was protected.

These campaigns brought significant benefits. Yaws was almost wiped out by the mid-1960s and Gunther noted that communities seemed generally healthier after their dose of antibiotics (Gunther 1972: 753). The anti-yaws campaign, in PNG and elsewhere in the Pacific, may have been a major, if unsung, contributor to general health improvements, because it simultaneously impacted on other infections, broke disease synergies and included the most disadvantaged (Roizen 1996: 267, 268–271). BCG vaccination against TB also detracted from disease synergies and benefited the most vulnerable, and by the early 1970s special tuberculosis hospitals were deemed no longer necessary (Wigley 1990: 198). Malarial infestation also dropped in the worst areas (Parkinson and Tavil 1973: 167).

But success was qualified. By the late 1960s, yaws was rebounding while syphilis began spreading among populations to which yaws had formerly conferred cross-immunity (Bell 1973b: 385). Tuberculosis had appeared beyond the 'vaccine barricade' in the highlands and was still being disseminated from such centres as urban settlements and colleges (Wigley 1990: 195). Antimalarial spraying had mixed results and by the late 1960s was beset by problems – including popular resistance and changing biting habits of mosquitoes (Aitken 1991: 34; Parkinson and Tavil 1973: 168).

Lives were also saved by the increasing accessibility of improved medical assistance. Gunther oversaw the development of a three-tiered network of health delivery: village-level aid posts; district-level hospitals; and provincial-level hospitals.[14] Most of the killer diseases could be treated effectively at village level with antibiotics, choloroquine and asprin administered by an aid-post orderly in what Bryant Allen calls a 'spraygun' approach (Allen 1989: 61). But patients could also be referred to centres with superior medical provision. The increased cadre of trained and/or experienced staff was vital here and from the early 1950s, European refugees whose medical qualifications were not recognized in Australia became the 'backbone' of PNG's medical service (Gunther 1990: 60).

By the end of the colonial period, a health service that Denoon describes as possibly one of the best in the developing world had been built rapidly from very little (Denoon 1989: 5). A valuable capacity for applied research was also fostered in the Institute of Medical Research, headquartered in Goroka. It strengthened local efforts against malnutrition, TB, malaria, pneumonia, goitre, pigbel (nectrotizing enteritis, common in the highlands) and kuru (a degenerative disease found among the Fore people) and made distinguished contributions to global public health (Alpers 1999).[15] Yet any tendencies to exaggerate the accessibility and quality of medical services in this 'golden age' should be checked by graphic personal recollections of the opposite (see, e.g. Taylor 2006: 59–67); and by the late 1960s certain shortfalls were becoming clear. More infants and children could be saved – particularly though immunizations and the supervision of childbirth (Bell *et al.* 1973: 491). The latter would save mothers too, who continued to miss out. Maternal mortality, though largely unrecorded, was high, and few women had antenatal care or trained assistance in labour. Even for women who attended MCH (maternal and child health) clinics, Johnson wryly noted that in many places there was 'very little "M"' (Johnson 1973: 486). The availability of modern family planning was similarly scant (Muirden 1973: 481). Sexually transmitted infections were largely uncontrolled (see Maddocks 1973b: 234–236).

The militaristic campaigns against specific diseases appeared to have reached their limits. They highlighted the need to coordinate services and resources at the local level and to equip communities to play a greater role in the management of their health interests. As Robert Black indicated, such campaigns had been successful in spite of the fact that they were conducted without the support or understanding of the people they were intended to benefit: yet for consolidation and further progress, informed and self-directed popular participation was needed (Black 1958: 1).

Nor could public health services claim all the credit. Other factors contributed to health gains. Despite certain negative consequences of dietary change, wider access to purchased foodstuffs was probably of net benefit in PNG, providing many people with crucial extra protein and calories that strengthened resistance to disease, as some studies of child health have stressed (Heywood 1983). Better transport and communications along with resources they could mobilize, managed by agencies committed to people's welfare, often mitigated the effects of famine and other natural disasters (Binns 1976; Gunther 1972: 751–752). Finally, the post-war boom in public health provision coincided with possibly a natural waning of the effect of introduced diseases on populations that had experienced them for several generations. Some observers supposed that TB, for instance, had already reached and passed its epidemic peak among lowland communities (Wigley 1990: 201).

Independence to present

Disorderly transitions

Using the model of epidemiological transition, one might have predicted that in the decades following independence in 1975, overall life expectancy in PNG would continue to lengthen and infant mortality rates (IMRs) decline; the burden of infectious disease would diminish and that of NCD increase; population would grow but fertility rates would fall. Such predictions would have also accorded with the general optimism of the 1970s about health (reflected in Omran's model) and the high hopes surrounding independence.

Certain features of this prognosis have been realized, but the picture is more disorderly and disconcerting. Population has grown, but at a rate exceeding most earlier predictions, more than doubling between 1975 and 2005.[16] Although infant and child mortality rates today are lower, and life expectancy higher, than they were at independence, these improvements are more modest than those of PNG's closest Melanesian neighbours to the east – the Solomon Islands and Vanuatu, where life expectancy is higher and, in Vanuatu, where IMR is lower – and much smaller than those of most Polynesian and Micronesian states and territories (see Table 13.1). Successes in some of PNG's southeast Asian neighbours dwarf them (Ahlburg and Flint 2001: 3).

Nor have PNG's reductions in infant mortality been steady. Rates regressed in the 1980s and 1990s; and though some overall progress has been reported more recently (Duke 2004), this small upward turn masks extreme local variation.[17] In parts of PNG, particularly where health services have ceased, uncounted lives that would have been saved before by medical intervention have been lost.

The burden of infectious disease has not declined. In fact, infections known under colonial rule have resurged, further introductions have occurred, and the bulk of PNG's morbidity and mortality is still due to infection. Pneumonia is the largest single cause of reported death, often as a complication of other infections. Malaria has become more extensive and epidemiologically complex, with the severest strain, falciparum, now predominating and largely chloroquine resistant. While pneumonia and malaria together account for 30% of recorded deaths in PNG, TB ranks in the top five causes and is increasing (PNG MOH 2000, Vol. 3, pt 1: 34–35). One contributing factor is the spread of HIV, since AIDS commonly expresses as TB in PNG. Nonetheless, most TB sufferers in PNG are HIV-free.

HIV is the best known of the 'new' post-independence infections and piggy-backs on an exuberant epidemic of other STIs (Jenkins and Passey 1998). AIDS was first reported in 1987; the spread of HIV shifted from 'slow burn' to 'explosive growth' in the early 1990s; and in 2003 PNG was the first Pacific country and the fourth (after Thailand, Cambodia and Myanmar) in the wider Asia-Pacific region to be classed as having a generalized epidemic, meaning that HIV is widely disseminated geographically and found outside so-called high risk groups. Approximately 2% of PNG's population is estimated to be HIV positive (UNAIDS 2006: 61). Although the capital Port Moresby, other towns and development enclaves have generally higher prevalence, some reports suggest that levels of HIV may be much higher than anticipated in many isolated areas, where 30% to 40% of some populations, normally beyond the reach of medical facilities and testing, are reportedly infected (Anon 2006a). Most observers predict that HIV in PNG will follow a course similar to the severe sub-Saharan epidemics, with destructive long-term effects for PNG's health, demographic structure, economy and social capital (HEMIS 2006: 12–80).

In PNG the classic 'diseases of modernization' have a low profile – in contrast to their predominance in the majority of PNG's Pacific neighbours (Coyne 2000). Yet their toll on 'the young, economically productive and elite workforce' is particularly heavy (PNG MOH, Vol. 2: 35). Diabetes mellitus, ischaemic heart disease and hypertension have increased among urban and periurban populations, while the first signs of changing tolerance to glucose have been noted in the highlands (Flew 1996: 1; King 1992: 369; Naraqi et al. 2003: 8). The prevalence of cancers also seems to be increasing. The most common are of the cervix, liver, breast and mouth (PNG MOH 2000, Vol. 2: 37).

Yet other ills that could more loosely be termed 'diseases of modernization' are escalating. PNG is experiencing an 'epidemic of trauma' (Watters and Lourie 1996). Injury is the fourth leading cause of hospital admissions in PNG and accounts for 4% of hospital deaths (PNG MOH 2000, Vol. 3, pt 1: 34). Car accidents and work accidents are increasing. So too is 'tribal warfare', along with the use of guns, thus multiplying fatalities (Mathew 1996). Several studies suggest that family and gender violence is increasing too (Bradley 2001): some international surveys rate PNG among the highest for intimate partner violence (WHO 2002: 90); research indicates a wide acceptance of and participation in pack rape (see, e.g. NSRRT; Jenkins 1994; 102); and research also indicates that children are increasingly vulnerable to sexual abuse and violence (HELP 2005). While family and gender violence can cause immediate bodily injury, other physical consequences (such as pregnancy, infertility, HIV infection) may ensue from sexual assault. A factor in this 'epidemic of trauma' is alcohol abuse, which continues to be a massive public health problem, while more recently cannabis abuse, also implicated with violence, has attracted publicity (Marshall 1990; and see, e.g. Anon 2006b).

Some of PNG's fertility characteristics still sit uncomfortably with Omran's model of transition. TFRs, at 4.6, have scarcely declined. While urban fertility tends to be lower than rural, highlands fertility is still the lowest in the country (Lavu 1997: 33, 35). Although PNG's TFRs remain relatively high, among the factors keeping them below the possible maximum, sterility caused by STIs probably rivals both modern contraception, which is only used by 8 per cent of women (PNG MOH 2000, Vol. 2: 51) and residual respect for traditional customs, such as the post-partum taboo, that favour birth-spacing. High maternal mortality also continues with levels in PNG, estimated at 370 per 100,000, among the world's worst (PNG MOH 2000, Vol. 2: 46, 48). Finally, contrary to the global norm, during the 1990s male life expectancy in PNG overall exceeded female (Jorari and Kalamoroh 1997: 4). Recent figures suggesting that female life expectancy is now slightly ahead (see Table 13.1) raise the question whether women's health has so significantly improved, or whether the health of adult men – who appear to be more prone to death from growing causes such as injury and heart disease – has recently deteriorated relative to women. In either case increasing AIDS, because it tends to kill women in PNG at a younger age than men (as is the pattern in epidemics driven largely by heterosexual transmission), may in the future erode any slight female lead.

Public health breakdown

A generation after independence, the Ministry of Health described the health system as collapsed (PNG MOH 2000, Vol. 1: 2). Although other providers have come to play a role (private practitioners and overseas medical treatment are used by elites; while some large mining companies offer health services to local people), the government is still the main provider.

The most obvious sign of deterioration is shrinking geographic coverage. Despite in-principle commitment to rural health services, from the mid-1980s village visits by health workers ceased and aid posts and health centres in many areas closed (PNG MOH 2000, Vol. 1: 2). An accurate figure for the number of closed aid posts, health centres and hospitals is elusive, while some classed officially 'open' are not in fact, but in 1998 almost one fifth of the nation's aid posts were declared no longer operating (PNG MOH 2000, Vol. 3, pt 2: 160–162). In 2006, according to another estimate, about half the aid posts that were functioning 30 years earlier had closed (Nelson 2006: 3). The repertoire and quality of services from open facilities has also, in practice, diminished. Only some of the reasons for this decay can be flagged here.

Fundamentally, PNG has experienced a 'dysynergy' of public health intervention, population growth and development. In some developing countries, health measures arguably delivered in falling mortality, combined with fertility reductions, a 'demographic bonus' of workers who could be harnessed by development, which in turn generally raised living standards and amplified health provision (Ahlburg and Flint 2001: 9–10).

But in PNG population growth has not combined with strong fertility declines nor has it been harnessed by PNG's kind of 'elite and enclave' development.[18] The living conditions of the majority have not improved enough (for many, at all) to facilitate further great gains in health conditions. Indeed, population pressure in some locations has placed a strain on subsistence. With respect to basic health services, the financial base cannot support the extension, let alone maintenance of pre-existing coverage, while simultaneously health needs have diversified and become more complex. In the late 1960s, PNG's per capita investment in health ranked much higher than that of many developing countries (Bassett and Bell 1973: 548) but it declined from the 1980s. Compared with the other main Pacific Island states and territories, PNG's inputs, as a percentage of gross national product and on a per capita basis, are now the lowest; while donors (chiefly Australia) provide approximately 20% of health funding (PNG MOH 2000, Vol. 3, pt 1: 2; WHO 2005). Among other shortfalls, absolute declines of qualified personnel combined with demographic increase could, according to the minister of health, leave most people in PNG without basic health services within ten years' time (Anon 2006a). Thus population growth has helped undermine the medical services that engineered it.

If, in public health 'it is almost all administration that counts',[19] PNG's system has suffered pervasive failings, though some areas, including services administered by churches, function better than others (Crouch-Chivers 1998: 98). But the policy of decentralization, foreshadowed in the late colonial period, implemented in the 1980s and 1990s, and intended to improve the responsiveness and coordination of health services within local conditions, has proven massively counterproductive (PNG MOH 2000, Vol. 1: 2). Though the case for decentralization was strong and pressed by international donors, by the early 1990s devolution had clearly failed rural health, that is, the health of the majority, and especially women and children (Newbrander et al. 1991: 75; Thomason et al. 1991). Nationally, the IMR rose from 72 in 1981 to 82 in 1991 and female life expectancy dropped behind that for males (Jorari and Kalamoroh 1997: 4). Further devolution in the mid-1990s was no remedy. Broadly speaking, there are two explanations for its failure: decentralization was not properly done (and health provision suffered a similar fate to that of other decentralized services); or was basically doomed, since the best interests of health, at the provincial or local level, cannot compete with others.

Broader conditions, some already mentioned, continue to challenge public health provision. Although it is trite to stress difficulties of transport and communication among a culturally diverse people dispersed across daunting terrain, these remain fundamental difficulties nonetheless, and airlines, shipping and roads have declined (Hanson et al. 2001: 13). While it can be argued too that the health system, despite culturally sensitive and innovative training for health workers (Duke et al. 2004), has failed in public health education, this also involves broader questions – including those relating generally to education in a country where half the women and nearly half the men are illiterate (PNG 2003: 42). While bettering women's health and empowering women as health providers within their families and communities are recognized internationally as pivotal for improving a population's health, in PNG women remain comprehensively disadvantaged (Macintyre 1998). PNG's grave and worsening 'law and order problem' is another example of social conditions that simultaneously affect both people's health and the department's ability to respond. Much crime and violence inflates, through injuries and sickness, demands for care while simultaneously impeding services: by preventing patients and staff (especially women) from travel; by forcing some facilities to close; and, in other ways, by vitiating health services from within.[20]

Shortcomings of the health system have directly contributed to shortfalls in the people's health over recent decades, but both health conditions and public health provision are subject to broader factors that the department has limited potential to fix. Within current means and circumstances, the area of provision where the department has the best opportunities to 'score' impressively for the nation's health indices is perhaps in the arena of past successes: infant health, particularly through the restoration and expansion of immunization services (Duke 2000: 1–2; Shann 2000: 24). Yet, without appropriate development and concomitant falls in fertility, such measures will exacerbate the problems of population growth.

Three final questions

How does PNG's experience illuminate that of the wider Pacific? PNG accounts for most of the Pacific's Islands land and people, and contains within it many Pacific microcosms. But in national terms, its history of changing health and modern health provision resembles most closely that of its easterly neighbours, the Solomon Islands and Vanuatu, while suggesting perhaps as many differences as similarities with the rest. Despite their variation, most other Pacific Island countries shoulder a greater and faster growing burden of NCD, with many demonstrating more vividly than PNG the 'double burden' of NCD and infectious disease. Nevertheless, all indigenous Pacific populations have participated in a transition into the global disease pool; some elements of the history and cultural dynamics of health change and health intervention during the colonial and independence periods outlined here for PNG will be recognizable elsewhere; and many of PNG's difficulties in raising health conditions and providing public health services resonate more widely.

What good was and is public health? Before World War II, measures by colonial administrations failed to negate the ill effects of colonial change, including the introduction of metropolitan infections, or make much headway against local diseases. And retrospectively it seems doubtful that colonial health services could have made a significantly bigger difference for the better at that time. After the war, in PNG and throughout the Pacific, falls in infant mortality and consequent extensions in life expectancy were largely due to effective health campaigns.

268 *Vicki Luker*

Though such saving of life is always a transcendental good, PNG and most Pacific Island states and territories have been variously challenged by the subsequent mismatch between medically triggered population growth and patterns of development. The circumstances created by these latter complicate and multiply the demands on health systems while making, in many parts of the Pacific, the provision of basic services to everyone more difficult.

Finally, so varied and disorderly are the current health transitions in PNG that one could be forgiven for asking: are they all heading in the one direction? The metaphor of epidemiological transition is robust and elastic, and can figuratively be widened, protracted, even balkanized to accommodate PNG's variety of transitions. Yet these nevertheless disconcert two of the comforting promises implied in the model: progress and convergence on ultimately a better state of health. Similar questions can be posed for the Pacific, indeed the world, at large.

Notes

1 'Papua New Guinea' properly designates the nation state that came into being in 1975. When I use this term or its acronym for any time prior to independence, it refers merely to the geographic entity.
2 For a fuller treatment of much of the material discussed here, see Denoon (1989).
3 See, for example, Denoon (1989) and Hattori (2004), perhaps the two pre-eminent books in the historiography of colonial health in the Pacific Island.
4 The Indonesian province of Papua, in the western half of the island of New Guinea, is omitted from this discussion for no good geographic, cultural or epidemiological reasons. However, because of colonial accident and current politics, in many contexts it is not counted as a 'Pacific country'.
5 See, for example, Moore (2003: 41–53).
6 McNeill frequently invoked the figure of the 'disease pool'; see, for example, his chapter title 'Confluence of the Civilized Disease Pools of Eurasia...' (McNeill 1979: 78).
7 See, for example, Rallu (1991).
8 German New Guinea and British New Guinea were founded in 1884. The latter became the Australian Territory of Papua in 1906. German New Guinea was occupied by Australian forces in 1914 and administered by the military until 1921, when the territory became a League of Nations Mandate under Australia. After World War II Australia ruled both territories under a single administration, but New Guinea was a Trust Territory of the United Nations.
9 While not disputing that colonialism spread TB, some scholars are open to the possibility that TB pre-dated 'first contacts' with 'Europeans' in PNG. See, for example, Wigley (1990: 167).
10 Scragg's research on depopulation in New Ireland highlighted the 'slow and pernicious effect' of reduced fertility due to gonorrhoea (Scragg 1957: 118). Disease-induced infertility has been further stressed by Stannard in his work on Hawaii (Stannard 1990) and in Crosby's comparative treatment of Hawaiian and Amerindian depopulation (Crosby 1992). Pirie also identified a range of factors – including infertility and perennially raised mortality due to introduced diseases – as potentially contributing to depopulation (Pirie 1972).
11 A major theme of Denoon's study is that the new discipline of 'tropical medicine' captured colonial public health and, in 'disregard for European history', gave more status to doctors and laboratory medicine than to engineers and sanitary works (Denoon 1989: 20–21).
12 See also the most comprehensive history of medical missionary work in PNG by the former missionary nurse, Kettle (1978).

13 I use the terms 'Melanesia', 'Polynesia' and 'Micronesia' in a purely geographical sense.
14 Initially, the district was known as the 'sub-district'; the province as the 'district'.
15 Perhaps the best known feat of medical research in PNG, though it impacted on fewer lives than much of the Institute's work, was into the cause of kuru, which won Dr Carleton Gajdusek the Nobel prize. See Nelson (1996).
16 In 1986, for example, the health department made three projections (low, medium and high) for population growth. The high variant, assuming gradual mortality declines and no change in fertility, projected a population of 4.9 million by 2000 (PNG DOH 1986, 15). The population enumerated in the 2000 census exceeded this (see Table 13.1).
17 See PNG MOH 2000, vol. 3, pt II for regional breakdowns of health data. For a broader analysis of provincial and district variation, including health, see Hanson et al. (2001).
18 For a recent critique of development in PNG, see Baxter (2001); also Hughes (2003).
19 Sir William Refshauge, interview, quoted in Denoon (1989: 74).
20 Peter A. Sims, professor of public health medicine at the School of Medicine in Port Moresby, has pleaded for law and order as the first requirement for the restoration of medical services and outreach (Sims 2003: 165).

References

Ahlburg, D. A. and Flint, D. J. (2001) 'Public Health Conditions and Policies in the Asia Pacific Region', *Asian-Pacific Economic Literature*, 15(2): 1–17.

Aitken, I. W. (1991) 'The Health Services of Papua New Guinea', in J. A. Thomason, W. C. Newbrander and R.-L. Kolemainen-Aitken (eds), *Decentralization in a Developing Country: The Experience of Papua New Guinea and its Health Service*, Canberra: National Centre of Development Studies, Australian National University, 23–35.

Allen, B. J. (1989) 'Infection, Innovation and Residence: Illness and Misfortune in the Torricelli Foothills from 1800', in S. Frankel and G. Lewis (eds), *A Continuing Trial of Treatment: Medical Pluralism in Papua New Guinea*, Dordrecht: Kluwer Academic Publishers, pp. 35–68.

—— (1983) 'A Bomb or a Bullet or the Bloody Flux? Population Change in the Aitape Inland, Papua New Guinea, 1941–45', *Journal of Pacific History*, 18(3–4): 218–235.

—— (2002) 'Health and Environment in the Tari Area', *Papua New Guinea Medical Journal*, 45(1–2): 1–7.

Alpers, M. J. (1999) 'Past and Present Research Activities of the Papua New Guinea Institute of Medical Research', *Papua New Guinea Medical Journal*, 42(1–2): 35–51.

ANGAU (Australian New Guinea Administrative Unit) (1944) 'Medical Services in Papua and New Guinea' (TS held in main collection of the National Library of Australia, Canberra).

Anon (2006a) 'HIV/AIDS Prevalence Could Be Higher', *PNG Post-Courier*, 26 September, 7.

—— (2006b) 'Health Worker Shortage Worries PNG Minister', *PNG Post-Courier*, 2 May, 3.

Bakker, M. L. (1986) *Fertility in Papua New Guinea: A Study of Levels, Patterns, and Changes based on Census Data*, Port Moresby: National Statistics Office.

Barton, C. (1904) 'Report on Central Division', in Commonwealth of Australia, *Report on British New Guinea for the year ending 30 June, 1903*, Melbourne.

Bassett, J. and Bell, C. O. (1973) 'Resources – Financial', in C. O. Bell (ed.), *The Diseases and Health Services of Papua New Guinea: A Basis for National Health Planning*, Port Moresby: Department of Public Health, 546–556.

Baxter, M. (2001) *Enclaves or Equity: The Rural Crisis and Development Choice in Papua New Guinea*, International Development Issues no. 54, Canberra: Australian Agency for International Development (AusAID).

Bell, C. O. (1973a) 'Vital Statistics', in C. O. Bell (ed.), *The Diseases and Health Services of Papua New Guinea: A Basis for National Health Planning*, Port Moresby: Department of Public Health, 132–145.

—— (1973b) 'Yaws', in C. O. Bell (ed.), *The Diseases and Health Services of Papua New Guinea: A Basis for National Health Planning*, Port Moresby: Department of Public Health, 385–386.

Bell, C. O., Lane, W. R. and Mercado, R. (1973) 'Immunization Programme and Policy', in C. O. Bell (ed.), *The Diseases and Health Services of Papua New Guinea: A Basis for National Health Planning*, Port Moresby: Department of Public Health, 491–507.

Biddulph, J. (1970) 'Longitudinal Study of Children Born in a Periurban Papua Village – A Preliminary Report', *Papua New Guinea Medical Journal*, 13(1): 23–27.

Binns, C. W. (1976) 'Famine and the Diet of the Enga', *Papua New Guinea Medical Journal*, 19(4): 231–235.

Black, R. H. (1957) 'The Epidemiology of Malaria in Southwest Pacific: Changes Associated with Increasing European Contact', *South Pacific*, 9(6): 417–422.

—— (1958) 'Health Education in Papua and New Guinea', *South Pacific*, 10(1): 1–7.

Bradley, C. (2001) *Family and Sexual Violence in Papua New Guinea: An Integrated Long-Term Strategy*, Port Moresby: Institute of National Affairs.

Burton, J. (1983) 'A Dysentery Epidemic in New Guinea and its Mortality', *The Journal of Pacific History*, 18(3–4): 236–261.

Caldwell, J. C. (2001) 'Population Health in Transition', *Bulletin of the World Health Organization*, 79(2): 159–170.

Cilento, R. W. (1927) 'Report on the Public Health of The Territory of New Guinea 1925–1926', in Commonwealth of Australia, *Report to the Committee of the League of Nations on the administration of the Territory of New Guinea, 1 July 1925–30 June 1926*, Melbourne.

—— (1928) *The Causes of the Depopulation of the Western Islands of the Territory of New Guinea*, Canberra: Government Printer.

Commonwealth of Australia (1923) *Report to the League of Nations on the Administration of the Territory of New Guinea from 1 July, 1921 to 30 June, 1922*, Melbourne.

—— (1938) 'Health Aspects of the Hagen-Sepik Patrol', in *Report to the Committee of the League of Nations on the Administration of the Territory of New Guinea, 1 July to 30 June 1937*, Canberra.

—— (1947) *Report to the General Assembly of the United Nations on the Administration of the Territory of New Guinea from 1 July, 1946 to 30 June, 1947*, Canberra.

Connell, J. (1997) 'Health in Papua New Guinea: A Decline in Development', *Australian Geographical Studies*, 35(3): 271–293.

Coyne, T. (2000) *Lifestyle Diseases in Pacific Communities*, Noumea: Secretariat of the Pacific Community.

Crosby, A. W. (1992) 'Hawaiian Depopulation as a Model for the Amerindian Experience', in T. Ranger and Paul Slack (eds), *Epidemics and Ideas: Essays on the Historical Perception of Pestilence*, Cambridge: Cambridge University Press, 175–201.

—— (1997) 'Papua New Guinea, its Demographic History and Infectious Diseases', in H. J. Hiery and J. M. MacKenzie (eds), *European Impact and Pacific Influence: British and German Colonial Policy in the Pacific Islands and the Indigenous Response*, London: I.B. Tauris Publishers, 151–167.

Crouch-Chivers, P. R. (1998) 'Editorial: The Public Health Imperative in Papua New Guinea', *Papua New Guinea Medical Journal*, 41(3–4): 97–100.

Denoon, D. (with Kathleen Dugan and Leslie Marshall) (1989) *Public Health in Papua New Guinea: Medical Possibility and Social Constraint, 1884–1984*, Cambridge: Cambridge University Press.

Duke, T. (2000) 'Editorial: A Movement for the Protection of Infancy: What We Must Do to Lower Child Mortality in Papua New Guinea', *Papua New Guinea Medical Journal*, 43(1–2): 1–4.

—— (2004) 'Slow But Steady Progress in Child Health in Papua New Guinea', *Journal of Paediatrics and Child Health*, 40(12): 659–724.

Duke, T., Tefuarani, N. and Baravilala, W. (2004) 'Getting the Most of our Health Education in Papua New Guinea', *Medical Journal of Australia*, 181(11/12): 606–607.

Firth, S. (1982) *New Guinea under the Germans*, Melbourne: Melbourne University Press.

Flew, S. J. and Paika, R. L. (1996) 'Health and Major Resource Developments in Papua New Guinea: Pot of Gold or Can of Worms at the End of the Rainbow?' *Papua New Guinea Medical Journal*, 39(1): 1–5.

Foley, W. A. (1992) 'Language and Identity in Papua New Guinea', in R. D. Attenborough and M. P. Alpers (eds), *Human Biology in Papua New Guinea*, Oxford: Clarendon Press, 136–149.

Frankel, S. and Lewis, G. (1989) 'Patterns of Continuity and Change', in S. Frankel and G. Lewis (eds), *A Continuing Trial of Treatment: Medical Pluralism in Papua New Guinea*, Dordecht: Kluwer Academic Publishers, 1–34.

Garner, M. F., Hornabrook, R. W. and Backhouse, J. L. (1972) 'Treponematosis along the Highlands Highway', *Papua New Guinea Medical Journal*, 15(3): 139–141.

Gillett, J. E. (1990) *The Health of Women in Papua New Guinea*, Papua New Guinea Institute of Medical Research Monograph no. 9, Goroka: Papua New Guinea Institute of Medical Research.

Gunther, J. D. (1972) 'Medical Services, History', in P. Ryan (ed.), *Encyclopedia of Papua and New Guinea*, Melbourne: Melbourne University Press.

—— (1990) 'Postwar Medical Services in Papua New Guinea: A Personal View', in B. G. Burton-Bradley (ed.), *A History of Medicine in Papua New Guinea: Vignettes of an Earlier Period*, Kingsgrove, NSW: Australasian Medical Publishing Co, 748–756.

Hanson, L. W., Allen, B. J., Bourke, R. M. and McCarthy, T. J. (2001) *Papua New Guinea: Rural Development Handbook*, Canberra: The Australian National University.

Hattori, Anne Perez (2004) *Colonial Disease: US Navy Health Policies and the Chamorros of Guam, 1894–1941*, Honolulu: Hawai'i University Press.

Hawai'i (2001) *The State of Hawai'i Data Book 2001*. Online. Available <http://www.state.hi.us/dbedt/stats.htm> (accessed 12 December 2002).

HELP (2005) *A Situational Analysis of Child Sexual Abuse and the Commercial Sexual Exploitation of Children in Papua New Guinea*, HELP Resources, Inc., [n.p.]

HEMIS (HIV Epidemiological Modelling Impact Study) (2006) *Impacts of HIV/AIDS 2005–2025 in Papua New Guinea, Indonesia and East Timor: Final Report of the HIV Epidemiological Modelling Impact Study February 2006*, Canberra: AusAID.

Heywood, P. (1983) 'Growth and Nutrition in Papua New Guinea', *Journal of Human Evolution*, 12: 133–143.

—— (1992) 'Iodine-Deficiency Disorders in Papua New Guinea', in R. D. Attenborough and M. P. Alpers (eds), *Human Biology in Papua New Guinea: The Small Cosmos*, Oxford: Clarendon Press, 355–362.

Heywood, P. F. and Jenkins, C. (1992) 'Nutrition in Papua New Guinea', in R. D. Attenborough and M. P. Alpers (eds), *Human Biology in Papua New Guinea: The Small Cosmos*, Oxford: Clarendon Press, 249–267.

Hughes, Helen (2003) 'Aid has Failed the Pacific', *Issue Analysis* No. 33. St Leonards, NSW: The Centre for Independent Studies.

Jenkins, C., Dimitrakakis, M., Cook, I., Sanders, I. and Stallman, N. (1989) 'Culture Change and Epidemiological Patterns among the Hagahai, Papua New Guinea', *Human Ecology*, 17(1): 25–57.

Jenkins, C. and Passey, M. (1998) 'Papua New Guinea', in T. Brown, R. Chan, D. Mugrditchian, B. Mulhall, D. Plummer, R. Sarda and W. Sittitrai (eds), *Sexually Transmitted Diseases in Asia and the Pacific*, Armidale: Venereology Publishing, 230–254.

Johnson, D. J. (1973) 'Obstetric Services in Papua New Guinea', in C. O. Bell (ed.), *The Diseases and Health Services of Papua New Guinea: A Basis for National Health Planning*, Port Moresby: Department of Public Health, 486–490.

Jorari, A. and Kalamoroh, J. (1997) 'Introduction', in *Papua New Guinea Demographic and Health Survey 1996: National Report*, Port Moresby: National Statistical Office.

Kettle, E. (1978) *That They Might Live*, Sydney: F.P. Leonard.

Kiki, A. M. (1968) *Kiki: Ten Thousand Years in a Lifetime: A New Guinea Autobiography*, Melbourne: F.W. Cheshire.

King, H. (1992) 'The Epidemiology of Diabetes Mellitus in Papua New Guinea and the Pacific: Adverse Consequences of Natural Selection in the Face of Sociocultural Change', in R. D. Attenborough and M. P. Alpers (eds), *Human Biology in Papua New Guinea: The Small Cosmos*, Oxford: Clarendon Press, 363–372.

Knauft, Bruce M. (1987) 'Reconsidering Violence in Simple Human Societies: Homicide among the Gebusi of New Guinea', *Current Anthropology*, 28(4): 457–482.

Lavu, E. (1997) 'Fertility', in *Papua New Guinea Demographic and Health Survey 1996: National Report*, Port Moresby: National Statistical Office, 33–44.

Lindenbaum, Shirley (1979) *Kuru Sorcery: Disease and Danger in the New Guinea Highlands*, Palo Alto: Mayfield Publishing.

Macintyre, M. (1998) 'The Persistence of Inequality: Women in Papua New Guinea since Independence', in L. Zimmer-Tamakoshi (ed.), *Modern Papua New Guinea*, Kirksville, MO: Thomas Jefferson University Press, 211–230.

McNeill, W. H. (1979) *Plagues and Peoples*, Harmondsworth, UK: Penguin.

Maddocks, D. L. and Maddocks, I. (1977) 'The Health of Young Adults in Pari Village', *Papua New Guinea Medical Journal*, 20(3): 110–116.

Maddocks, I. (1973a) 'History of Disease in Papua New Guinea', in C. O. Bell (ed.), *The Diseases and Health Services of Papua New Guinea*, Port Moresby: Department of Health, 70–74.

—— (1973b) 'Venereal Diseases', in C. O. Bell (ed.), *The Diseases and Health Services of Papua New Guinea*, Port Moresby: Department of Health, 234–237.

Marshall, M. (1990) 'Alcohol as a Public Health Problem in Papua New Guinea', in B. G. Burton-Bradley (ed.), *A History of Medicine in Papua New Guinea: Vignettes from an Earlier Period*, Kingsgrove, NSW: Australasian Medical Publishing, 101–117.

Mathew, P. K. (1996) 'Changing Trends in Tribal Fights in the Highlands of Papua New Guinea: A Five Year Review', *Papua New Guinea Medical Journal*, 39(2): 117–125.

Meggitt, M. (1977) *Blood is their Argument: Warfare among the Mae Enga Tribesmen of the New Guinea Highlands*, Palo Alto: Mayfield Publishing Company.

Moore, C. (2003) *New Guinea: Crossing Boundaries and History*, Honolulu: University of Hawai'i Press.

Muirden, N. (1973) 'Family Planning', in C. O. Bell (ed.), *The Diseases and Health Services of Papua New Guinea: A Basis for Health Planning*, Port Moresby: Department of Public Health, 392–396.

Murray, J. H. P. (1923) 'The Population Problem in Papua', a paper read before the Pan-Pacific Conference, at Melbourne, 21 August 1923, Port Moresby: Government Printer.

Naraqi, S., Feling, B. and Leeder, S. R. (2003) 'Disease and Death in Papua New Guinea: Infectious Diseases are Still the Dominating Cause of Death', *Medical Journal of Australia*, 168: 7–8.

Nelson, Hank (1976) *Black, White and Gold: Goldmining in Papua New Guinea 1878–1930*, Canberra: Australian National University Press.

—— (1996) 'Kuru: The Pursuit of the Prize and the Cure', *Journal of Pacific History*, 31(2): 178–201.

—— (2006) 'Governments, States and Labels', *State, Society and Governance in Melanesia Discussion Paper* 2006/1, Canberra: State, Society and Governance in Melanesia Project, Research School of Pacific and Asian Studies, The Australian National University.

Newbrander, W. C., Aitken, I. W. and Kolemainen-Aitken, R.-L. (1991) 'Performance of the Health System under Decentralization', in J. A. Thomason, W. C. Newbrander and R.-L. Kolemainen-Aitken (eds), *Decentralization in a Developing Country: The Experience of Papua New Guinea and its Health Service*, Canberra: National Centre of Development Studies, Australian National University, 23–35.

New Zealand (2005a) Quick Facts – People. Online. Available <http://www.stats.govt.nz> (accessed 19 September 2005).

—— (2005b) Quick Facts – Lands & Environment. Online. Available <http://www.stats.govt.nz> (accessed 19 September 2005).

—— (2005c) Demographic Trends 2004, pt 2. Online. Available <http://www.stats.govt.nz> (accessed 19 September 2005).

NSRRT (National Sex and Reproduction Research Team) and Jenkins, C. (1994) *National Study of Sexual and Reproductive Knowledge and Behaviour in Papua New Guinea*, Goroka: Papua New Guinea Institute of Medical Research.

Omran, A. R. (1971) 'The Epidemiological Transition: A Theory of the Epidemiology of Population Change', *The Milbank Memorial Fund Quarterly*, 49(4): 509–538.

Parkinson, A. D. and Tavil, N. (1973) 'Malaria', in C. O. Bell (ed.), *The Diseases and Health Services of Papua New Guinea: A Basis for National Health Planning*, Port Moresby: Department of Public Health, 385–386.

Pirie, P. (1972) 'Population Growth in the Pacific Islands: The Example of Western Samoa', in R. G. Ward (ed.), *Man in the Pacific Islands: Essays on Geographical Change in the Pacific Islands*, Oxford: Clarendon Press, 189–218.

PNG DOH (Department of Health) (1986) *Papua New Guinea National Health Plan 1986–1990*, Boroko: Department of Health.

PNG MOH (Ministry of Health) (2000) *National Health Plan 2001–2010: Health Vision 2001–2010*, 4 Vols, [Port Moresby]: Ministry of Health.

PNG NSO (National Statistical Office) (2003) *Papua New Guinea 2000 Census*, Port Moresby: National Statistical Office.

Porter, D. (1994) 'Introduction', in D. Porter (ed.), *The History of Public Health and the Modern State*, Amsterdam: Editions, Rodopi B.V, 1–44.

Rallu, J.-L. (1991) 'Population of the French Overseas Territories in the Pacific, Past, Present and Projected', *Journal of Pacific History*, 26(2): 169–186.

Riley, I. (1983) 'Population Change and Distribution in Papua New Guinea: An Epidemiological Approach', *Journal of Human Evolution*, 12: 125–132.

—— (2000) 'It's Everyone's Problem: HIV/AIDS and Development in Asia and the Pacific: Lessons from Sexually Transmitted Disease Epidemics', paper prepared for Australian Agency for International Development (AusAID) special seminar, Canberra,

22 November 2000. Online. Available <http://www.ausaid.gov.au/ publications/pdf/riley.pdf> (accessed 14 January 2002).

Roizen, J. A. (1996) 'Explaining the Fijian Mortality Decline: Trends, Levels and Government Response', unpublished thesis, London School of Hygiene and Tropical Medicine, University of London.

Scragg, R. F. R. (1957) *Depopulation in New Ireland: A Study of Demography and Fertility*, [Port Moresby]: Administration of Papua and New Guinea.

—— (1971) 'The Eyes of the Crocodile: Inaugural Lecture', [Port Moresby]: The University of Papua New Guinea.

—— (1977) 'Historical Epidemiology in Papua New Guinea', *Papua New Guinea Medical Journal*, 20(3): 102–109.

—— (1990) 'Medical Tul-Tul to Doctor of Medicine', in B. G. Burton-Bradley (ed.), *A History of Medicine in Papua New Guinea: Vignettes of an Earlier Period*, Kingsgrove, NSW: Australasian Medical Publishing Company Ltd, 15–46.

Serjeantson, S., Board, P. C. and Bhatia, K. K. (1992) 'Population Genetics in Papua New Guinea: A Perspective on Human Evolution', in R. D. Attenborough and M. P. Alpers (eds), *Human Biology in Papua New Guinea: The Small Cosmos*, Oxford: Clarendon Press, 198–233.

Shann, F. (2000) 'Immunization – Dramatic New Evidence', *Papua New Guinea Medical Journal*, 43(1–2): 24–29.

Shlomowitz, R. (1988) 'Mortality and Indentured Labour in Papua (1995–1941) and New Guinea (1920–1941)', *Journal of Pacific History*, 23(1): 70–79.

Sims P. A. (2003) 'Papua New Guinea Needs Law and Order', *BMJ*, 326(7381): 165 (letter).

Sinnett, P. F. Kevau, I. H. and Tyson, D. (1992) 'Social Change and the Emergence of Degenerative Cardiovascular Disease in Papua New Guinea', in R. D. Attenborough and M. P. Alpers (eds), *Human Biology in Papua New Guinea: The Small Cosmos*, Oxford: Clarendon Press, 373–386.

SPC (Secretariat of the Pacific Community) (2005) Pacific Island Populations, pts 1 and 2, 'New 2004 Date'. Online. Available <http://www.spc.org.nc/demog> (accessed 16 September 2005).

Stannard, D. (1990) 'Disease and Infertility: A New Look at the Demographic Collapse of Native Populations in the Wake of Western Contact', *Journal of American Studies*, 25(3): 325–350.

Taylor, G. (2006) *A Kiap's Story: An Australian Patrol Officer's Life and Work in Papua New Guinea*, Adelaide: privately published.

Thomason, J. A., Newbrander, W. C. and Kolemainen-Aitken, R.-L. (1991) 'Introduction', in J. A. Thomason, W. C. Newbrander and R.-L. Kolemainen-Aitken (eds), *Decentralization in a Developing Country: The Experience of Papua New Guinea and its Health Service*, Canberra: National Centre of Development Studies, Australian National University, 3–7.

Tomkins, S. M. (1992) 'The Influenza Epidemic of 1918–19 in Western Samoa', *The Journal of Pacific History*, 27(2): 181–197.

Turner, O. (1905) 'Report, Resident Magistrate's Office, Samarai, Eastern Division 20th July 1906', in Commonwealth of Australia, *Report on British New Guinea for the Year ending 30 June 1905*, Melbourne.

UNAIDS (2006) *2006 AIDS epidemic update*, [Geneva]: Joint United Programme on HIV/AIDS (UNAIDS) and World Health Organization. Online. Available <http://data.unaids.org/pub/EpiReport/2006/> (accessed 3 March 2007).

Watters, D. A. K. and Lourie, J. A. (1996) 'Editorial: Trauma in Papua New Guinea: An Epidemic Out of Control', *Papua New Guinea Medical Journal*, 39(2): 91–93.
Watts, G. (1996) 'Looking to the Future', in Roy Porter (ed.), *The Cambridge Illustrated History of Medicine*, Cambridge: Cambridge University Press, 342–372.
WHO (2002) *World Report on Violence and Health*, Geneva: United Nations. Online. Available <www5.who.int> (accessed 5 December 2002).
Wigley, S. C. (1990) 'Tuberculosis in New Guinea: Historical Perspectives, with Special Reference to the Years 1871–1973', in B. G. Burton-Bradley (ed.), *A History of Medicine in Papua New Guinea: Vignettes of an Earlier Period*, Kingsgrove, NSW: Australasian Medical Publishing Co. Ltd, 167–204.
Williams, F. E. (1933) *Depopulation of the Suau District*. Anthropology Report No. 13, Port Moresby: [Territory of Papua].
World Bank (2005) Data by Country. Online. Available <http://www.worldbank.org> (accessed 19 September 2005).
Zimmet, P. and Whitehouse, S. (1981) 'Pacific Islands of Nauru, Tuvalu and Western Samoa', in D. P. Burkitt and H. C. Trowell (eds), *Western Diseases: Their Emergence and Prevention*, Cambridge, MA: Harvard University Press, 204–224.

14 History of public health in Pacific Island countries

Richard Taylor

Introduction

This chapter considers the main population health issues and public health responses since colonization began in the Pacific Island region; a region that includes the recognized geo-ethnic boundaries of Polynesia, Melanesia and Micronesia. Some states are now politically 'independent', although the functional meaning of this requires examination for many entities, even prior to the recent extensive Australian interventions in Papua New Guinea, the Solomon Islands and Nauru.

Some Pacific Island states are dependencies of other countries: American Samoa and Guam (the United States); and New Caledonia, French Polynesia, and Wallis and Futuna (France). Other states have close political, economic and migration ties with Pacific Rim metropolitan countries: the Cook Islands, Niue and Tokelau with New Zealand; and the Marshall Islands, Federated States of Micronesia, Palau and Northern Marianas with America. There are Pacific Islands previously populated only by Pacific Island peoples that are included within, or constitute, Pacific Rim countries: Hawaii (a state of the United States); west Irian (a province of Indonesia); and Aotearoa (now called New Zealand). Furthermore, there are significant migrant Pacific Island populations in Hawaii and Guam, New Zealand,[1] and to a lesser extent Australia.

There are considerable populations of migrants from outside of the Pacific Islands who now live within the region, some for many generations. Partly as a consequence of native population decline, indentured labourers were brought from British India (especially Gujarat) to work on the Fiji sugar plantations.[2] Indo-Fijians still constitute a significant proportion of the Fijian population, even after considerable emigration of the elite following successive military coups led by ethnic Fijians in the 1980s and 1990s. There is a significant population of Europeans in Melanesian New Caledonia, both locally born *caldoche* and *metropoles* (born in France), as well as migrants from Indo-China and other former French colonies, and Polynesians from other French Pacific territories – many second or more generation Caledonians.[3] On Guam, the local Chamorro population, which is an admixture of Micronesian and Spanish (since the original colonizers slaughtered most of the men), also supports considerable populations from Asia (especially the nearby Philippines), other northern Micronesian states formerly part of the US-administered UN Trust Territory of the Pacific Islands (TTPI), and mainland Americans.

Finally there are social divisions based on ethnic admixture, mostly with Europeans. This occurs especially in French Polynesia where the sizable '*les demis*' (Euro-Polynesians) usually align themselves politically with the relatively small European (French) minority.

Australian Aborigines are not considered part of the geo-ethnic categories of Pacific Island peoples; they came from Asia much earlier than Austronesian speakers and are not admixed with them. Torres Strait Islanders are closely related to Papua New Guinea (PNG) Melanesians, and the Australian border that encompasses these islands extends to within a few kilometres of the New Guinea mainland. Neither Australian Aborigines nor Torres Strait Islanders will be considered in this chapter (see Chapter 12 on Australia). Cursory reference only will be made to native Hawaiians, West Irian Melanesians, New Zealand Maori and Pacific Island migrants to the United States, New Zealand and Australia. The health status of Pacific Island populations dwelling within countries of the Pacific Rim is closely bound up with the local situations in these countries, and their social and economic positions within them. Since a separate chapter is devoted to Papua New Guinea (which is proper since it is a large country of the region in terms of population), this state will not receive the attention here its size deserves.

The present chapter will cover the history of the settlement of Pacific Island countries and the population health and demographic situations that evolved, and the public health and health services responses to these situations. The approach will be mainly chronological, considering various Island populations at a particular time without focusing excessively on any one Island state.

The first period extends from the arrival on Pacific Islands of *Homo sapiens* to European contact. Human diseases and health conditions during this period are largely conjectural, although there are distributions of diseases and vectors which have obviously existed for a very long time (*Anopheles* mosquitoes and malaria, for example), and absence of disease can be inferred from the sequelae of European contact.

The second period extends from the sixteenth century, and the disastrous effects of the introduction of hitherto inexperienced infectious diseases of Eurasian origin, to the eve of World War II, by which time depopulation had stabilized and even been reversed in some places, and public health efforts based on germ theory were applied in what had become a patchwork of colonies of European, American and Asian powers.

World War II was a short interlude, and led to severe privations for some Islanders, but it was also a time of great excitement and temporary affluence for those behind the lines who serviced the troops in Polynesia and southern Melanesia. The war also spawned public health and medical advances first used on troops then later applied to populations.

The fourth period consists of the decades of development and political independence from the end of Word War II through to the end of the cold war in 1990. This period saw extensive focused programmes by colonial and independent governments, and bilateral, international and non-governmental agencies, to improve health status in Pacific Island populations; these, in concert with parallel social and economic development, bore considerable fruit. The consequent demographic and health transitions that occurred in many populations also brought non-communicable diseases to the fore, leading to new public health challenges.

The last period, beginning in 1990, has seen a continuation of both infectious disease and non-communicable disease problems in different populations, with HIV/AIDS becoming prominent in some populations, especially that of PNG. The winding-back of external assistance in the 1990s, implosion of governance in some countries, coupled with 'terrorism' threats since 2001, have led to a relaunch of large-scale Australian aid and interventions in PNG, the Solomon Islands and Nauru. General conclusions will be drawn at the end concerning the evolution and control of major public health issues in Pacific Island countries, and lessons that can be learnt from this experience.

Prehistory

The Pacific Island region was populated by successive waves of migration from Asia. The first wave of *Homo sapiens* came probably via land bridges and over short sea stretches that could be traversed by raft during the last ice age, around 60,000 to 40,000 before the present (BP). From these hunter-(fisher)-gatherer populations came the Melanesians and Australian Aborigines. Melanesians reached the southern Solomons by 10,000 BP, south-east of which there are no land animals, except those carried by humans. While coastal and island Melanesians are admixed with subsequent Polynesian diasporas, PNG highlanders are the most closely related to the original migrants, and are credited with one of the earliest independent establishment of agriculture (around 10,000 BP).

The second wave of migrants was of Austronesian speakers (Malay and Polynesian languages), originally from Taiwan. There are still Aboriginal hill tribes in Taiwan that speak Austronesian, survivors of the Han Chinese invasion of 500 BP. These people developed important maritime technology, especially triangular sails and the outrigger for (dugout) canoes (which provided stability in the open sea), and methods of navigation using knowledge of winds, currents and stars. The migration started from Taiwan around 5,500 BP, and the Philippines was reached by 5,000 BP, then Indonesia and Malaya 4,000 BP, the Melanesian chain 3,600 BP, Central/Eastern Polynesia 3,200 BP, Hawaii and Easter Island 1,500 BP, and finally New Zealand 1,000 BP. Importantly, these people were farmers, as well as fishers, and animal husbanders, and brought with them root crops, breadfruit, coconut, pigs and fowl. This wave of migration intermingled with existing coastal and island populations in Melanesia, and then populated what is now called central and eastern Polynesia, north to Hawaii, south to New Zealand (via the Cook Islands), and east to Easter Island. These people used tools of stone, wood, shell and bone (but not metal), made twine and cloth, and pottery (Lapida style). Micronesia was settled by Austronesian-speaking peoples who reached the Philippines and eastern Indonesia, and then went on to occupy western Micronesia (the Marianas) by 3,000 BP, and from there spread eastwards. Thus, Micronesians are only distantly related to Polynesians.

Successive diasporas of humans brought their co-evolved disease species. Malaria would have descended the Melanesian chain with the earliest human migrations, and could be spread by local *Anopheles* mosquitoes. These are distributed across Southeast Asia and Australia, and down the Melanesian chain to Vanuatu (but not south to New Caledonia nor further east). The principal species are *Anopheles faraunti, A. kolienses* and *A. punctulatus* (complex) in Australia, New Guinea and Pacific Islands. The Buxton line marks the eastward extent of *Anopheles* species and passes between Futuna and Aneityum (longitude 170 degrees) in the southern tip of the Vanuatu archipelago. Humans have an uncomfortable relationship with malaria. A long period of co-evolution has led to the development of variants of haemoglobin that render erythrocytes (red cells) less susceptible to parasitism (Bowden *et al.* 1987: 357–361; Clegg and Weatherall 1999: 278–282; Ubalee *et al.* 2005: 544–549); this connection was first made by the British biologist J. B. S. Haldane in the 1940s. These abnormal haemoglobins are widespread in malarious Melanesia as heterozygotes (affecting one chromosome of the pair), and although providing some protection from the effects of malaria can lead to debilitating effects of their own, especially as homozygotes (affecting both chromosomes). Recurrent infection with malaria provides a measure of immunological resistance, so long as the child survives the first few attacks.[4] It is for this reason that epidemic (episodic) malaria (Mueller *et al.* 2005: 554–560) can be more dangerous than endemic (continuous) malaria because the latter leads to a more advantageous adjustment of the host–parasite relationship and less illness and mortality from waning immunity then reinfection. Early European observers often noted the resistance of adults to malaria but underestimated its effect on children. No doubt malaria limited populations in Anopheline regions, especially where settlement began to become dense and sessile because of agriculture and animal husbandry, and fishing on the coast.

Plasmodium falciparum is now the predominant form of malaria in PNG (Muller *et al.* 2003: 253–259) and the southwest Pacific; it produces large numbers of parasites in the blood and causes serious illness and even death in the non-immune, especially children. *Falciparum* malaria needs to do this because it has only one chance to transmit as there is no recurrent phase; it thrives in dense populations of human hosts. *Plasmodium vivax*, formerly more common, is more adapted to sparse human populations, and has recurrent phases from a liver cycle that can provide multiple opportunities for transmission, and thus episodes of illness, over many years in the same infected individual. Until recently, Melanesia has been population poor, and women are valued through bride prices (not dowry) because they produce progeny, as well as providing agricultural and domestic labour. Malaria was probably one of the reasons restricting population, especially through its effect on the mortality of children under five. This was not immediately obvious to early European observers because of the complex interactions of malaria with pneumonia, diarrhoea and under-nutrition in this age group, and because their observations were more likely to focus on prevalent illness rather than death. Family limitation, especially as a response to food scarcity, could be ensured by sexual abstinence (especially postpartum), infanticide and induced abortion.

By migrating east across the Buxton line, humans escaped the clutches of malaria because they escaped the extent of distribution of the *Anopheles* vector. *Anopheles* will not breed in artificial containers aboard ship or land transport, and can only be carried as adults (of each sex) in sufficient quantities to establish breeding colonies in a suitable new habitat. Despite extensive human travel, including air travel, and massive troop movements during war, *Anopheles* mosquitoes have never been introduced outside of their range in the western Pacific to date, except into Guam, probably during World War II and the war in Vietnam by extensive military aircraft activity (Nowell 1987: 259–265).

The other co-evolved, vector-borne human disease to hitch a ride to a new life is a species of filariasis, *Wuchereria Bancrofti*.[5] The resulting medical condition is sometimes called elephantiasis from the swollen deformities consequent on lymphatic blockage caused by the effects of adult worms that live for years. These worms periodically release microfilariae into the blood to be picked up by feeding mosquitoes and transmitted to other humans. Bancroftian filariasis is exquisitely adapted to its vectors by producing microfilariae at the precise biting times of the locally prevalent mosquito involved in transmission. *Wuchereria Bancrofti* has a near continuous distribution from its undoubted home in central Africa through the Middle East, South Asia, Indo-China, Southeast Asia, thence New Guinea, northern Australia (formerly), and the Pacific Islands through to eastern Polynesia. In this instance it was not possible for humans to outrun the disease vector, for *Wuchereria Bancrofti* proved very flexible, and has adapted to numerous mosquito species for transmission, including *Anopheles* malaria vectors in Melanesia, but also local *Aedes* and *Culex* species across Melanesia and Polynesia, which are much less fastidious breeders than *Anopheles*. Infection with Bancroftian filariasis leads to disease in only a small proportion of cases producing deformity and handicap rather than death. Nevertheless, asymptomatic cases are capable of spreading the disease to others.

Other fellow travellers with early humans would have been intestinal worms. Hookworm[6] can cause significant iron deficiency anaemia depending on the intensity of infection, concurrent iron loss from other sources (especially in women), and dietary iron intake. The eggs that pass out in the faeces require development in the soil to become infective larvae which then penetrate the bare feet of unsuspecting pedestrians. Hookworm anaemia produces tiredness and reduces productivity. The locally endemic variety, possibly brought by early humans is necator americanis, whereas ankylostoma duodenale may have been introduced by Asian immigrants (Hermant *et al.* 1929: 53). *Ascaris lumbricoides*, a parasite only of humans, with transmission by ingestion of eggs from the faeces of other infected humans, is usually asymptomatic. However, it can cause some direct illness, and also compete for calories and protein in the host gut, precipitating overt signs of under-nutrition in those (especially children) on a marginal diet.

It may have been brought by original humans or introduced. Intestinal worms are still considerable problems in Pacific Island countries (Hughes et al. 2004: 163–177).

Parasitic zoonoses (from animals) are infrequent in PNG and further east in the Pacific Islands, except those from imported pigs and dogs, because of the paucity of large mammals (Owen 2005: 1–14). Australasian fauna extends east from the Wallace line between Lombok and Bali and Borneo and Sulewesi. A new species of *Trichinella* (*papuae*) has been described in wild pigs in PNG with evidence of human infection – which presumably dates back to prehistory (Owen, Gomez Morales, Pezzotti and Pozio 2005: 618–624). The pig tapeworm (*Taenia solium*), which causes cysts in many organs (including the brain) in humans, was introduced to pigs in west Irian via Indonesia only in the 1970s, according to Desowitz, in his classic story of New Guinea tapeworms and Jewish grandmothers (Desowitz 1981).[7] Other intestinal infections also probably accompanied the early human diasporas, although not those that require large dense populations for sustenance. Perhaps salmonella was a traveller because it can infect poultry, pigs, dogs and humans, and produces episodes of diarrhoea.

Of endemic infections, yaws and hepatitis B were probable companions. Yaws, a bacterial treponemal infection (related to syphilis), is transmitted by direct contact between children, or adults and children, with open sores from the infection, usually on the legs. The infection can progress to disfigurement. Significant proportions of skeletal lesions in prehistoric samples of bones from the Solomon Islands and the Marianas are considered to be consequent to yaws (Buckley and Tayles 2003: 303–324; Pietrusewsky, Douglas and Ikehara-Quebral 1997: 315–342). Those infected with yaws are immune to venereal syphilis, a phenomenon that is initially advantageous, but leads to problems following yaws eradication. Tropical ulcers (non-yaws) due to infection of minor scratches or insect bites are likely to have been a major source of morbidity since this was the case following contact, especially in PNG (Spencer 1998: 261–267).

The liver virus infection, hepatitis B, is also transmitted by direct contact from sores and open wounds (but not due to the disease), especially amongst children, but also from mother to infant at birth, through sexual activity from adolescence, and through ritual scarification and tattooing, the latter being common in Polynesia. The diversity of a specific genotype (C) in Pacific Island populations, with specific base sequences in the nuclear material in some island populations, suggests a long evolutionary history (Jazayeri et al. 2004: 139–146). Hepatitis B infection can result in a carrier state for decades (during which transmission of infection can occur) and lead eventually to liver cirrhosis and liver cancer, the latter being one of the most common cancers in Pacific Island countries (Blakely et al. 1999: 204–210; Srivatanakul et al. 2004: 118–125).

As at least as important as the infectious diseases that humans brought with them to Pacific Islands are the diseases that they did not; in particular, the 'crowd' diseases, spread by the respiratory route, that require hundreds of thousands of people in close proximity in order to sustain themselves. The childhood viral exanthemata[8] produce large numbers of cases of generally symptomatic and immunizing infections, and spread to new cohorts of non-immune children (continually being born) during the acute phase only, since there is no carrier state or prolonged infection. In many instances these viral diseases of childhood produce more severe effects when non-immune adults are infected. Adult respiratory illnesses such as influenza and other viral infections share a similar epidemiology. This is a fragile existence for a microorganism trying to perpetuate its genetic material, and one way around it is to mutate frequently as influenza does so that previous immunizing infections are rendered useless; and huge numbers of new susceptibles are thereby created. None of these diseases has developed mechanisms for maintaining itself in sparse and isolated populations. Furthermore, as far as is known, prior to European contact there was no tuberculosis or leprosy in Pacific Island populations, nor smallpox (*variola*), nor gonorrhoea and bacillary dysentery except in parts of PNG where there were introductions of *variola* and leprosy from Malay and Chinese incursions prior to European contact (Spencer 1998: 25–44).

A small tribe in PNG, first contacted in 1984, showed evidence of endemic Bancroftian filariasis, malaria, diphtheria (*C. diphtheriae*), cytomegalovirus, HTLV-1, the Ross River arbovirus and several viruses associated with the common cold, and recent evidence of mumps, influenza A and hepatitis B since contact, but they had not been affected by TB or measles (Jenkins 1988: 97–106).

Probably of greater moment than disease was under-nutrition. Away from the coast in inland Melanesia, especially the PNG highlands, protein has always been scarce. Most root crops are low in protein content as is sago. There is little in the way of animals or birds to hunt, and pigs are infrequently consumed, and then only on ceremonial occasions, mostly by men. Perhaps in part as a consequence, cannibalism was widely practiced and in the Fore language group led to the transmission of the infective agent, now called a prion,[9] of the neurological disease, kuru (Gajdusek and Zigas 1957: 974–978). Recent genetic studies show evolutionary adaptation and resistance to kuru amongst surviving Fore from times when kuru was prevalent, and such genetic patterns in other populations may reflect previous human adaptation to the disease risks of a cannibalistic past (Mead *et al.* 2003: 640–643).

Protein–calorie malnutrition leads to illness and death, often through increased susceptibility to infection, especially in children, but also in women weakened through repeated instances of childbearing. Childhood malnutrition is marked by small frame size and short stature into adulthood – part of the instantly recognizable physique of a PNG highlander. Diminutive frame size has been considered to be adaptive in areas where shortage of food supply will be a lifelong predicament.

On the volcanic high islands near the coast, life is not necessarily hard. Food crops grow well and there are fish, cephalopods and crustacea to catch, and molluscs to be collected. However, there are hardships, especially the regular cyclones with winds that flatten and uproot food crops, strip coconut trees of their nuts, and waves and tidal surges (also *tsunami* from undersea earthquakes) which inundate lowlying food crops with sea water. This can lead to serious mass starvation until food crops can recover.

While coastal life on the high islands can be something like 'subsistence affluence' (Fisk 1982: 1–12; Sahlins 1972), human habitation on atolls, especially near the equator, requires fortitude and considerable ingenuity. Atolls are indeed desert islands where few food-producing plants besides coconut and pandanus grow naturally. Root crops are grown in pits dug down to the water table and fed by mulching; these giant taro take years to grow and are harvested and eaten on ceremonial occasions, much like pigs in the PNG highlands. South American plants such as papaya did not reach atoll countries until taken there as food plants by European colonizers. Lack of green leafy vegetables and yellow/orange fruits lead to vitamin A deficiency causing increased susceptibility to infection, especially in children, and night blindness and eye disease. A previous focus on explicit signs of eye disease (*xeropthalmia*) as indicative of clinical vitamin A deficiency masked the more widespread effects of infection and death due to subclinical deficiency. When looked for, significant vitamin A deficiency has been found in several Pacific Island countries, especially the atoll countries of Kiribati and the Marshall Islands (Anonymous 2001: 667–668; Schaumberg *et al.* 1995: 311–317), and may well partly explain some of the infant and childhood mortality found there.

Atolls in the doldrums near the equator are particularly difficult for human habitation because of drought which can last for years. Although fresh water from rain filters through the atoll sand and floats above the sea water of the subterranean water table as a 'lens'[10] that can be reached by shallow wells or galleries, the lens can be rendered brackish and undrinkable by overuse without replenishment (through rain). Fresh well water for human consumption may become polluted with animal or human excrement from adjacent taro pits (also dug down to the water table), and later, from pit latrines (a European invention). Without sufficient rain, the sap ('toddy'), which is usually collected daily from the cut spathe of the coconut tree, ceases to flow. This provides one of the few sources of thiamine (vitamin B1) for atoll dwellers. Thiamine deficiency leads to beriberi which produces neurological and cardiovascular complications. Drought-induced beriberi on the central Pacific Island of Nauru in the 1920s was countered by emergency supplies of the yeast extract, Vegemite (or Marmite) brought from Australia (Grant 1933: 113–118).

The other major category of premature mortality and handicap in the traditional situation would have been external causes: injury from falls, agricultural work, violence, and drowning. Tree climbing for coconuts and harvesting toddy must have occasioned falls, also the use of (stone) tools in agriculture and construction of dwellings and boats. Furthermore, there was always the risk of drowning in coastal areas, especially for children, but also for fishermen swept away or upturned in their flimsy fishing craft.

While much is made of the observations by early European explorers of the wonderful physique of the natives they encountered, they were coast-dwellers, and it was mostly fit, male warriors who came to meet the strangers on the beach. Furthermore, they were the survivors of considerable child mortality, especially in malarious areas.

European contact, depopulation and colonization

It fell to the Atlantic Europeans (and Chinese) to develop sturdy ocean-going vessels for intercontinental exploration and conquest. Pacific Island populations were contacted by Spanish, Dutch, Portuguese, French and English explorers and traders from the sixteenth century. The Spanish administered the Philippines across the Pacific from Mexico, and sweet potato brought there from South America soon found its way to PNG (Spriggs 1997: 52–68). Further diffusion of new flora to Pacific Islands followed, such as papaya from South America.

Europeans started with trade and missionary activities. The British, Australians and New Zealanders were active in parts of New Guinea, the Solomon Islands, Vanuatu, New Caledonia and Fiji, in Kiribati and Tuvalu (formerly the Gilbert and Ellis Islands), and in Tonga, Samoa and the Cook Islands. France was active in eastern Polynesia, New Caledonia, Wallis and Futuna, and Vanuatu. Germany was active in parts of New Guinea, central and northern Micronesia, and Samoa. With Europeans came Asian indentured or free workers and traders, especially in Fiji. European powers and later America competed for spheres of influence then created protectorates and colonies. All German Pacific colonies were captured by Britain, Australia, New Zealand or Japan at the outbreak of war in 1914, and the US occupied parts of German Micronesia and Samoa. While the small islands were easy to colonize, much of Melanesia proved difficult to penetrate because of the rugged terrain and endemic malaria which devastated the non-immune European colonists (Eckart 1999: 1389–1391). The highlands of PNG were not contacted by Europeans until the 1930s, and then by airplane.

The initial result of European contact was devastating epidemics of infectious diseases, especially respiratory diseases (often called 'ship fever', because they struck whenever a ship visited), to which these isolated populations had no immunity. In the late 1600s, epidemics occurred in the Marianas with the arrival of each trans-Pacific galleon. Measles (*morbilli, rubella*), chicken pox (*varicella*), whooping cough (*pertussis*), influenza, tuberculosis and leprosy (*mycobacteria tuberculosis; mycobacteria leprae*), smallpox (*variola*) and bacillary dysentery (*shigellosis*) were introduced. A large measles outbreak in Fiji in 1874 led to 40,000 deaths in a population of 150,000 (27%) within weeks. There were also many deaths from epidemics along the Papuan coast. Dysentery epidemics plagued the goldfields in PNG (Spencer 1998: 106–120). The 1919 influenza pandemic in western Samoa killed 20% of the population (Denoon 1997: 218–252). Not one case occurred in American Samoa, just across the water, as a consequence of a two-year quarantine imposed by naval blockade. This is a striking example of the success of quarantine, enforced by military means and assisted by the geography.

Another factor was the advent of guns. Guns and European adventurers turned relatively innocuous warfare into a deadly business, with much increased deaths from violence between warring factions in many Island populations.

Reduced fertility occurred from tubal obstruction due to rampant venereal infections (*gonorrhoea; clamydia*) – the 'false fertility transition'. The noxious combination of excess mortality and lowered fertility led to the well-documented declines in populations in accessible Pacific Islands and was accentuated in some places near Australia (especially Vanuatu and New Caledonia) by emigration under indentured labour schemes to the Queensland canefields.

This phase resulted in the New Hebrides (Vanuatu) losing half of its population, and New Caledonian Kanaks were reduced by two-thirds by 1900. The population of almost all Polynesian populations fell by at least half, and much more in some island groups, such as the Marquesas. There was significant depopulation in Micronesia. Huge depopulations (up to 90%) of native peoples occurred in Hawaii and New Zealand (and in Australia) (Denoon 1997: 218–252). The effects were much less substantial in some Melanesian countries (especially PNG) where rugged terrain and health hazards (especially malaria) limited the advance of colonizers. However, significant depopulation (by more than half) of the western islands of PNG is recorded in the early 1900s due primarily to the introduction of malaria from the PNG mainland, but also introduced were tuberculosis, influenza, pneumonia and dysentery, and there were underlying nutrient deficiencies. The social disruption, violence and warfare that often followed the initial depopulation then accentuated it (Cilento 1928: 82).

European commentators thought that indigenous populations were headed for extinction. This opinion, based on observations of extensive illness and population decline in native peoples, was buttressed by theoretical support from the social version of Darwinism that had considerable currency in the late nineteenth and early twentieth centuries. According to this widely held view, Island populations declined because the native peoples were inferior to the colonizers as a consequence of inherited traits and these led to immoral behaviours. Eugenics became a prominent discourse in public health and medicine, giving rise to support for restriction of breeding of 'inferior' human stock and to measures to improve the quality of the white 'race' (Bowler 2003: 274–324). Laws for the sterilization of the mentally and morally unfit were enacted in several American states and European countries in the 1920s and 1930s, and the movement reached its zenith in Germany under National Socialism.

Stabilization

By the 1890s 'tropical medicine' emerged as a discipline with strong scientific input from microbiology and vector biology, and with a focus on public health interventions including quarantine, water supply and sanitation, personal and family hygiene, vector control, nutrition and vaccination (against smallpox), many of which had also been found to be empirically effective in European and North American populations. Many diseases deemed 'tropical', then and now, were formerly considerable problems in Europe (Porter 1999: 462–492) – such as malaria, plague, cholera and leprosy; and also malnutrition and vitamin deficiencies. But there were also new conditions: *filariasis, schistosomiasis, trypanosomiasis* (sleeping sickness), to name a few. This new specialty produced a steady stream of trained practitioners and informed policy advice for colonial administrators which was then implemented within an authoritarian and military context, firstly for the protection of the health of expatriates, then of the local population (for the benefit of expatriates), and eventually for health improvement in the whole population.

International quarantine was implemented with varying efficacy and enthusiasm depending upon the legal framework and the organization of colonial administrations. Quarantine in most cases only delayed the introduction of diseases rather than permanently protecting populations. Quarantine also was applied to importation of infected animals and may have restricted entry of exotic zoonoses, especially of pigs and cattle. Internal quarantine of infected areas could be practiced on the larger islands, and within island groups. Segregating diseased individuals with acute infections (for example, dysentery) and chronic infections (for example, leprosy and tuberculosis) probably has some effect in containing spread.

Probably the most important actions were to separate water for human consumption from human and animal excreta – the traditional task of public health. However, this was not easy in many situations whether in shanty settlements or rural villages. Pit latrines were dug these could contaminate underground water supplies. Water sources were protected from human and animal contamination. Personal hygiene also depended on water supply, but changing behaviour was not easy in local populations who saw no connection between these activities and disease believed to be due to supernatural forces. Furthermore, clean water supplies and sanitation require funds for construction and maintenance.

Following the discovery of the life cycle of the malaria pathogen and the role of the *Anopheles* mosquito, endeavours were made to control breeding sites including surface water oiling and the use of larvivorous fish of the *Gambusia* species in contained water sources. For expatriates there was the possibility of residential screening and bed nets. Similar anti-mosquito measures could also be taken against vectors of filariasis and dengue. Quinine was available for treatment of malaria,but this was available only for restricted, mostly expatriate populations and would have had no effect on the epidemiology of the disease.

Proper nutrition could also be recommended and to some extent enforced, not only sufficiency of calories and proteins, but also sufficient of the newly discovered micronutrients, especially thiamine, which was removed from polished rice during milling; removal led to beriberi in indentured labourers and others dependent on a restricted diet of imported food.

Targeting hookworm became a near obsession for the Rockefeller Foundation in its international health programmes of the early twentieth century (from 1910) (Birn and Solorzano 1999: 1197–1213; Brown 1976: 897–903). This was particularly curious because there were much greater problems than hookworm (such as malaria). Hermant and Cilento noted that throughout Melanesia in 1928 hookworm was almost universal but of little significance except in the New Hebrides (now Vanuatu). They dutifully quote Dr S. M. Lambert of the Rockefeller Foundation: 'hookworm disease is widespread and has disastrous effects in lowering the vitality of the race, in lowering resistance to.... inter-current disease.' Rockefeller was convinced that 'education and health.... rather than indiscriminate charity, would make philanthropy produce dividends'.[11] He wanted to target something that affected large numbers of people, was curable and preventable, and 'of which the cause could be seen'[12] (Heiser 1936: 266–268) Hookworm led to anaemia and reduced productivity (a plausible explanation for the well-known 'laziness' of Southern US blacks and indigenous peoples in a wide variety of countries). It could be diagnosed and the prevalence measured (by eggs in the stool), treated individually or *en masse* by a 'magic bullet' (medication), and also prevented though hygienic measures. Against this must be balanced the conscious use of hookworm eradication as an 'entering wedge' to the establishment of permanent public health institutions by doctors and administrators involved in campaigns (Warren and Schad 1990: 3–14). Mass treatment (even with modern drugs) has little long-term effect in helminthic disease in the absence of sanitation because of prompt reinfection; and the effectiveness of the early quite toxic treatments (thymol, chenopodium and beta-naphthol) is questionable (Boccaccio 1972: 30–53). There was very little research on the effectiveness of all the activity and expenditure related to hookworm control in the Pacific Islands or elsewhere (Warren and Schad 1990: 3–14). Modern control efforts employing effective anti-helminthic drugs would usually involve at least two distributions per year; and without sanitation, there is no agreement on whether there would have an effect on anaemia and hence productivity without iron supplements (Stoltzfus *et al.* 1997: 223–232). By the late 1920s, it was understood that hygienic improvement for hookworm eradication required broad-based economic and social development with physical sanitary infrastructure, and Rockefeller switched focus to funding public health and medical schools at Johns Hopkins, Harvard, London, Sydney and other universities.

Prior to World War II, there was very little in the way of effective medical treatment. Venesection (bleeding) and purging were on offer, but no doubt made the patients worse rather than better. Quinine was effective against malaria and supplies became more abundant following cultivation of the tree (a native of South America) in India and the East Indies. Sanatoria for lepers and tuberculosis patients may have helped immune responses through adequate food and relief from manual labour, but their main public health effect was quarantine of obviously infectious patients. Medical treatments had little or no effect. And there were the toxic arsenicals for syphilis which were also effective against yaws. Gonorrhoea was treated with urethral or vaginal lavage with solutions of potassium permanganate, silver nitrate and the like, and this was said to be effective. Hookworm was treated with chenopodium oil. Tropical ulcers responded to cleaning and topical antiseptic solutions such as iodide.

The above was the sum total of the public health and medical armamentarium. Then, as now, medical doctors tended to exaggerate the effectiveness of their treatments, and medical activity in treating the ill does not necessarily translate into substantial changes in the natural course of illness in individuals, let alone disease control or mortality decline in populations. Nevertheless, this armamentarium was not ineffective, especially the public health component. By the late 1930s, life expectancy in Australia had risen to 64 years for males and 68 years for females, with cardiovascular disease significantly exceeding infection as a cause of death (Taylor et al. 1998a: 27–36; Taylor et al. 1998b: 37–44).

The importance of formal colonization was that public health measures and even mass treatments could be mandated through law and enforced through the police and courts if necessary. Before colonization there were anarchic situations of interference by expatriate adventurers who brought guns and alcohol (as well as disease), a patchwork of competing missionary influences (with hinterlands and outer islands virtually untouched), and uncontrolled trading and exploitation by European commercial companies and planters which were unable to exercise control and were concerned predominantly with profit. Colonialism in the Pacific Islands provided law and pacification and a legislative framework for quarantine, water supply and sanitation, food hygiene, vector control and labour regulation (including nutrition and housing). Colonization also supplied many dedicated administrators and medical personnel who, while recognizing commercial realities, had some independence of action and were not mostly motivated by profit. In 1921, the PNG chief medical officer finally convinced plantation owners and managers it was in their own best interests to provide adequate nutrition and living conditions for their Papuan workers (Spencer 1998: 189–194).

From 1889, native medical practitioners were trained in Fiji and engaged in certain limited tasks, especially vaccination. From the late 1800s, native medical assistants were trained in both British and German New Guinea. From 1929, the School of Medicine in Fiji graduated doctors with a diploma in medicine. Students were drawn from Fiji and several other English-speaking colonies in the Pacific; after graduation they worked in Fiji or returned to their islands of origin to provide medical care and public health advice. Nurses were trained in hospitals in many places in the Pacific Islands.

Christian missionaries helped promote hygiene ('Cleanliness is next to godliness') and offered some medical services. Importantly, they provided education in European languages (chiefly English and French) and in the vernacular. Literacy has uses as anyone who has ever tried health promotion amongst the illiterate well knows.

Despite the worst predictions, Pacific Island populations stabilized by the first quarter of the twentieth century after previously epidemic diseases had become endemic, armed conflict ended, food supplementation in marginal areas and in times of emergency was provided, and rudimentary public health measures, especially water supply and sanitation in towns and vector control, were introduced. The last great epidemic was influenza in 1918. Although the population of Fiji finally started to increase during World War I after continuous decline from at least 1891, the influenza epidemic dealt another blow; by 1927 the population had only recovered to that of a decade earlier (Hermant et al. 1929: 34–35).

In 1928, the mortality situation in malarious Melanesia (Papua New Guinea, the Solomon Islands and Vanuatu) was that the major causes of death were: malaria, especially in children, followed by pneumonia, then tuberculosis, dysentery and under-nutrition (including beriberi, especially in indentured labourers). Along with tropical ulcer, these also contributed to morbidity. Yaws was common, but no syphilis was reported. Filariasis was multi-focal, and hookworm almost universal but of little clinical significance. In non-malarious Melanesia (New Caledonia and Fiji) there were: pneumonia, dysentery, enteric fevers (typhoid and so on), filariasis, yaws, childhood infections, tuberculosis, leprosy and syphilis amongst immigrant 'Asiatics' (unexposed to yaws) but not in Melanesians. Quarantine was strenuously undertaken in the non-malarious countries to prevent introduction of *Anopheles* mosquitoes and cases of malaria[13] as well as other infectious diseases. In 1928, PNG infant mortality was given as 176 per 1,000 births in districts monitored (variation of 120 to 420), and in Fiji, 158 per 1,000; and maternal mortality varied from 1.8% to 6.5% (Hermant *et al.* 1929: 69–71).

World War II

The Pacific Islands were pushed to the forefront as a major theatre of operations in World War II. Many Micronesians were shipped as forced labour to Truk (in the now Federated States of Micronesia), the site of a large Japanese naval base.[14] Great hardships were suffered by both local and expatriate Micronesians on Truk and on other islands in Micronesia under Japanese control. Twelve hundred male Nauruans were taken to Truk as forced labour; a third returned to Nauru after the war. It may be suggested that this process accentuated the selection pressure for the 'thrifty genotype' (Neel 1999a: 692–703; Neel 1999b: S2–S9) as the underlying reason for the propensity for diabetes mellitus (adult onset or type II) found in Nauruans and other Pacific Islanders. Pacific Islanders were also affected by the fighting and starvation in New Guinea and the Solomons.

Troop movements facilitated the spread around the Pacific of *Aedes Aegypi*, the principal vector for dengue. They also distributed malaria cases around the Pacific region but transmission could only occur within the distribution of the *Anopheles* vector. Such was the seriousness of troop casualties from malaria, responsibility for control through personal protection, vector control (including Dichloro-Diphenyl-Trichloroethane (DDT) from 1943) and suppressive treatment (atebrin) passed from medical officers to field commanders (Fenner 1998: 55–63; Spencer 1992: 33–66) with considerable success. Malaria transmission from returning troops via local *Anopheles* species at the end of the war occurred as far south as Melbourne in Australia (Black 1981: 146).

In order to protect troops various measures were introduced: improved hygiene, including water supply and sanitation; vector control, including chemical insecticides such as DDT (from 1943); new antimalarial and antibiotic chemotherapy; and improvements in surgery and blood transfusion. These would be used after the war to benefit Island populations.

Development, independence and dependence

The post-war period marked the beginning of serious population-wide economic and social development for the Pacific, and the application to populations of the public health methods, and new drugs and insecticides, that had been developed during the war.

This period also marked the beginning of extensive modernization, especially in urban areas, with growth of government bureaucracy, school education and moneterization of the economy, more trade and food imports, tourism, mechanization of sea and land transport, and a decline in subsistence living in many areas. These changes were more prominent in Polynesia and Micronesia than in Melanesia.

During the 1960s and 1970s, political independence was granted or thrust upon many Pacific Island countries. By 1980 the current political geography had been established. Some states were completely independent, some continued with significant ties to previous colonial powers, and some remained as territories of France or the United States. International aid became available in huge quantities on a per capita basis. A large impact could be produced for relatively small amounts of money. Tourism that catered to Western tastes developed in some accessible places. Modernization *in situ* continued apace, and extensive migration to 'metropolitan' countries, especially the United States and New Zealand, also ensured acculturation to Western norms.

Population

With significant declines in mortality, populations increased, especially since most states showed little inclination to reduce fertility. To some extent this high fertility is due to real and perceived previous depopulation and current underpopulation, especially in Melanesia, but also to the considerable opportunities for out-migration available in some states such as Tonga and Samoa, reinforced by a strong pronatalist culture and the important role of children in the subsistence economy.

Tonga was one of the first countries in the Pacific officially to accept family planning precisely because of its small land area and the requirement of an allocation of land to each adult male; a regional agency that focuses on family planning, the South Pacific Alliance for Family Health (SPAFH), was established there.

Increased population on small main atolls (supported by wages and imported food) such as Tarawa (Kiribati) or Majuro (Marshall Islands) soon led to overconsumption (and hence brackishness) of the freshwater lens and also pollution of the underground fresh water supply from human and animal faeces. This has required pumping and piping of water from distant sparsely populated parts of the atoll or catchments on airport runways, then road tanker delivery or rationed reticulation, supplemented by roof catchments. Roof catchment requires expensive large storage tanks, metal roof sheeting, gutters and piping, and maintenance of these. It provides a wonderful environment for mosquitoes to breed. During times of drought, external delivery of water by ship is needed (Nauru and Christmas Island in Kiribati). The development of saltwater flush sewage systems relying on non-rustable mostly plastic materials is a great boon for urbanized atoll populations where freshwater is in limited supply. However, these require significant capital investment and maintenance as well as intensive communication, information, and education programmes to ensure their correct use.

Communicable disease control

Yaws eradication by mass penicillin administration is one of the more spectacular ventures of the early post-war era. But without the immunity provided by yaws the next generation would be susceptible to venereal syphilis (Willcox 1980: 204–209). In Marshallese women in the 1980s, the bimodal serological pattern of treponemal infection by age reflected yaws infection in the older women and syphilis in the young (Gershman et al. 1992: 599–606; Levy et al. 1989: 46, 61).

In 1955 the World Health Organization adopted malaria eradication as a global strategy (Trigg and Kondrachine 1998: 11–16). Eradication had proved possible in areas where the disease was seasonal and focal, such as in southern Europe. A concerted attack on the *Anopheles* vector using all means possible (including DDT) was employed to reduce transmission plus comprehensive detection and treatment of all cases. Since there is no animal reservoir, once the disease is eradicated from humans, anti-mosquito measures are no longer required. By 1967 malaria had been eradicated from all developed countries. While there was considerable success in reducing mortality and morbidity, global eradication proved to be beyond reach. Tropical climates combined with rural populations to ensure continued exposure to *Anopheles* mosquitoes. *Anopheles* became selected to a predominance of strains that fed outdoors at dusk and daybreak, rather than night-biting indoors and then alighting on DDT sprayed walls leading to certain death. Also some *Anopheles* became relatively resistant to DDT, as did the malaria parasite to the effects of antimalarial drugs, especially chloroquine (al-Yaman et al. 1996: 16–22).

Moreover, with political independence, populations could no longer be forced to comply with anti-mosquito measures, as they had been by colonial regimes. Non-cooperation with such government public health measures was often part of a more general rejection of government authority because of political, ethnic or religious conflict with the regime in power. Newly independent nations often lacked the will, expertise and resources to pursue vigorously malaria eradication. By 1993, eradication formally gave way to control as WHO policy (Trigg and Kondrachine 1998: 11–16), with the objective of reducing and controlling morbidity and mortality from the disease by personal protection though bed nets (impregnated with insecticide) and treatment of symptomatic cases with antimalarials. Malaria declined in the Solomon Islands during the 1990s from a combination of DDT spaying, insecticide-impregnated bed nets and health education (Over et al. 2004: 214–223).

While Bancroftian filariasis was reduced with vector control, and with periodic mass treatment to reduce micro-filaria in the blood (and interrupt transmission) using DEC (diethylcarbamazine), elimination proved elusive even in French Polynesia where considerable resources were allocated (Esterre et al. 2001: 190–195). The introduction of the more efficacious drug, ivermectin, may prove effective for elimination (Ichimori and Crump 2005: 441–444).

Antibiotics became available and cure for previously untreatable diseases could be offered: pneumonia, tuberculosis and leprosy, intestinal infections, meningitis, as well as malaria. Furthermore, vaccines became available, especially for childhood diseases: diphtheria, pertussis, poliomyelitis, tetanus and later measles and hepatitis B. For diarrhoeal diseases, there was oral rehydration salts since most are viral and unresponsive to antibiotics and mortality is due to dehydration. However, these medical marvels had to be made available to the population at large to be effective and the largely treatment-oriented urban health services were ill-equipped to deliver these to most of the population. Primary health care as expounded at the Alma-Ata Conference came to the rescue.

Population under-nutrition diminished with improvements in food distribution, supplemented by extensive imports in some countries, and nutritional monitoring and education, especially as part of organized government maternal and child health (MCH) services; these included food and micronutrient supplementation where necessary. Under-nutrition is an important underlying factor in morbidity and mortality from communicable disease.

The other important interventions were water supply and sanitation, and domestic and personal hygiene, which continued to improve in both urban and rural areas.

Medical and health worker training

In Fiji, Melanesian vaccinators (against smallpox) were trained from 1879 and 'native medical practitioners' were produced by the Suva Medical School from 1888 after a three-year course. From 1917, Islanders from other Pacific states attended. In 1928, when there were 50 native medical practitioners at work (Hermant et al. 1929: 33), a new Central Medical School (renamed Fiji School of Medicine in 1961) was constructed, financed largely through the Rockefeller Foundation; and the training period was extended to four years. Graduates were called 'assistant medical practitioners', then 'medical officer' from 1972. An advantage of the local diploma qualification was that it had limited international recognition and thus precluded out-migration of these doctors to Pacific Rim or distant metropolitan countries. The Fiji medical qualification was upgraded in 1982 to a Bachelor of Medicine/Bachelor of Surgery awarded by the University of the South Pacific; it enjoyed more general recognition (Penington 1984: 314–318). This facilitated emigration, especially by Indo-Fijian doctors, prompted partly by racially-based political coups in 1987 and 2000. In any case, the medical workforce had become somewhat skewed towards Indians because in a period in the 1980s entry became based on merit (secondary school results) before re-institution of racial quotas for Fijians. Between 1987 and 2002, 510 doctors left the Fiji government health service, while 284 graduates for Fiji were produced (Baravilala and Moulds 2004: 602).

In Papua New Guinea medical assistant training began in the early years of the twentieth century, with three months of training of medical assistants, variously called 'doctor boys', dressers and medical orderlies. There were over 2,000 by 1928 (Hermant et al. 1929: 25). This was upgraded after World War II when orderlies were armed with penicillin (for most infections), chloroquine (for malaria), aspirin (for pain and fever) and gentian violet (for skin ulcers). The PNG system was reputedly used as an exemplar by the architects of primary health care at the Alma-Ata Conference in 1979. It was not until 1961 that the Papuan Medical College was established in Port Moresby to train doctors for a diploma of medicine and surgery in line with the Fijian model. In 1965 the University of PNG was established, and the Medical College was incorporated as a faculty, with students graduating as Bachelor of Medicine/Bachelor of Surgery from 1973 (850 graduates to 1999); some students were from other Pacific Island states. In 1999, health sciences (pharmacy, dental therapists, post-basic nurses, and so on.) became part of the faculty, having been separate since its inception in 1974. The Master of Medicine programme to train specialists started in 1974 (Sapuri 1999: 59–62).

In much of the former American Micronesia – the Marshall Islands, Federated States of Micronesia (FSM) and Palau – and in American Samoa, the deficiency of local medical doctors was perceived to be a problem by the 1980s, and a five-year medical officer degree was developed and delivered by the Pacific Basin Medical Officer's Training Programme, a satellite of the University of Hawaii School of Medicine, based in Ponape FSM. The successful model of the Fiji School of Medicine diploma was embraced to produce a cohort of locally trained medical doctors who could provide basic medical care only in the jurisdictions (mentioned above) where they were licensed to practice. Around 15 per year were graduated, with a total of 70 by 1998 (Dever 1994: 71–72).

The unsung heroines of health services in many Pacific Island states are nurses and midwives, generally trained in hospitals and clinics to certificate level. Very little is written about nursing training and services in the Pacific, although nurses have often provided the backbone of primary health care in many Island states such as Fiji.

Health services

Health services after World War II often concentrated disproportionately on provision of medical and surgical clinics and hospital services since many conditions were amenable to curative treatment, especially infections. Individualized treatment and care of the ill were enthusiastically supported by expatriate Christian churches as part of their mission. For those able to reach services, care was supplied by expatriate doctors, although there was often a lack of coordination between government and mission services and between missions of different Christian denominations. At the same time, there was also a paucity of services in most rural and remote areas, and a lack of focus on more mundane public health issues such as clean water and sanitation, vector control, nutrition and immunization (when this became available).

The situation was nowhere more preposterous than in the English–French condominium of the New Hebrides (now Vanuatu) where two competing hospitals existed in Port Vila (one Anglophone, the other Francophone); there was a rural health service (supposedly combined Anglo-French) in addition to competing mission hospitals and health centres (English Protestant; French Catholic) in some of the outer islands.[15] Such situations were not sustainable once political independence supervened. It was the existence of such residual colonial medical superstructures that led, in part, to the Primary Health Care initiative at the Conference in Alma-Ata in 1976 (World Health Organization 1978: 409–430).

Following independence it was apparent in many Island countries that expensive hospital- and doctor-based medical services could not be sustained at former levels, and, coinciding with the Primary Health Care (PHC) initiative of Alma-Ata, many outer-island hospitals were consolidated or closed and replaced by PHC centres staffed by nurses or other primary health-care workers.

With the development of public health and medical services that involved evacuation for secondary and tertiary care, the archipelagic nature or rugged terrain of some Pacific Island states present significant problems. In scattered atoll and mountainous island states such as central and eastern Micronesia, eastern Polynesia and Island Melanesia (especially Vanuatu), inaccessibility of the population outside of the main Island poses great problems for the provision of health and other services. Boat transport is rendered difficult by lack of harbours and in many cases only small boats can cross the reef, and then only at high tide. On atolls there are considerable problems in moving between populated islets which are broken up by passages of seawater. In Melanesia, the rugged terrain makes land transport difficult, particularly away from the coast where there is no possibility of waterborne transport. All this leads to a dependence on aeroplanes which are expensive to purchase and maintain and have very small carrying capacity.

In some US-associated states, especially the Marshall Islands and American Samoa, there has been general expectation of evacuation to Hawaii, mostly to the Military Hospital (Trippler) for serious illness, or even investigation for less serious illness. A significant proportion of the health budget has been spent on these evacuations, which often included family members for support, and have been, in some instances, allocated according to connections with the ruling elite. This produces a huge distortion in health-care expenditure.

Non-communicable disease

In some Island states consumption patterns changed significantly, coincident with imported food, alcohol, and tobacco, and exercise decreased. This was more evident in urban than rural areas, on main islands rather than outer islands, and in Polynesia, Micronesia and parts of Melanesia (Fiji), rather than in malarious Melanesia. Tobacco consumption had been implanted in many countries for a very long time, and tobacco had been used as exchange by visiting sailors in the Gilbert Islands (now Kiribati) from the early nineteenth century.

By the 1970s, non-communicable diseases, such as cardiovascular disease and diabetes, were an evident cause of significant morbidity and mortality in adults in many Island populations. This was a result of a real increase in these conditions, as well as the decline in infectious diseases and under-nutrition as important health issues. Numerous studies showed non-communicable disease to be greater problems in modernized and urban areas, and less important in other places, especially in Melanesian malarious countries (Taylor et al. 1992: 283–293). In some instances the rise of non-communicable conditions led to a decline or plateau in life expectancy, which had previously been rising, because of the control of infection and under-nutrition.

Injuries

Motor vehicle accidents (MVA) are prominent as a cause of death in many Pacific Island countries, especially when expressed as a rate per vehicle registered. MVA deaths and injuries are often a consequence of alcohol intoxication, and the frequent use of motorcycles (without helmet use) results in vulnerability of the rider (Watters and Dyke 1996: 121–125).

Domestic violence (against children and wives) has been common in many Pacific societies, although seemingly only noticed by anthropologists since the 1980s (Counts 1990: 1–5).

Suicide in young men in some Island populations (FSM (Chuk), Guam, Fiji Indians, western Samoa) show very high rates internationally, and in western Samoa and Fiji Indians female rates exceed those of males (1988–1992 data). Furthermore there is evidence of increases in suicide over three decades to 1990 (Booth 1999: 433–448). One explanation posits tensions between the traditional and the modern, with such tensions less in both highly traditional (and isolated) and in very modernized cosmopolitan situations.

Excessive alcohol intake ('binge drinking') is rife in young men when they have access, and is associated with accidents, interpersonal violence and domestic violence; older men frequently do not provide sober role models.

Nuclear weapons testing

Remoteness is a comparative advantage for nuclear weapons testing, especially before it was shown that radioactivity from atmospheric testing soon becomes globalized. Remote Pacific Islands under colonial control were ideal places for nuclear weapons testing following the dawn of the nuclear warfare age at Hiroshima and Nagasaki. Bikini and Enewetak atolls in the Marshall Islands were used for nuclear testing by the US (1946–1958) and exposure occurred to inhabitants of Rongerik atoll from fallout from the 1954 atmospheric test on Bikini with suggestions of acute radiation sickness. A result has been thyroid cancer (Takahashi et al. 2003: 99–107). A consequential continuing issue has been the jealousies created by the United States' providing of unlimited medical care to the few exposed Islanders compared to the inadequate medical services for the majority of the population. The United States then moved nuclear testing underground in remote and favourable geological environments on the US mainland.

France conducted atmospheric tests in 1966–1974 at Mururoa and Fangataufa atolls in French Polynesia and, subsequently, underground testing until 1996. Previous reports suggested that doses from fallout were 5–10% of the average natural background radioactivity exposures in Tahiti and New Zealand; however, rain-out events on specific days in Samoa in 1966 and Tahiti 1974 recorded much higher levels.[16] Nevertheless, the conclusion has been that there are no perceptible health effects because of insufficient exposure although some of the calculations were based on French exposure data. Cancer registry data based on small numbers revealed no anomalies (New Zealand Ministry of Foreign Affairs 1984: 166). With the Polynesian opposition having been elected in French Polynesia, recent investigations have found significant exposures of populations from atmospheric tests (especially Mangareva in the Gambier group) – these were known but not revealed by French authorities – as well as significant exposures of workers involved in nuclear testing and clean-up (Commission d'enquête sur le conséquences des essais nucléaires 2005). A report of higher thyroid cancer incidence (1985–1995) in Polynesians of French Polynesia compared to Polynesians of Hawaii or New Zealand (not attributed by the authors to radioactive exposure) (de Vathaire *et al.* 2000: 59–63; Le Vu *et al.* 2000: 722–731) as well as claims of higher cancer incidence in veterans of nuclear tests compared to the general population (Commission d'enquête sur le conséquences des essais nucléaires 2005: 174–176) have been reported.

Overall, the evidence for a significant health effect from radioactive fallout from testing in the Pacific is slim. However, in the Marshalls and French Polynesia, nuclear testing and associated militarization was associated with large expenditures on expatriate personnel and infrastructure that spread through the society. There was considerable support for nuclear testing within French Polynesia because it provided jobs and affluence, although it was a Faustian bargain in the view of many. The main health effects of these programmes were the hastening of the disease transition with the evolution of non-communicable disease from changes in diet and exercise and increases in tobacco and alcohol consumption. There were also the usual results, in terms of sexually transmitted infections, from an influx of males of military age with money.

By 1980, and continuing through to the new millennium, it was evident that Pacific Island populations are quite heterogeneous with respect to health and mortality: the demographic and epidemiological transitions are at quite different stages in various populations, with the less developed states still affected by endemic infectious disease and under-nutrition with relatively high mortality (especially in children), and other states with relatively high life expectancy and a predominance of non-communicable disease and accidents (in adults), but with other Island countries located in the middle, with double burdens and divergence between rural and urban areas. Cross-sectional patterns mirror the longitudinal progression of the demographic and health transitions (see Figures 14.2 and 14.3).

Despite huge efforts to eradicate malaria, by the 1980s it was recognized that this could not be accomplished in endemic areas, especially with the decline in government authority following political independence, so reversion to malaria control became official policy, as elsewhere in the world.

The new realities

Following the end of the cold war in 1990, foreign aid (which had been to a significant extent 'geopolitical rent') declined substantially, and independent and partially independent countries struggled with the realities of their actual resource base, fluctuating demands for products and services (sugar, tourism, labour and so on) and their remoteness from the larger populations of Asia, Australasia and the Americas. The USAID office in Suva closed in 1994 but reopened in the wake of the events of 11 September 2001.

Rent for deep sea fisheries access in exclusive economic zones could be obtained, but not without the military aerial surveillance capacity of metropolitan countries. The technological sophistication required to operate and service the complex equipment[17] required for modern competitive deep sea fishery industries was beyond the capacity of most states even apart from the capital costs involved in such ventures. Many Pacific Island countries maintained their standard of living (and non-communicable disease rates) with the help of large cash remittances from relatives living abroad – the 'transnational corporations of kin'.

In retrospect, the age of independence was over in Pacific Island states by 1980. Nevertheless, there were further accommodations that had to be worked out in the French territories where civil disturbances in New Caledonia and French Polynesia[18] mixed demands for better government services and employment opportunities with demands for political independence and for socialist transformation. These conflicts were as much within these societies as between them and France. Some of the results were significant increases in prosperity in indigenous populations with coincident acceleration of the epidemiological transition; and a considerable improvement in health and other services resulting in significant declines in infant and child mortality (Institute de la Statistique et des Études Économiques 2006; Institut Statistique de Polynésie Française 2006).

Repeated coups in Fiji, and government implosion in Solomon Islands and partial implosion in PNG, are as much symptomatic of the disarray in governance including health services as they are factors which produce these circumstances. This is not a suitable environment for the critical analysis of health problems and the orderly implementation of interventions and services. This situation is compounded by the woeful lack or inaccuracy of health statistics in many Pacific Island states which prevents proper population health assessment, monitoring and evaluation; for example, mortality and life expectancy in Fiji and elsewhere (Taylor *et al.* 2005: 207–214).

The events and aftermath of 11 September 2001 in the United States, in association with ethnic and political implosions, produced concerns in Australia and elsewhere of the possible consequences of failed states in the neighbouring Pacific region which could be used as possible bases for terrorist activity and money laundering for financing terrorism, as well as transit havens for illegal migration, and even sources of infectious disease for mainland Australia (especially HIV and TB). These events have produced a context within which a considerable increase in Australian involvement in PNG, and the Solomons in particular, has occurred. This includes extensive health sector activity but with an open-ended programmatic approach rather than limited project focus, considerable use of expatriate staff, and a focus on governance as well as technical issues. The results of these new endeavours are awaited.

The 1990s saw the introduction of health-sector reform in many Pacific Island states prompted by the World Bank and its interest in the health sector dating from its report on Investing in Health in 1993 (The World Bank 1993). This was coincident with structural adjustment economic policies pushed by the International Monetary Fund (IMF) and the World Bank. This occurred in the context of changing economic ideologies in Western countries from the late 1970s,[19] and was reinforced by the introduction of significant market mechanisms in several centrally planned economies ranging from Eastern Europe and the former USSR to China and Vietnam, and the collapse of the Soviet Union in 1990. Health sector reform involved a downsizing of government services and a focus on user-pays, cost-recovery insurance schemes and 'close-to-client' services. By 1990 primary

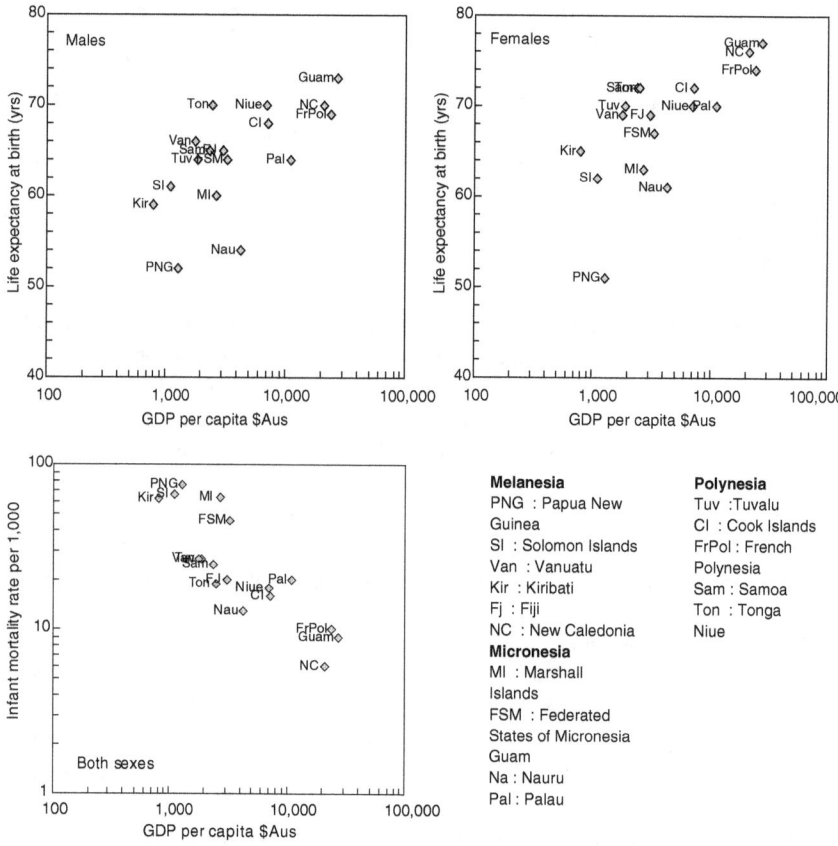

Figure 14.1 Life expectancy and infant mortality in Pacific Island states *c.*2000 in relation to GDP per capita.

Sources: Taylor, Bampton and Lopez (2005: 207–214); Secretariat of the Pacific Community (2004).

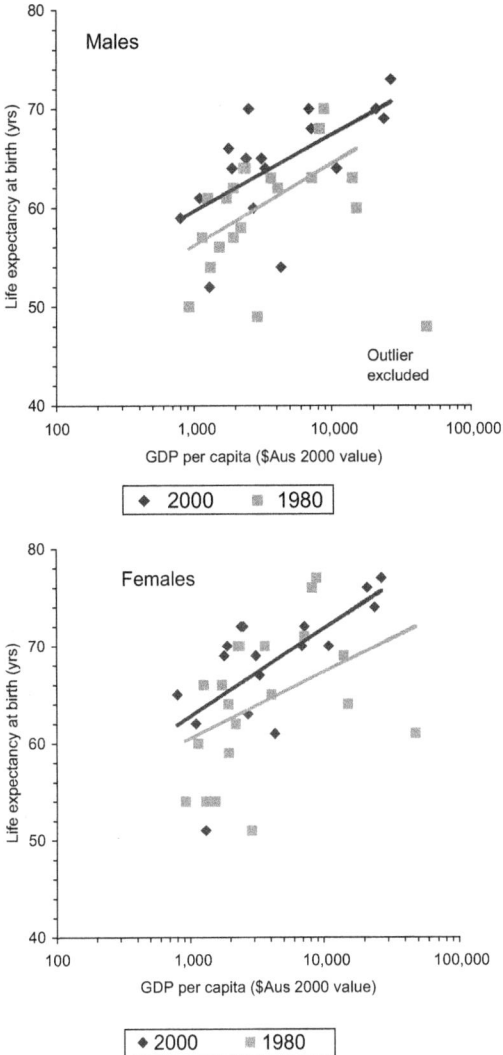

Figure 14.2 Life expectancy in Pacific Island states in 1980 and 2000 in relation to GDP per capita.

Sources: Secretariat of the Pacific Community (2004); Taylor *et al.* (2005: 207–214); Taylor *et al.* (1989: 634–646); Taylor *et al.* (1991: 207–221).

health care was officially declared a failure and the words expunged from most of the WHO lexicon (World Health Organization 2000).

The period since 1990 has seen the continuation of the transition from infectious diseases in children to non-communicable disease in adults as major causes of morbidity and mortality. Although there are continuing improvements in health

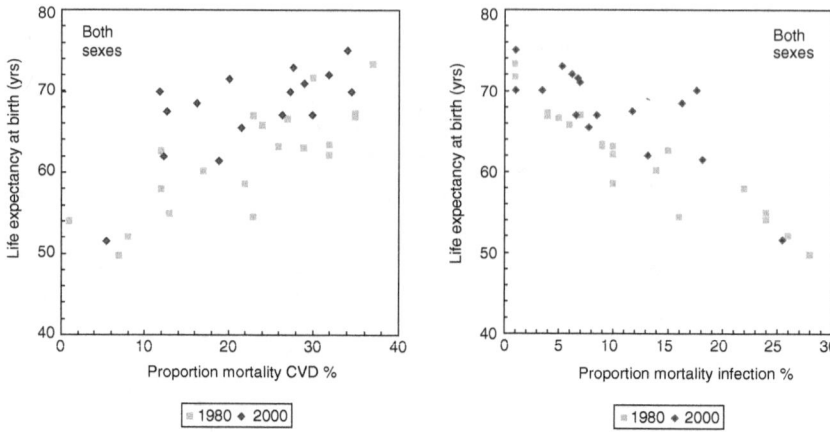

Figure 14.3 Life expectancy in Pacific Island states in 1980 and 2000 in relation to proportional mortality from cardiovascular disease (CVD) and infection.

Sources: Taylor *et al.* (2005: 207–214); Taylor *et al.* (1989: 634–646); Taylor *et al.* (1991: 207–221). Cause of death data abstracted from multiple country sources for *c.*1980 and *c.*2000.

status in the most developed areas, there is also evidence of less improvement at relatively high levels of mortality in the least developed countries still afflicted by communicable disease and under-nutrition, and in some mid-level mortality countries with a significant burden of both infectious and non-communicable disease. The stagnation of improvement in life expectancies in some Pacific Island states is likely to be a consequence of intractable epidemics of non-communicable disease, especially cardiovascular disease and diabetes (see Figures 14.1–14.3).

HIV/AIDS has increased spectacularly, especially in PNG, and a situation not unlike sub-Saharan Africa could well develop there (Hauquitz 2004: 39–49).

Conclusions

This survey illustrates the ecological relationships between humans and their diseases, both infectious and non-communicable, and injuries. These relationships have been evident from earliest times and were first formed in the Pacific Islands through the successive waves of human migration from Asia and the biogeographical context they encountered in the Melanesian chain and the smaller isolated islands of Micronesia and Polynesia. The survey describes again the consequences of contact between isolated and immunologically naive populations and the later waves of Europeans and Asians which led to disastrous mortality and depopulation in Pacific Islands, probably aided by diminished fertility because of sexually transmitted infections. This scenario was also evident in the Americas and Australia.

Subsequent disease patterns and their effects in Pacific Island countries can be understood in the context of geography, history, and social, economic and political developments. The pattern of colonization in the Pacific, while partly a result of chance and inter-power rivalry, has been also a consequence of: the perceived interests of colonial powers, their geographical location and hence strategic interests; the integration of Europeans with the local population, and their number along with the alienation of land, the economic resources available and uses to which Pacific Islands could be put; and the barriers to colonization such as endemic disease (especially malaria), rugged terrain, far-flung and remote archipelagoes, and relatively large indigenous populations. During the wave of decolonization in the 1960s and 1970s the British and Australians left early although they continued to own important assets; the New Zealanders left but continued to have organic connections with many Polynesian states through extensive Islander migration to New Zealand; the French stayed in nickel-rich New Caledonia where there is also agricultural land and tourism, and in French Polynesia which was used for nuclear testing and also has a viable tourist industry; the United States stayed in several guises; it uses Guam as an important military base close to Asia and controls the foreign and defence policies of the Micronesian chain between there and Hawaii. Micronesia was formerly used by the United States for nuclear testing and is still used for missile tests; inhabitants have migration rights to the United States and can join the armed forces. As previously mentioned, the present arrangements are to a large extent mutually beneficial and demands for complete independence have waned with improvement in living standards, improved service provision and better employment opportunities, underwritten to a considerable extent by the metropolitan power. Furthermore, the decline in quality of governance, political coups and administrative implosion in some independent Pacific states has not passed unnoticed by previous *Independentists*.

There are presently significant differences between Pacific Island countries in health status, with a large range in life expectancy and child mortality and a significant variation in cause of death and morbidity patterns. The historical evolution of disease in Pacific Island states, and the demographic and health transitions, are mirrored by contemporary cross-sectional patterns. The less developed states, as crudely measured by GDP per capita, have higher mortality compared to the more developed, with a linear relationship between GDP/capita (on a logarithmic scale) and life expectancy and infant mortality. Not only has income per capita increased over the period 1980 to 2000, associated with higher life expectancy, but the linear relationship between GDP per capita and life expectancy has also moved upwards indicating the contribution of social development including health services; this secular phenomenon was first described by Preston in 1975 (Preston 1975: 231–248).

The public health and medical response can be understood in the context of knowledge and technology available, the magnitude and nature of the problems, the difficulties of implementation (islands, terrain and so on), the resources available (personnel, facilities and finance), and issues of governance in some countries. Colonial administrators, and their few medical officers trained in the fundamentals of tropical medicine and public health, were faced with a disastrous situation in terms of infectious mortality and depopulation. Some were reconciled to the extinction of many Island populations. By the 1930s, population stabilization had occurred and excess mortality had come under control. While some of this was due to the end of immunological naivety, public health and medical efforts are likely to have had some effect especially through provision of clean water and sanitation, vector control, domestic and personal hygiene, nutritional improvements, medical treatment (for the small number who could avail themselves of the few effective therapies available) and possibly quarantine (although this delayed disease introduction rather than prevented it).

Following World War II, coincident with economic and social development, there was extensive implementation of public health and medical measures with substantial reduction in communicable disease and under-nutrition in many Island states, but with much lesser effects in malarial areas and in inaccessible and dispersed populations in Melanesia and Micronesia.

The response to epidemics of non-communicable disease (especially cardiovascular disease and diabetes) has been more problematic because primary prevention involves active independent contributions from non-governmental organizations, universities and professional associations, sophisticated health promotion strategies and structural changes in marketing and advertising of potentially health-damaging products. Governments and their health departments are seriously handicapped in control of non-communicable disease by understandable reluctance to act to change individual behaviours which lack obvious direct effects on others (unlike infectious diseases) and attribution of consumption behaviour solely to individual 'choice'; reluctance to intervene in markets through price manipulation of healthy and unhealthy products because of the prevailing neoliberal economic orthodoxy; and links to large national and transnational corporations that produce unhealthy products for consumption. Furthermore, evaluation of the non-communicable disease epidemic is difficult because of unreliable (or nil) statistics on population risk factors and non-communicable disease mortality. Nevertheless, some of the more developed Pacific Island countries appear to have enjoyed improving life expectancy over the period 1980 to 2000, despite significant proportional mortality from non-communicable disease, implying a reduction in the death rates from these causes, while others manifest a more modest improvement, with a heavier burden of non-communicable disease and injury mortality as possibly the main reason.

The future of health status in the Pacific Islands depends on their own continuing social and economic development and retention of their trained human capital (rather than loss through migration), but also, importantly, especially for microstates, the policies and interactions with international and regional agencies and neighbouring and distant metropolitan powers.

Notes

1 Auckland is the largest Polynesian city in the world when immigrant Polynesians are added to local Maori. The vast majority of Niueans and Tokelauans live in

New Zealand as do around half of Cook Islanders; there are also considerable numbers of Samoans and Tongans.
2. The first indentured labourers from India arrived in 1879 in the wake of the disastrous measles epidemic of 1875 that resulted in 40,000 Fijian deaths.
3. Producing a 'société sectoriseé' ('sectorized' or segmented society), although no more so than Fiji.
4. 'That which does not kill us makes us stronger' Nietzsche (Hollingdale and Tanner) (1968).
5. After Dr Joseph Bancroft, a Queensland medical practitioner, who described Bancroftian filariasis in Queensland in 1876.
6. So called because of the hooks that it uses to attach to the insides of the host intestine where it sucks blood.
7. The grandmother part concerns the fish tapeworm, *Diphyllobothrium latum*.
8. Measles (*morbilli; rubella*), chicken pox (*varicella*), whooping cough (*pertussis*).
9. Mad Cow Disease (*bovine spongiform encephalopathy*) is also caused by a prion and transmitted in a similar manner.
10. So called because of its shape floating atop the more dense saltwater.
11. Fully congruent with human capital theory propositions concerning education and health as human-factor inputs to economic production.
12. 'Nothing so vague as microscopic bacteria but something visible to the naked eye' (Heiser 1936: 268).
13. It was still not known whether a competent mosquito vector for malaria existed in New Caledonia and/or Fiji.
14. Now an important tourist attraction for recreational scuba diving.
15. Described as 'Condominium or Pandemonium'. See Grubb (1999).
16. Ten times the peak historic dose registered from northern hemisphere fallout.
17. Large, fast and sophisticated trawlers with the latest navigational electronics and onboard helicopters for locating schools of fish and other purposes.
18. '*Les troubles*' in New Caledonia; and according to a famous headline in *Le Monde*, 'Des emertes en paradis' (Riots in Paradise) in French Polynesia.
19. Exemplified by the election of Ronald Reagan in the United States and Margaret Thatcher in the United Kingdom.

References

al-Yaman, F., Genton, B., Mokela, D., Narara, A., Raiko, A. and Alpers, M. P. (1996) 'Resistance of Plasmodium Falciparum Malaria to Amodiaquine, Chloroquine and Quinine in the Madang Province of Papua New Guinea, 1990–1993', *Papua and New Guinea Medical Journal*, 39(1): 16–22.

Anonymous (2001) 'From the Centers for Disease Control and Prevention: Vitamin A Deficiency among Children: Federated States of Micronesia, 2000', *JAMA*, 286(6): 667–668.

Baravilala, W. R. and Moulds, R. F. (2004) 'A Fijian Perspective on Providing a Medical Workforce', *Medical Journal of Australia*, 181(11–12): 602.

Birn, A. E. and Solorzano, A. (1999) 'Public Health Policy Paradoxes: Science and Politics in the Rockefeller Foundation's Hookworm Campaign in Mexico in the 1920s', *Social Science & Medicine*, 49(9): 1197–1213.

Black, R. (1981) *Malaria in Australia*, Canberra: Australian Government Publishing Service.

Blakely, T. A., Bates, M. N., Baker, M. G. and Tobias, M. (1999) 'Hepatitis B Carriage Explains the Excess Rate of Hepatocellular Carcinoma for Maori, Pacific Island and Asian People Compared to Europeans in New Zealand', *International Journal of Epidemiology*, 28(2): 204–210.

Boccaccio, M. (1972) 'Ground Itch and Dew Poison; the Rockefeller Sanitary Commission 1909–14', *Journal of the History of Medicine and Allied Sciences*, 27(1): 30–53.

Booth, H. (1999) 'Pacific Island Suicide in Comparative Perspective', *Journal of Biosocial Science*, 31(4): 433–448.

Bowden, D. K., Hill, A. V., Weatherall, D. J. and Clegg, J. B. (1987) 'High Frequency of Beta Thalassaemia in a Small Island Population in Melanesia', *Journal of Medical Genetics*, 24(6): 357–361.

Bowler, P. J. (2003) *Evolution: The History of An Idea*, Berkeley and Los Angeles: University of California Press.

Brown, E. R. (1976) 'Public Health in Imperialism: Early Rockefeller Programs at Home and Abroad', *American Journal of Public Health*, 66(9): 897–903.

Buckley, H. R. and Tayles, N. (2003) 'Skeletal Pathology in a Prehistoric Pacific Island Sample: Issues in Lesion Recording, Quantification, and Interpretation', *American Journal of Physical Anthropology*, 122(4): 303–324.

Cilento, R. (1928) *The Causes of the Depopulation of the Western Islands of the Territory of New Guinea*, Canberra: Government Printer.

Clegg, J. B. and Weatherall, D. J. (1999) 'Thalassemia and Malaria: New Insights into an Old Problem', *Proceedings of the Association of American Physicians*, 111(4): 278–282.

Commission D'enquête sur le Conséquences des Essais Nucléaires (2005) *Les Polynésiens et les essaies nucléaires: Indépendance nationale et dépendance polynésienne*, Assemblée de la Polynésie Francaise.

Counts, D. A. (1990) 'Introduction. Special Issue: Domestic Violence in Oceania', *Pacific Studies*, 13(3): 1–5.

De Vathaire, F., Le Vu, B. and Vathaire, C. C. (2000) 'Thyroid Cancer in French Polynesia between 1985 and 1995: Influence of Atmospheric Nuclear Bomb Tests Performed at Mururoa and Fangataufa between 1966 and 1974', *Cancer Causes Control*, 11(1): 59–63.

Denoon, D. (1997) 'New Economic Orders: Land, Labour and Dependency', in D. Denoon, M. Meleisea, S. Firth, J. Linnekin and K. Nero (eds), *The Cambridge History of Pacific Islanders*, New York: Cambridge University Press, 218–252.

Desowitz, R. (1981) *New Guinea Tapeworms and Jewish Grandmothers: Tales of Parasites and People*, New York: W.W. Norton.

Dever, G. (1994) 'Pacific Basin Medical Officers Training Program: An Alternative Training Program in the Pacific', *Pacific Health Dialog*, 1(1): 71–72.

Eckart, W. U. (1999) '[German New Guinea: "Grave of the White Man". Early Malaria Reports in the Deutsche Medizinische Wochenschrift]', *Deutsche Medizinische Wochenschrift*, 124(46): 1389–1391.

Esterre, P., Plichart, C., Sechan, Y. and Nguyen, N. L. (2001) 'The Impact of 34 Years of Massive DEC Chemotherapy on *Wuchereria Bancrofti* Infection and Transmission: The Maupiti Cohort', *Tropical Medicine & International Health*, 6(3): 190–195.

Fenner, F. (1998) 'Malaria Control in Papua New Guinea in the Second World War: From Disaster to Successful Prophylaxis and the Dawn of DDT', *Parasitologia*, 40(1–2): 55–63.

Fisk, E. (1982) 'Subsistence Affluence and Development Policy', *Regional Development Dialogue*, Special Issue: 1–12.

Gajdusek, D. C. and Zigas, V. (1957) 'Degenerative Disease of the Central Nervous System in New Guinea; the Endemic Occurrence of Kuru in the Native Population', *The New England Journal of Medicine*, 257(20): 974–978.

Gershman, K. A., Rolfs, R. T., Larsen, S. A., Zaidi, A. and Palafox, N. A. (1992) 'Seroepidemiological Characterization of a Syphilis Epidemic in the Republic of the Marshall Islands, Formerly a Yaws Endemic Area', *International Journal of Epidemiology*, 21(3): 599–606.

Grant, A. (1933) 'A Medical Survey of the Island of Nauru', *Medical Journal of Australia*, 1(4): 113–118.

Grubb, J. (1999) 'British and French Administration of the New Hebrides, 1904–1910: Condominium or Pandemonium'?, unpublished paper, Department of History, University of Otago.

Hauquitz, A. C. (2004) 'Looking Down the Barrel of a Cannon: The Potential Economic Costs of HIV/AIDS in Papua New Guinea', *Papua and New Guinea Medical Journal*, 47(1–2): 39–49.

Heiser, V. G. (1936) *An American Doctor's Odyssey: Adventures in Forty-five Countries*, New York: Norton.

Hermant, P., Cilento, R. and League of Nations Health Organization (1929) *Report of the Mission Entrusted with a Survey on Health Conditions in the Pacific Islands*, Geneva: League of Nations Health Organization.

Hughes, R. G., Sharp, D. S., Hughes, M. C., Akau'ola, S., Heinsbroek, P., Velayudhan, R., Schulz, D., Palmer, K., Cavalli-Sforza, T. and Galea, G. (2004) 'Environmental Influences on Helminthiasis and Nutritional Status among Pacific Schoolchildren', *International Journal of Environmental Health Research*, 14(3): 163–177.

Ichimori, K. and Crump, A. (2005) 'Pacific Collaboration to Eliminate Lymphatic Filariasis', *Trends in Parasitology*, 21(10): 441–444.

Institut Statistique de Polynésie Française (2006) 'Indicateurs démographiques de la population de la Polynésie française depuis 1975', in P.i.d.d. à. 2005 (ed.), Online. Available <http://www.ispf.pf>, Papeete: Institut Statistique de Polynésie Française.

Institute de la Statistique et des Études Économiques (2006) 'Décès: Évolution du nombre de décès, Historique depuis 1965', Online. Available <http://www.isee.nc/tec/popsociete/popdeces.html>, Noumea: Institute de la Statistique et des Études Économiques, Nouvelle Calédonie.

Jazayeri, M. S., Basuni, A. A., Cooksley, G., Locarnini, S. and Carman, W. F. (2004) 'Hepatitis B Virus Genotypes, Core Gene Variability and Ethnicity in the Pacific Region', *Journal of Hepatology*, 41(1): 139–146.

Jenkins, C. L. (1988) 'Health in the Early Contact Period: A Contemporary Example from Papua New Guinea', *Social Science & Medicine*, 26(10): 997–1006.

Le Vu, B., De Vathaire, F., De Vathaire, C. C., Paofaite, J., Roda, L., Soubiran, G., Lhoumeau, F. and Laudon, F. (2000) 'Cancer Incidence in French Polynesia 1985–95', *Tropical Medicine & International Health*, 5(10): 722–731.

Levy, S., Taylor, R., Higgins, I., Gillet, D., Grafton, D., Whitemore, J., Bach, F., Deroeck, D., Halkena, J., Maddison, M. and Le Brun, J. (1989) *Marshall Islands Women's Health Survey 1985*, Noumea: South Pacific Commission.

Mead, S., Stumpf, M. P., Whitfield, J., Beck, J. A., Poulter, M., Campbell, T., Uphill, J. B., Goldstein, D., Alpers, M., Fisher, E. M. and Collinge, J. (2003) 'Balancing Selection at the Prion Protein Gene Consistent with Prehistoric Kurulike Epidemics', *Science*, 300(5619): 640–643.

Mueller, I., Namuigi, P., Kundi, J., Ivivi, R., Tandrapah, T., Bjorge, S. and Reeder, J. C. (2005) 'Epidemic Malaria in the Highlands of Papua New Guinea', *American Journal of Tropical Medicine and Hygiene*, 72(5): 554–560.

Muller, I., Bockarie, M., Alpers, M. and Smith, T. (2003) 'The Epidemiology of Malaria in Papua New Guinea', *Trends in Parasitology*, 19(6): 253–259.

Neel, J. V. (1999a) 'Diabetes Mellitus: A "Thrifty" Genotype Rendered Detrimental by "Progress"? 1962', *Bulletin of the World Health Organization*, 77(8): 694–703; discussion 692–693.

—— (1999b) 'The "Thrifty Genotype" in 1998', *Nutrition Reviews*, 57 (5 Pt 2): S2–S9.

New Zealand Ministry of Foreign Affairs (1984) *Report of a New Zealand, Australian and Papua New Guinea scientific mission to Mururora Atoll*, Wellington: Ministry of Foreign Affairs.

Nietzsche, F. W. (Hollingdale, R. J. (translator) Tanner, M. (ed.)) (1968) *Twilight of the Idols and the Anti-Christ*, Harmondsworth: Penguin.

Nowell, W. R. (1987) 'Vector Introduction and Malaria Infection on Guam', *Journal of the American Mosquito Control Association*, 3(2): 259–265.

Over, M., Bakote'e, B., Velayudhan, R., Wilikai, P. and Graves, P. M. (2004) 'Impregnated Nets or DDT Residual Spraying? Field Effectiveness of Malaria Prevention Techniques in Solomon Islands, 1993–1999', *American Journal of Tropical Medicine and Hygiene*, 71(2 Suppl.): 214–223.

Owen, I. L. (2005) 'Parasitic Zoonoses in Papua New Guinea', *Journal of Helminthology*, 79(1): 1–14.

Owen, I. L., Gomez Morales, M. A., Pezzotti, P. and Pozio, E. (2005) 'Trichinella Infection in a Hunting Population of Papua New Guinea Suggests an Ancient Relationship between Trichinella and Human Beings', *Transactions of the Royal Society of Tropical Medicine and Hygiene*, 99(8): 618–624.

Penington, A. H. (1984) 'The Fiji School of Medicine: A Brief History', *Hawaii Medical Journal*, 43(9): 314–318.

Pietrusewsky, M., Douglas, M. T. and Ikehara-Quebral, R. M. (1997) 'An Assessment of Health and Disease in the Prehistoric Inhabitants of the Mariana Islands', *American Journal of Physical Anthropology*, 104(3): 315–342.

Porter, R. (1999) *The Greatest Benefit to Mankind: a Medical History of Humanity from Antiquity to the Present*, London: Fontana Press.

Preston, S. H. (1975) 'The Changing Relation between Mortality and Level of Economic Development', *Population Studies*, 29: 231–248.

Sahlins, M. (1972) *Stone Age Economics*, Chicago: Aldine-Atherton.

Sapuri, M. (1999) 'Introduction of a New Curriculum Method of Teaching Known as Problem-Based Learning to the University of Papua New Guinea Medical School', *Papua and New Guinea Medical Journal*, 42(3–4): 59–62.

Schaumberg, D. A., Linehan, M., Hawley, G., O'Connor, J., Dreyfuss, M. and Semba, R. D. (1995) 'Vitamin A Deficiency in the South Pacific', *Public Health*, 109(5): 311–317.

Secretariat of the Pacific Community (2004) 'Selected Pacific Economies – A Statistical Summary (SPESS)', Online. <Available <http://www.spc.int/statsen/English/Publications/Spess14/Spess_Main_Page_E.htm> (accessed on January 2005) Noumea, New Caledonia: Secretariat of the Pacific Community.

Spencer, D. M. (1998) *The Early Development of the Health Services of Papua New Guinea, 1870–1939*, Brisbane: Tropical Health Program of the Australian Centre for International and Tropical Health and Nutrition, University of Queensland.

Spencer, M. (1992) 'The History of Malaria Control in the Southwest Pacific Region, with Particular Reference to Papua New Guinea and the Solomon Islands', *Papua and New Guinea Medical Journal*, 35(1): 33–66.

Spriggs, M. (1997) 'Recent Prehistory (The Holocene)', in D. Denoon, M. Meleisea, S. Firth, J. Linnekin and K. Nero (eds), *The Cambridge History of Pacific Islanders*, New York: Cambridge University Press, 52–68.

Srivatanakul, P., Sriplung, H. and Deerasamee, S. (2004) 'Epidemiology of Liver Cancer: An Overview', *Asian Pacific Journal of Cancer Prevention: APJCP*, 5(2): 118–125.

Stoltzfus, R. J., Dreyfuss, M. L., Chwaya, H. M. and Albonico, M. (1997) 'Hookworm Control as a Strategy to Prevent Iron Deficiency', *Nutrition Reviews*, 55(6): 223–232.

Takahashi, T., Schoemaker, M. J., Trott, K. R., Simon, S. L., Fujimori, K., Nakashima, N., Fukao, A. and Saito, H. (2003) 'The Relationship of Thyroid Cancer with Radiation Exposure from Nuclear Weapon Testing in the Marshall Islands', *Journal of Epidemiology*, 13(2): 99–107.

Taylor, R., Badcock, J., King, H., Pargeter, K., Zimmet, P., Fred, T., Lund, M., Ringrose, H., Bach, F., Wang, R. L. and Sladden, T. (1992) 'Dietary Intake, Exercise, Obesity and Noncommunicable Disease in Rural and Urban Populations of Three Pacific Island Countries', *Journal of the American College of Nutrition*, 11(3): 283–293.

Taylor, R., Bampton, D. and Lopez, A. D. (2005) 'Contemporary Patterns of Pacific Island Mortality', *International Journal of Epidemiology*, 34(1): 207–214.

Taylor, R., Lewis, M. and Powles, J. (1998a) 'The Australian Mortality Decline: All-Cause Mortality 1788–1990', *Australian and New Zealand Journal of Public Health*, 22(1): 27–36.

—— (1998b) 'The Australian Mortality Decline: Cause-Specific Mortality 1907–1990', *Australian and New Zealand Journal of Public Health*, 22(1): 37–44.

Taylor, R., Lewis, N. D. and Levy, S. (1989) 'Societies in Transition: Mortality Patterns in Pacific Island Populations', *International Journal of Epidemiology*, 18(3): 634–646.

Taylor, R., Lewis, N. D. and Sladden, T. (1991) 'Mortality in Pacific Island Countries around 1980: Geopolitical, Socioeconomic, Demographic and Health Service Factors', *Australian Journal of Public Health*, 15(3): 207–221.

The World Bank (1993) *World Development Report 1993 – Investing in Health*, New York: Oxford University Press.

Trigg, P. I. and Kondrachine, A. V. (1998) 'Commentary: Malaria Control in the 1990s', *Bulletin of the World Health Organization*, 76(1): 11–16.

Ubalee, R., Tsukahara, T., Kikuchi, M., Lum, J. K., Dzodzomenyo, M., Kaneko, A. and Hirayama, K. (2005) 'Associations Between Frequencies of a Susceptible TNF-Alpha Promoter Allele and Protective Alpha-Thalassaemias and Malaria Parasite Incidence in Vanuatu', *Tropical Medicine & International Health*, 10(6): 544–549.

Warren, K. S. and Schad, G. A. (1990) *Hookworm Disease: Current Status and New Directions*, London: Taylor & Francis.

Watters, D. A. and Dyke, T. (1996) 'Trauma in Papua New Guinea: What Do We Know and Where Do We Go?', *Papua and New Guinea Medical Journal*, 39(2): 121–125.

Willcox, R. R. (1980) 'Venereal Diseases in the Islands of the South Pacific', *British Journal of Venereal Diseases*, 56(4): 204–209.

World Health Organization (1978) 'The Alma-Ata Conference on Primary Health Care', *World Health Organization Chronicle*, 32(11): 409–430.

—— (2000) *World Health Report 2000. Health Systems: Improving Performance*, Geneva: World Health Organization.

Index

Note: References to illustrations and tables are in bold type.

Aborigines, health of: in Australia 235, 239, 277, 278; and National Aboriginal Health Strategy 240; and NSW Aborigines Welfare Board 239–240; and Northern Territory Aboriginal Department 239–240; in Malaysia 173, 174
abortion: in Australia 239; in Pacific Island states 280; in Singapore 197, 200
Ackroyd, W. R. 151n
Adams, Tony 238
aging population and the elderly 4; in Hong Kong 21, 45, 46; in Japan 68–69, 71; in Korea 71; in Singapore 200
Aglipay, Father 216
Alba y Martin, D. R. 207
alcohol, abuse and control of: in Australia 233–234, 235, 240; in Pacific Island states 288, 295–296; in Papua New Guinea 260, 265; in the Philippines 212; in Thailand 114, 118; *see also* motor vehicle accidents
Alice Memorial Hospital 12, 15
Allen, Bryant 262
Allen, Horace N. 75
Alma-Ata Declaration 2, 68, 111, 292, 293, 294; *see also* World Health Organization
American Bureau for Medical Aid 32
Anand Panyarachun 117
Andrews, Vernon 216
anklylostomiasis 171
antibiotics, fish contaminated with 44; resistance to 292; in treatment of diseases 65, 67, 69, 70, 87, 151, 229, 261, 262, 291; *see also* penicillin

anti-helminthic drugs 82, 287
Anti-Rightist campaign 33
Aquino, Corazon 218
Arab-Islamic medicine 6, 188
Arita, Isao 88
Armstrong, W. G. 225, 227
Ascaris lumbricoides 82, 280–281; *see also* parasites
Assistance Médicale Indigène 124
Atienza, Lito 219
Atlee, Louis 208
Australia: public health developments and the modern mortality decline in 222–232; public health and the second epidemiological transition in 232–240; public health and HIV/AIDs in 240–242; public health and its future in the Asia-Pacific region and 242–244
Australian Academy of Health 238
Australian and Asian Tobacco Documents Project 242
Australian and New Zealand Society for Epidemiology and Research in Community Health (ANZEACH) 238–239
Australian Federation of Aids Organizations 214
Australian Institute of Health 238
Australian International Development Assistance Bureau (AIDAB) 241
Australian National Council on AIDS 242
Australian Public Health Association 239
Australian Society for Epidemiology and Research in Community Health (ASERCH) 238
avian influenza 41, 47, 69, 116, 118, 181, 202, 243n, 244n; *see also* bird flu; H5N1

Avison, O. R. 76
Ayurveda college 111
Ayurvedic medicine 6, 106–107, 111, 119n, 188

BCG (Bacillus Calmette-Guérin), vaccinations: in China 34; in Hong Kong 22, 32; in Japan 65; in Korea 80; in Malaysia 179; in Papua New Guinea 261; in Vietnam 128, 136n; *see also* tuberculosis
bacteriology, Hong Kong institute of 18; Melbourne department of 225; Pasteurian 123; science of 94, 227
Bancroftian filariasis 282
Barbezieux, Georges 126–127
Basic Law (of Hong Kong) 10, 37, 48
Beau, Paul 124
Bekedam, Hank 47
Belos, Carlos 161, 164
Bentley, C. A. 94
beriberi: in Hong Kong 18, 20; in Japan 58, **59** 61; in Malaysia 171, 172; in Pacific Island states 283, 286, 288; in the Philippines 207; in Singapore 193, 194
bidan 149–150, 151n, 192, 193; *see also* midwifery
biomedicine 3, 33, 107, 112, 118, 135, 193, 195, 196
Bioyee Pharmaceutical (Guangdong) 48
bird flu 2, 10, 41–42, 47, 48; *see also* avian influenza; H5N1
birth control 19, 30, 35, 96, 164; use of condoms for 164; use of intrauterine device (IUD) for 98, 200; *see also* family planning
Black, Robert 262–263
Black May 110–111
Blewett, Neal 237
blood, alcohol in 233; cholesterol in 114; donors of 24, 165, 240; parasites in 279, 280, 291, 303n; pressure, high 47, 200, 237; products of 69; sales of 24, 39, 40; transfusions of 229, 289; venesection, of 287
Bombay Improvement Trust 93
Bourns, Frank 213
Bradley, Dan Beach 107
Bridges-Webb, Charles 236
British empire 7, 10, 94; *see also* colonization
British Leprosy Mission 80
British Medical Association 230
British Medical Research Council (BMRC) 22

British National Birth Control Association 19; *see also* birth control
British National Council for Combatting Venereal Diseases 18–19
Buddhism 107, 110, 111, 133
Bumiputra 176
Buxton line 280
Byuk Yeok Shin Bang 74

Cai Hangang 48
Caldwell, J. C. 250
cancer 4, 5; in Australia 223, 232–233, 237; in China 46; in Hong Kong 21, 24, 25; in Japan 67; in Malaysia 180–181; in Pacific Island states 281, 295–296; in Papua New Guinea 264; in Singapore 198, 199, 203n; in Thailand 112, 114; in Vietnam 124
Canos, Rodolfo 217–218
Carter, E. C. 207
Catholic Church: hospitals in China 27; in Korea 83; NGOs in Vietnam 132, 133; in Pacific Island states 294; in the Philippines 215, 216; in Timor-Leste 160–162, 166
Central Field Station (China) 28
cerebrospinal meningitis 18, 19, 155
cerebrovascular disease 4, 21, 57, 65, 181, 223; *see also* heart disease
Chadwick, Edwin 15
Chadwick, Osbert 15–16, 17
Chamberlain, Joseph 190
Chamorro 276
Chan, Margaret Fung Fu-chun 42, 48
Chartchai Choonhavan 110
Che Chung Won (hospital) 76
Cheewajit 112
China: cross-border public health issues in 42–47, emerging infectious diseases in 42–43; international transfer of modern medicine and public health to 11–12; during the Nationalist decade 28–32; plague and public health development in 26–27 politics of public health in 33–35; during the reform period 35–42; wartime public health of 32–33; *see also* Hong Kong
China Medical Association 28
The China Medical Journal 28
The China Medical Missionary Journal 28
Chinese Center for Disease Control and Prevention (CDC) 36, 46, 48
Chinese Medical Council 25
Chinese University of Hong Kong 25
Choe Han-ki 74–75

Cholera 6, 7; in Australia 224, 254; in China 19–20, 24, 31, 32, 34, 35; El Tor 24, 35, 217–219; in Hong Kong 6, 14, 24, 31, 35, 37; in India 88, 89, 90–91, 92, 93, 97; in Japan 56, 64; in Korea 74, 76, 77; in Malaysia 171–172, 173, 181, 189; in Pacific Island states 285; in the Philippines 206–219; in Singapore 197; in Thailand 107, 108; treatment with Benzozone 211; in Vietnam 123
Choquan Hospital 139
Chosen Society for Preventing Tuberculosis 80; *see also* tuberculosis
Chosen Wangjo Shilok 73–74
Choy, Paul D. 79
Chulalongkorn, King 107
Church, Thomas 189
Cilento, Raphael 228, 256
Closer Economic Partnership Agreement (CEPA) 38
Colonial Development and Welfare Act 174
Colonization 3, 4, 166; of Australia by Britain 222–228; of Hong Kong by Britain 3, 6, 10–25, 37; of India by Britain 87, 88–95; of Indonesia by the Dutch 146–150 *passim*; of Korea by Japan 73, 77–81; of Malaysia by Britain 171–174; of Malaysia by the Portuguese 170–171; of Pacific Island states 276, 284–289, 301; in Papua New Guinea by Germany, Britain and Australia 254–263 *passim*; of the Philippines by America 206–207, 208–217 *passim*; of the Philippines by Spain 207–208; of Singapore by Britain 188–195; of Timor-Leste by the Portuguese 153–157, 166; of Vietnam by the French 123–180 *passim; see also* European expansionism
Commonwealth Tuberculosis Act 221
Communist insurgency 7, 173
Communist party: in China 10, 20, 21, 29, 32–35, 48; in Japan 62; in Thailand 110–111
Confucianism 24, 73, 76, 85
Constitution of Pacifism and Democracy 65
Contagious Diseases Ordinance 14
convergence theory 25–26, 37–39
Cook Islands **252**–253, 276, 278, 284, **298**, 303n

Court of Final Appeal 45
Crosby, Alfred 255
Cumpston, J. H. L. 228
Curzon, Lord 93
Cytomegalovirus: HTLV-1 282; Ross River arbovirus 282

DALYs (Disability Adjusted Life Years) 7
Darling, Samuel T. 142
Darling Commission Report 142
Davidson, Lindsay 236–237
Davisakd Puaksom 107, 108
Dayrit, Manuel 218
DDT *see* Dichloro-Diphenyl-Trichloroethane
De Bevoise, Ken 206, 207, 208
De May, C. F. 210
demographic transition 21–22; 88, 100, 101
dengue fever 153, 162, 181, 286, 289
Deng Xiaoping 48
Denoon, Donald 258
dental services 66, 173, 179, 196, 228, 231, 260, 293
Depo-Provera 162; *see also* birth control
Dew, Harold 230
diabetes mellitus 5n, 46, 84, 101, 181, 200, 260, 264, 289, 294, **300**, 302
diarrhoeal disease: in Australia 222, 223–224; in India 88; in Japan 66; in Pacific Island states 279, 282, 292; in the Philippines 218–219, 220; in Timor-Leste 153, 156, 163
Dichloro-Diphenyl-Trichloroethane (DDT) 64, 113, 261, 289; *see also* malaria and mosquitos
Dick, Robert 225, 230
Dili Hospital 156, 159, 167n
diphtheria: in Australia 230; in China 31; in Hong Kong 23; in Japan 64, 65; in Malaysia 179; in Pacific Island states 292, 293; in Thailand 113
DPT (diphtheria, pertussis, tetanus) 113, 179, 284, 292
Direct Observed Treatment Scheme (DOTS) 98
Dominican friars 154
Donaldson, P. J. 109
Donghu Hospital 47
Doumer, Paul 123, 124
drugs: addiction to 33, 40, 115, 116, 135, 233–236, 241, 243n; anti-tuberculosis

22, 67, 98; fake 44–45, 49n; guilds 29; legislation of 66, 44, 179, 216, 226; oriented medical profession 111–112; manufacture of 28, 63; in the treatment of disease 36, 97, 261, 287, 290, 291; in the treatment of HIV 102, 131; resistant diseases 2, 5, 8, 22, 98, 181; *see also* IDUs
Dubois, Frank 214
Duffy, John 211
Dysentery: amoebic 154–155; in China 31; in Hong Kong 12, 14, 18; in India 88; in Japan 56; in Malaysia 171, 173; in Pacific Island states 282, 284, 285, 286, 288, 289; in Papua New Guinea 256, 258, 259

East Timor 1, 4, 6, 153, 158, 161–167, 167n; *see also* Timor-Leste
East Timorese Ministry of Health 164
E. coli 218; *see also* water supplies
Elkington, J. S. C. 228
Ellis, Constance 227
Emerson, Bert 212
Encephalitis 113
English Public Health Act 224
enteric fever 171
environment: adaptability of the 177; authorities on 8, 219; degradation of 8, 19, 42–43, 44, 45, 93, 118; determinants of 1, 4, 5, 8, 10, 234; health and 2, 3, 7, 55, 66, 124, 238; sanitation of 1, 3, 11, 15, 31, 82, 89, 95, 96, 101, 142, 179, 180; urban 16–19, 114, 133
epidemiological transition 4, 5n; in Australia 232–242; in Hong Kong 20–25; in India 88, 101; in Pacific Island states 296, 297; in Papua New Guinea 250–268;
Erwin, C. H. 80
eugenics 35, 285
Eugenics League 19
European expansionism: in Asia 1, 3, 78, 87–89, 90–91, 140, 170–171, 190–191, 200, 222, 228, 255–256, 268n, 279, 283–289; *see also* colonization
eye diseases 25, 58, 88, 125, 284

Fabian socialism 226
family planning: in China 36; in Hong Kong 19, 45; in India 95, 96, 98, 99–100; in Korea 83, 85; in Malaysia 176; in Pacific Island states 290; in Papua New Guinea 260, 262; in the Philippines 217; in Singapore 196–197, 200; in Timor-Leste 161–162, 166; *see also* birth control; eugenics
Faust, Ernest Carroll 31
fertility: in China 35; in Hong Kong 21, 45; in India 98; in Pacific Island states 284–285, 290, 300; in Papua New Guinea 257, 260, 263, 265–266, 267, 268n, 269n; in Singapore 197
Fiji 276, 284, 288–289, 292–**298** *passim*; 303n
Fiji Medical School 292
Filariasis 153
Fletcher, A. G. 80
food safety: in China 31; in Hong Kong and China 43–45; in Japan 69; of milk supply in Australia 226; and Pure Food Act in Australia 226; and Pure Foods and Drugs Act in the Philippines 216
Fore people 262, 282
'Fortress Australia' 228
Foucault, Michel 111
Four Modernizations 35
Four Pests Campaign 34
Fox, Wallace 22
Fraternité Viêt Nam 132
Freer, Paul 209
Fretilin 157, 158, 159
fungal infections 254

Gajdusek, Carlton 269n
Gandhi, Mahatma 95–96
Gaoqiao district health station 30
Gao Yaojie 40
Garcia, Rachel 219
gastroenteritis 98, 217, 218, 219
gentian violet 293
geopathology 6
germ theory 107–108, 277
Gleeck, Lewis 207, 211
Global AIDS Fund 40
Global AIDS Program 241
Global Fund for Malaria, Tuberculosis and HIV/AIDS 98
globalization, and public health 1, 2, 3, 5n 42, 83–85, 198–202, 201, 255, 295
goitre 262
Gold Plan 21 68–69
Gomez, Manuel 214

312 *Index*

gonorrhoea 256, 257, 259, 268n 282, 284, 287; *see also* sexually transmitted diseases (STDs)
Grant, John B. 30
Great Leap Forward (GLF) 22, 34
Great Proletarian Cultural Revolution (GPCR) 23, 34–35, 37
Guam 252–253, 276, 280, 295, **298**, 301
Guangzhou 12, 13, 15, 16, 17, 19, 20, 21, 26, 27, 31
Gunther, John 261, 262
Guomindang (Nationalist party) 20, 21, 26, 28–33, 35

Haldane, J. B. S. 279
Hall, Sherwood 79–80
Hamilton, Lord 93
hand, foot, and mouth disease 201, 203n
Hanoi School of Medicine 123–124
Hansen's bacillus 122; *see also* leprosy
Harty, Archbishop 215–216
Harvey, William 74
Hawaii 268n, 276, 277, 278, 285, 294, 296, 301
Hawke, R. J. L. 234, 238
Heaf, F. R. G. 22
health: campaigns: in Australia 230, 231, 234, 235; in China 31, 33–34; in Hong Kong 19–20, 23, 47; in India 88, 95, 97; in Indonesia 150; in Malaysia 172; in Pacific Island states 287; in Papua New Guinea 261–263, 267–268; policy development of 33, 65, 77, 88–101, 102, 108, 136, 179, 180; security of 6; in Thailand 113, 118; in Timor-Leste 166; in Vietnam 123, 124–125, 137n
health insurance: in Australia 230, 231, 235; in China 34, 36, 46; in Hong Kong 45; in India 97; in Japan 62, 63, 65–66, 69, 70; in Korea 84; in Malaysia 178, 179; in Pacific Island states 298
Healthy Japan 21 68
heart disease 4; in Australia 223, 232; in China 46, in Hong Kong 21; in India 101; in Japan 67; in Papua New Guinea 264; in Singapore 198, 203n; in Thailand 114; in Timor-Leste 210
Heiser, Victor 140, 207, 208, 215, 216
hemorrhagic fever (Korean) 81
Hennessy, John Pope 13
hepatitis 24, 88; type A 43; type B 24, 113, 179, 281, 282, 292; type C 48, 242; type D 24; type E 24

Herman, Meyer 210
H5N1, 2, 8, 10, 36, 41–42, 47, 116, 181; *see also* avian influenza; bird flu
Hobson, Benjamin 74
Hocquard, E. 133
Homo sapiens, migration to Pacific Islands 277, 278–284
Hong Kong: colonial and prewar public health development in 12–20; cross-border public health issues and problems with China 42–47; post-war epidemiological transition in 20–25; return to Chinese sovereignty 10, 47–49; sanitary reform and the built environment 15–16; *see also* China
Hong Kong Centre for Health Protection 47
Hong Kong College of Medicine for Chinese 13
Hong Kong flu (H3N1) 37
Hong Kong Ophthalmological Society 25
hookworm: in Indonesia 140–144, 145, 146; in Malaysia 172, 173; in Pacific Island states 280, 286–287, 289; in Papua New Guinea 258
hospitals 4, 7; in Australia 229, 230, 233, 235, 238; in China 26–48 *passim*; in Hong Kong 12–47 *passim*; in India 95, 98, 109; in Indonesia 139; in Japan 56, 57, **58**, **59**, 60, 61, 62, 63, 66, 67; in Korea 75–84 *passim*; in Malaysia 170–180 *passim*; in Pacific Island states 288, 293, 294; in Papua New Guinea 261, 262, 265; in Singapore 193–200 *passim*; in Thailand 109, 110, 111, 117, 118, 119n; in Timor-Leste 156, 157, 160, 163, 165; in Vietnam 124, 134, 137n; *see also* individual hospital names
Hospitals and Health Services Commission (HHSC) 235–236
housing, and public health: in Australia 223; in China 32; in Hong Kong 15, 17, 19, 23; in India 87, 89, 93, 96, 101; in Korea 74; in Malaysia 171, 172–173, **175**, 180; in Pacific Island states 288; in Singapore 191, 197–198, in Thailand 114; in Timor-Leste 163
Howard, John 243n
Howe, Brian 241
human rights 38–39
Hydrick, John Lee 140, 141
hygiene, as a health measure 1, 2; in Australia 226; in China 26, 27, 28, 44;

in Hong Kong 15, 18, 31–32, 44; in India 97, 100; in Indonesia 139–150 *passim*; in Japan 62, 73, 74–76; in Korea 78, 82; in Malaysia 173; in Pacific Island states 285, 286; in the Philippines 215; in Vietnam 127
Hygiene Mantri School 147–150

Ileto, Reynaldo 208
Illich, Ivan 111
immigration 6; to Australia 226, 235; to Hong Kong from China 4, 14; to Papua New Guinea 259; in Malaysia 171; to Singapore 189, 202n; to Timor-Leste 154
India: colonial health policy in 88–95; health policy after independence of 95–100; old and new health problems in 100–102
Indonesia: debates over reasons for modern mortality decline 139–140; evolution of public health in 140; the hookworm campaigns and the Rockefeller Foundation in 140–144; hygiene education and competing public health strategies in 147–151; hygiene propaganda in 144–147
infanticide 280
infant mortality: in Australia 223–224, 227, 239; in China 14; in Hong Kong 17, 19, 21, 22, 30; in India 101; in Indonesia 139; in Japan 62, **70;** Malaysia 172, 173, 180, **181**; in Pacific Island states **298**, 301; in Papua New Guinea 259, 260, 261, 263, 267, **252–253**, 289; in the Philippines 217; in Singapore 192, 194, 197; in Timor-Leste 153, 158, 161; *see also* mortality
influenza 7, 18, 23, 37, 92, 94, 155, 222, 223, 239, 254, 256, 258, 259, 282, 284, 285, 288; *see also* avian influenza; bird flu; H5N1
injecting drug users (IDUs) 39, 40, 115–116, 241
Inspection Générale de l'Hygiene et de la Santé Publique 124
Institute of Medical Research Goroka 262
International Bank for Reconstruction and Development 174–175
International Conference on Leprosy of Havanna 131
International Covenant on Civil and Political Rights 38

International Leper Union 80
International Monetary Fund (IMF) 298
International Sanitary Conference, Constantinople 19
iodine, deficiencies of 254
Isei (medical law) 56
Ishihara, Osamu 61

Japan: health developments during the Meiji restoration 55–58; industrialization and militarization and health in 58–63; post-war rehabilitation and health, in 63–66; rapid economic development and new health problems in 66–67; the turning point in primary health care and promotion in 68–71
Japanese occupation: of China 28, 32–33; of Hong Kong 19–20; of Korea 77–82, 85; of the Philippines 216; of Singapore 193–194; of Timor-Leste 155
Jeanselme, Edouard 125
Je Joong Won (hospital) 75
Jennerian cowpox vaccination 56, 91; *see also* vaccination
Johns Hopkins University Medical School 27, 287
Joseph Bhore Committee 95

Kai Ho Kai 15–16
kala-azar (*leishmania donovani*) 34
Kandang Kerbau Hospital 193
Kark, Sidney 235
Kerr, John C. 20
Kiribati **252–253** 283, 284, 290, 294, **298**
Kitasato, Shibasaburo 16
Kojong, Emperor 76
Korea: public health in the pre-modern period in 73–77; public health during the Japanese occupation of 77–82; public health during the post-war period in 81–82; public health problems in the 1960s and 1970s in 82–85
Korea Center for Disease Control and Prevention 83
Korea International Cooperation Agency (KOICA) 82
Korean Association of Parasite Eradication (KAPE) 82
Korean War 21, 33, 66, 73, 81, 82, 84, 85
kuru 262, 269n, 282
Kwang Je Won (hospital) 77

314   Index

Lambert, S. M. 286–287
Langton Clinic 233
League of Nations 7, 18, 28, 30, 32, 127, 226n, 228
Lee Kuan Yew 195
Lee Liming 36
Lee Yong-seul 79
leprosy 6; in Australia 224; in China 31; in Hong Kong 20; in India 95; in Japan 58, 60; in Korea 79–81, 82, 85; in Malaysia 176; in Pacific Island states 282, 284, 285, 286, 289, 291; in Papua New Guinea 256, 258, 261; in Singapore 197; in Thailand 113; in Timor-Leste 153, 154, 156; in Vietnam 122–137, 136n, 137n
Lian Zhenhui 48
life expectancy: in Australia 222, 287–288; in China 3, 35, 36, 223; in Hong Kong 3, 45; in India 4, 95 223; in Indonesia 223; in Japan 3, 63, 70, 222–223; in Korea 4, 83, **84**; in Malaysia 4, 180; in North Korea 4; in Pacific Island states 295–**298**, **299**, 300, 301; in Papua New Guinea 254, 255, 261–267 *passim*; in Singapore 4, 223; in Thailand 113; in Timor-Leste 153; in Vietnam 4
Lin, Ariston Bautista 214
Liu, Hung J. 30
London Board of Health 12
London Medical Missionary Society 12
London School of Hygiene and Tropical Medicine 94, 172, 190, 229
Luo Yunbo 43
Lysenkoism 33

MacGregor, William 190
McKeown, Thomas 139
McKinley, William 212
Mahidol University 110
Malaria 2, 3, 6: in China and Hong Kong 12, 14, 18, 19, 20, 31, 32, 37; fake drugs in the treatment of 45; in India 88, 92, 95, 87, 98, 100; in Indonesia 142, 151; in Malaysia 171, 172, 173, 176, 181; in Pacific Island states 277, 279, 280, 282, 284–293, 301–303n *passim*; in Papua New Guinea 254, 255, 256, 258, 259, 261, 262, 264; in the Philippines 216; in Singapore 191–192, 194, 195; in Timor-Leste 154, 158, 159; *see also* parasites
Malaysia: colonial health and medical services development in 171–174; decolonization and planning in 174–175; independence and development planning in 175–176; national development and public health planning in 176–177; reform of the medical and public health sector in 177–180; the state of health, in 180–181; trends and challenges in public health in 181–184
Manchurian Plague Prevention Service 26
Mann, Jonathan 39
Manson, Patrick 13
Maori 277, 302n
Mao Zedong 22, 33, 34, 35
Marchoux, Emile 127
Marcos, Ferdinand 218
Marianas 276, 279, 281, 284
Marshall Islands 276, 283, 290, 292, 293, 295, 296, **298**
Martin, James Ranald 89
Martin, S. H. 79
maternal and infant health care: in Hong Kong 21, 45; in China 35; in Singapore 192
Maurice, Frederick 192
Maus, L. M. 209, 213
Maxwell, W. E. 109
Meacham, Franklin 209, 214
measles, in Hong Kong 23; immunization in Malaysia 179; incidence among Aborigines 239; incidence in Thailand 114; increased incidence in North Korea 7; introduction into Pacific Island states 7, 282, 284, 303n; introduction into Papua New Guinea 254, 259
Medical Missionary Association 28
Medical Salvation Society 29
medical schools: in Australia 225; in China 25–26, 27, 28, 32, 33, 35, 36; in Hong Kong 13, 25, 27, 32; in Indonesia 150; in Japan 57–58, 62, 63, 67; in Korea 75, 77; in Malaysia 171; in Pacific Island states 287, 288, 292, 293; in the Philippines 207; in Singapore 191, 196; in Thailand 109, 119n; *see also* individual names
medicine, Western, introduction of: to China and Hong Kong 11–12, 13, 16; to India 91; to Japan 60; to Korea 74–77, 84, 85; to Vietnam 123; traditional: in China and Hong Kong 6, 11, 13, 21, 23, 25, 28–29, 30, 43; in India 92; in Indonesia 146; in Japan 60; in Korea 73, 74, 75, 76, 77, 79,

84, 85; in Malaysia 171, 179; in the
Philippines 207; in Singapore 188,
189, 193; in Thailand 106–113, 118; in
Timor-Leste 159; in Vietnam 126, 129,
134; *see also* Traditional Chinese
Medicine (TCM)
Melanesia 153, **252–253** 263, 269n,
276–302 *passim*
meningococcal meningitis 35
mental health 20, 58, 60–61,
114, 343n
Micronesia, **252–253** 260, 263, 269n,
276–302 *passim*
midwifery 30, 56, 107, 109, 148–150,
160, 192–193, 293
migration, of population 4, 5, 6, 15, 113,
115, 189, 240, 242, 278–283, 301, 302;
rural-to-urban 5, 8, 92, 114, 181
missionaries, medical: in China and Hong
Kong 12, 20, 25, 26, 27, 28, 31, 33; in
Japan 60; in Korea 74, 75, 76, 77, 79
80; in Pacific Island states 284, 288; in
Papua New Guinea 268n; in Thailand
107; in Vietnam 125, 134; *see also*
Catholic Church
Mongkut, King 107
mor muang 107
Morris, J. N. 230
mortality: child 108, 114, 153, 254, 263,
283, 297, 301; high 12, 16, 23, 29, 74,
87, 88, 92, 108, 190, 255, 296; maternal
21, 100, 113, 149, 180, **181**, 200, 217,
229, 262, 265, 289; modern decline of
3, 139, 222–223, 231, 257, 269, 287;
neonatal mortality 21, **71**, 181;
perinatal **71**, 222–223; premature 87,
153, 283; proportional **300**, 302;
see also infant mortality
mosquitoes 34, 64, 290; *Aedes* 280;
Anopheles 262, 279, 280, 289, 291;
Culex 280; species of *Anopheles*: *A.
dirus* 113, *A. faraunti* 279, *A. kolenses*
279, *A. minimus* 113, *A. punctulatus*
279; *see also* malaria
motor vehicle accidents (MVA): in
Australia 233; in Malaysia 180; in
Pacific Island states 295; in Thailand
114, 117
Moy, Gerald 43
Murray, Florence Jesse 79

Nagayo, Sensai 56
Nakajima, Hiroshi 68
National Better Health Program
(Australia) 37

National Campaign Against Drug Abuse
(NCADA) (Australia) 234
National Epidemic Prevention Bureau
(China) 32
National Federation of Thai
Medicine 112
National Health and Medical Research
Council (NHMRC) (Australia) 229
National Institute of Dermatology and
Venereology (Hanoi) 132
National Leprosy Control Program
(Vietnam) 131–132
National Public Health Partnership
(NPHP) (Australia) 239
National Quarantine Service (China) 22, 26
National Rural Health Mission (India) 100
National University of Singapore 196
Nehru, Jawaharlal 96
New Caledonia 276, 279, 284, 285, 289,
297, **298**, 301, 303n
New Zealand 239, 283, 290, 291, 296,
301, 303n
NGOs (non-governmental organizations)
2; in Australia 242; in India 100, 101;
in Thailand 111, 113, 115, 116, 117,
119n; in Timor-Leste 163, 164; in
Vietnam 131, 132
Nichols, Henry 216
Nightingale, Florence 90
nipah virus 201
Nippon Foundation 131
Niue **252–253**, 276, **298**, 302n
Novartis 131
NSW Royal Commission on the
Birthrate 227
nuclear weapons testing 295–296
nursing services 2; in Australia 227; in
China 28, 31, 32; in Japan 62, 66, 69;
in Malaysia 192; in Pacific Island states
288, 293, 294; in Papua New Guinea
258, 261; in Singapore 200–201; in
Thailand 109, 127, 132; in Timor-Leste
156, 157, 159, 160; in Vietnam 127,
132, 148, 149
Nutbeam, Don 237–238
nutrition 3, 4, 5; in Australia 224, 230,
237; in China and Hong Kong 18, 19,
20, 23, 32; in India 87, 95, 96, 97, 99,
100, 101; in Indonesia 139, 146, 151n;
in Korea 81, 84; in Malaysia 179, 180;
in Pacific Island states 279–296 *passim*;
in Papua New Guinea 252, 260, 262;
in Singapore 189, 190, 193, 194,
197; in Thailand 108, 113, 114;
in Timor-Leste 156–163 *passim*

316   Index

obesity 84, 114, 193, 198, 203n 261
occupational health 71, 179
Office International d' Hygiène Publique 228
Omi, Shigehiro 68
Omran, Abel 250, 255, 260; *see also* epidemiological transitions
one country, two systems 3, 10, 37, 38, 39, 47, 48
Opium War (1841–1842) 10
Organization for Economic Cooperation and Development (OECD) 84
Organization of Oil Exporting Countries (OPEC) 67

Pacific Island states: country data of **252–253**; health and population issues in 276–278; population migrations and disease spread during the prehistorical period of 278–283; public health, European contact,
depopulation and colonization of 284–289; public health issues, economic development and independence in 289–300; the relationship between ecology, diseases, human populations and health status in 300–303; *see also* Cook Islands; Fiji; Guam; Hawaii; Kiribati; Marshall Islands; Melanesia; Micronesia; New Caledonia; New Zealand; Niue; Palau; Polynesia; Samoa; Tokelau; Tonga; Tuvalu; Vanuatu; Wallis and Futuna
Padua, Allen 219
Padua, Regino 217
Palau **252–253**, 276, 293, **298**
Papua New Guinea: changing patterns of health in the pre-colonial period in 250–254; health during the colonial period in 254–258; public health and post-war epidemiological transitions in 259–263; public health problems and collapse after independence in 263–267; public health prospects of Pacific populations and 267–269
parasites 7, 63, 254, 256; *plasmodium falciparum* and *vivax* in malaria 279; surveys of 30–31, 64–65, 82, 113, 125, 146, 229
Pardo de Tavera, T. H. 214
Parkes, Harry Smith 59
Peking First Health Station 30
Peking Union Medical College (PUMC) 27, 31

penicillin 65, 156, 229, 261, 291, 292
Peverelli, P. 147
Philbun Songkhram 108, 118, 119n
Philippines: cholera during the Spanish colonial period in the 207–208; the 1960s El Tor epidemics in the 217–218; the cholera epidemics of 1902–1903 in the 208–211; the cultural conflict over control of cholera in the 211–215; ensuing epidemics under American rule in the 215–217; public health, culture and epidemics in the 218–219
pigbel (necrotizing enteritis) 262
pig tapeworm (*Taenia solium*) 281, 303n
Piot, Peter 40–41
plague 6, 7; bubonic in Australia 223, 334, 225; in China and Hong Kong 13, 14, 16–17, 26; in India 90, 91, 92, 93, 100; in Indonesia 145 in Japan 64; in Malaysia 171, 172; pneumonic in China 26–27, 32, 34; in Thailand 108; in Vietnam 123
policing, medical 7, 60, 106, 108, 191
poliomyelitis 4, 23, 64, 113, 179, 200, 231–232, 292
Pollitzer, R. 6
Polynesia 276–296 *passim*
Poorwo, Soedarmo 148–149, 150, 151n
population: growth of: in China 34, 36, 37; in Hong Kong 20, 21, 34; in India 90, 95, 98, 100, 101; in Japan 64; in Korea 79, 83, 85; in Malaysia 175, **182–183**; in Papua New Guinea 252–253, 255, 266, 267, 268, 269n; in the Philippines 208; in Singapore 188, 194, 196, 202n; in Thailand 109, 113; in Timor-Leste 156, 167n; decline of: in Pacific Island states 276, 285; in Papua New Guinea 257, 259
poverty, affects on health of 4, 6; in China and Hong Kong 13, 32; in India 98, 100, 101; in Malaysia 176, 177, 184; in the Philippines 219; in Timor-Leste 153, 156, 165, 167n; in Vietnam 124, 134
preventive medicine, definition of 1–8; *see also* public health
primary health care 2, 5; in Australia 240; in India 88, 96–97, 100–101; in Indonesia 139; in Malaysia 170, 179; in Pacific Island states 292–293, 294; in Thailand 111; in Timor-Leste 157, 159–160, 165–166
prostitutes *see* sex workers

public health: and the built environment 16–18, 197–198; in Australia 227, 232, 234–242 *passim*; in China 11, 28, 33, 35, 40; definitions of 1–2, 8–9n; education 2; in Hong Kong 16, 18, 22–23, 24, 26; in India 87, 94–98 *passim*; in Indonesia 140–150 *passim*; in Japan 56, 57, 61, 65, 68; in Korea 75, 82, 83, 85; in Malaysia 173, 175, 179–180; in Pacific Island states 286–287, 290, 291, 292, 303n; in Papua New Guinea 266–267; in the Philippines 215–218; in Singapore 193, 195, 198, 199; in Thailand 115; in Timor-Leste 157, 161; in Vietnam 124, 130; financing of: in China 29, 44–45; in Hong Kong 44; in India 94, 96–99; in Japan 81, 82; in Malaysia 170, 179–**180** 184; in Pacific Island states 294; in the Philippines 218; in Thailand 117–118, 119n; in Timor-Leste 166; in Vietnam 124, 127, 130, 132; legislation of: in Australia 224–236; in China 28, 29; in Hong Kong 16–18, 25, 26, 28, 47; in India 87, 89, 90; in Japan 57, 59, 60, 66; in Korea 84; in Singapore 191, 198; in Thailand 117, 118
Public Health and Building Ordinance 17
Puplick, Chris 242
Putiatin, Evfimii Vasilievich 59

Qing dynasty 18, 26, 27
quarantine, as a public health measure 7; in Australia 228; in China and Hong Kong 16, 20, 26, 44; in India 91, 93; in Japan 56, 57, 69; in Korea 76, 78; in Malaysia 172; in Pacific Island states 285–302 *passim*; in Papua New Guinea 257–258; in the Philippines 206–213 *passim*; in Vietnam 123, 125
quinine 172, 192, 255, 286, 287

rabies 113, 172, 197
Raffles, Stamford 148, 188, 202n
Red Cross Society, of Australia 159; in China and Hong Kong 18, 24, 32; International Committee of 164; hospital 77
Red Guards 35
Refshauge, William 269n
refugees, Chinese in Hong Kong 7, 19, 21, 22, 23, 31, 33, 34; European in Papua New Guinea 262; in Singapore 194
René Robin Hospital 129

Reproductive and Child Health Programme (India) 102
respiratory tract diseases 18, 21, 153, 156, 163, 281–282, 284
Rockefeller Foundation 7; China Medical Commission of 27–28; educational approach of, and hygiene and hookworm campaigns, in Indonesia 139, 140, 141 *passim*; financing of Fiji medical school 292; funding for London School of Hygiene and Tropical Medicine 94; funding for medical chairs in Hong Kong 18; and hookworm control in Pacific Island states 286, 287; International Health Board in Australia 228, 229; International Health Board in India 95, 97; and medicalizing of Thai society 109
Rockefeller Institute for Medical Research 18
Roe, Michael 226–227
Rohl, Timothy 235
Ross, Isabel Younger 227
roundworm 63, 65
Royal Australasian College of Physicians 196, 232
Royal Australasian College of Surgeons 196, 230, 232
Royal Brisbane Hospital 233
Royal Melbourne Hospital 233
rural health services: in China 26, 30–32, 34, 36, 46; in India 88, 91, 94, 96, 98, 99, 100, 101; in Indonesia 139, 140, 147, 148–149, 150; in Korea 82, 83; in Malaysia 172, 173, 174, 175, 176–177, 179, 184; in Pacific Island states 286, 291, 292, 293–294, 296; in Papua New Guinea 265, 266; in the Philippines 217; in Thailand 107, 109, 110, 111, 112, 116, 118; in Timor-Leste 157, 166, 170; in Vietnam 124, 125
Ruttonjee, Jehangir Hormusjee 22
Ruttonjee Sanitorium 22

Sadasivan, Balaji 202
Saint Anthony's Hospital 233
Saint Columban sisters 22
Saint Vincent's Hospital 231
Samoa **252–253**, 276, 284, 270, 293, 294, 295, 296, **298**, 303n
sanitation 1, 2, 3; in China 25, 28; in Hong Kong 15, 17, 19, 31; in India 88, 90–101 *passim*; in Indonesia 139, 142; in Japan 57; in Korea 82;

sanitation (*Continued*)
  in Malaysia 171, 176, 179, 180; in Pacific Island states 285–302 *passim*; in Papua New Guinea 258; in the Philippines 207, 216–217; in Singapore 201
San Lazaro Detention Camp 211
Santiago Hospital 212
SARS (severe acute respiratory syndrome) 2, 5, 8, 10; in Australia 243n; in China and Hong Kong 36, 41, 42, 43, 47, 48; in Japan 69; in Korea 83; in Malaysia 181; in Singapore 201; in Thailand 116
Sax, Sidney 235
schistosomiasis, in China 31, 34, 46; in Pacific Island states 285; in Papua New Guinea 254
school health services 61, 71, 173, 195, 227
Selwyn-Clarke, P. S. 20
Sepoy Mutiny 87
Service d'Assistance Sociale (AMI) 124
sexually transmitted diseases (STDs) 7; in Australia 229–230; in China 31, 34; in Hong Kong 13–14, 18, 19, 20; in India 95, 98 115; in Japan 58–59, 63, 65; in Malaysia 173; in Pacific Island states 284, 296, 300; in Papua New Guinea 254, 259, 262; in the Philippines 216; in Singapore 194; in Timor-Leste 162, 165; in Vietnam 124, 134; *see also* HIV/AIDS; gonorrhoea
sex workers, and STDs: in China 13, 14, 39; in Japan 59–60, 65; in Pacific Island states 254, 285; in Thailand 115; in Timor-Leste 165; in Vietnam 134
Shanghai, and public health 11–34 *passim*
Shin Ki Chon Hum 74
Siever, Doctor 212
silicosis 57
Simpson, W. J. 17, 190–191, 192
Sims, Peter A. 269n
Singapore: the absence of systematic health care in 188–182; colonial health provisions and sanitary reform in 189–193; the Japanese occupation and post-war health provision in 193–195; post-independence and healthcare in 195–198; public health and globalization in 198–203
Single, Eric 235
Sinho, Sanjay 47
Sino-British Joint Declaration 10, 36, 37

Sino-Japanese War 57
social capital 2, 264
Southern Federation of Thai Medicine 112
South Pacific Alliance for Family Health (SPAFH) 290
Small Deer Island (So Rok Do) leper asylum 80–81
smallpox 6, 7; in China and Hong Kong 13, 14, 18 19, 20, 23, 31, 34; in India 91–92, 95, 97; in Indonesia 150; in Japan 56, 64, 68, 74, 75; in Korea 74, 75; in Malaysia 171, 172; Pacific Island states 282, 284, 285, 292; in Papua New Guinea 254, 256; in the Philippines 207, 216; in Timor-Leste 155, 156; in Vietnam 123
smoking-related diseases and tobacco control 3; in Australia 232–233, 234, 242; in China 46–47; in Hong Kong 25, 47; in Japan 68; in Korea 84; in Papua New Guinea 260; in Malaysia 181; in Singapore 198–199
Solomon Islands 228, 258, 263, 267, 276, 278, 281, 284, 288, 291, 297, **298**
State Environmental Protection Agency (SEPA) (China) 43
State medicine 29–36, 73–77, 85, 184
State Secrets Law 40, 48
Streptococcus suis 44
Strong, Richard 207
Suharto 161
Sun Yat-sen 13
Suva Medical School 292

Tabar, Gregorio 212
Taft, Governor 214
Tai Lam Leper Hospital 31
Tai Ping Shan district 16
Tanabe, S. 112
Tan Tock Seng 189
Tan Tock Seng Hospital 189, 191, 193, 194
Thailand: traditional medicine in 106–107; modern medicine in 107–108; public health and the medicalization of the state in 108–110; public health and the status of epidemiological trends in 113–116; reform of public health in 116–118
Thaksin Shinawatra 116, 118
Timor-Leste: public health during the Portuguese colonial period in 153–157; during the Indonesian period in 157–162; during the UN transitional

Index 319

administration in 162–165;
and independence in 165–167
Tinbergen, Jan 37
Tokelau 252–253, 276, 302n
Tonga 252–253, 284, 290, **298**, 303n
Traditional Chinese Medicine (TCM) 3, 10, 11, 13, 22, 25; in Hong Kong, ambiguous status of 25; in China, status of 29, 34, 35; contamination of 43; in Japan renouncing of 57; medical theories of 193; practice in Korea 57; in Malaysia 171; in Singapore 189; in Vietnam 123
Traditional Medicine for Self-Curing Project 111
trauma: sexual and domestic 264–265
Trichinella (papuae) 281
tropical medicine 94, 172, 190, 191, 228, 268n, 286–287, 302; conferences on 129; and diseases 6, 254, 287, 288; and health 141, 239; schools of 27, 94, 129, 172, 190, 229, 156
trypanosomiasis 254
Tsang, Donald 44
tuberculosis 2, 8; in Australia 223, 226, 229, 231, 239; in China and Hong Kong 6, 7, 8, 19, 20–24, 31, 34, 37, 46; in India 93; in Japan 58–67 *passim*; in Korea 79–80; in Malaysia 6, 171, 173–174, 176, 181; in Pacific Island states 282–291 *passim*; in Papua New Guinea 256, 259, 262; in the Philippines 216, 217, 218; in Singapore 194, 195, 197, 200; in Timor-Leste 6, 153–158 *passim*; in Vietnam 124, 131; treatment with para-aminosalicyclic acid (PAS) 65
Tung Wah hospitals 12–13, 14, 20, 29
Tuvalu 252–253, 284
typhoid: in Australia 223, 224–225; in Hong Kong 18, 31; in India 88, 89; in Japan 64; in Pacific Island states 289; in the Philippines 218; in Singapore 194

Unequal Treaties 30, 55, 56, 57, 63
Union Indochinoise 123
United Kingdom General Medical Council 13
United Nations: admission of China to 35; Fund for Population Activities 161, 162; Security Council 163; Transitional Administration in East Timor 163–164; Trust Territory of the Pacific Islands (TTPI) 277; UNRRA 32; *see also* World Health Organization
United States Public Health Service 32, 215
Universal Declaration of Human Rights (UDHR) 38
University of Hong Kong 13, 25, 27, 32, 42
University of Tokyo Medical School 56, 57
urbanization 5, 8, 37, 87, 100, 106, 114, 186, 223

vaccination: in China 31, 32, 34, 48; in Hong Kong 18, 19, 22, 23–24; in India 91, 92, 95, 97; in Japan 56, 64, 65, 70, 75; in Korea 80; in Malaysia 173, 176; in North Korea 4; in Pacific Island states 285, 288; in Papua New Guinea 261; in Singapore 192, 197; in Timor-Leste 157; in Vietnam 123, 124
van Lonkhuyzen, J. J. 143–145
van Meerdervoort, Pompe 57, 59
van Noort, Doctor 142–143
Vanuatu 252–253, 263, 267, 279, 284, 285, 286, 288, 293, 294
venereal diseases *see* sexually transmitted diseases (STDs)
Vereniging van Indonesische Geneeskundigen 149
Vickers, W. J. 194–195
Vietnam: the discovery and impact of leprosy during the colonial period in 122–130; leprosy as a social problem in 130–131; post-colonial historical perspectives on leprosy in 131–132; exclusion of lepers as a continuing public health strategy in 132–136
Villarama, Antonio C. 216
Villegas, Antonio 217
vitamin A, deficiency of 283; *see also* eye diseases
vitamin B1, deficiency of 171, 283; *see also* beriberi

Wagner, Arthur L. 208
Wallis and Futuna islands **252–253** 276, 284
Wang Longde 46
Wang Ruotao 46
Wan Yanhai 40
water supplies: potable 4, 8, 9; in China and Hong Kong 15–16, 17, 19, 20, 26,

water supplies (*Continued*)
    31, 38, 42, 43; in India 87, 89, 96, 97, 98, 99, 100, 101; in Indonesia 139, 146; in Japan 61, 66, 71; in Korea 75, 76; in Malaysia 171, 172, 179, 150; in the Philippines 207, 209, 210, 212, 215; in Singapore 188, 191, 194, 197, 198; in Vietnam 124
Webster, Ian 236
Western Australia Health Act 226
White, Kerr 238
'White Australia' policy 226, 228
whooping cough 64, 239, 254, 256, 284, 303n
Winslow, Charles-Edward Amory 1–2, 8–9n
wi-saeng (weisheng) 11, 73
Wilson, R. M. 80
Worcester, Dean C. 206, 207
World Bank 164, 298
World Health Organization (WHO) 2, 5, 6, 7; and China and Hong Kong 22, 37, 39, 41–42, 43, 45, 46, 47, 48; Collaborating Center for Surveillance, Research and Training on Emergency Infectious Disease 47; Epidemiological Intelligence Station in Singapore 37; Expert Committee on Leprosy 131; Framework Convention on Tobacco Control 84; Health for All strategy 2, 5n, 68, 237; and India 98, 101; and Japan 68; and Korea 84; National Influenza Centre in Hong Kong 37; Ottawa Charter for Health Promotion 2; and Pacific Island states 291, 294, 299, 303; and Papua New Guinea 264, 266; and the Philippines 217; and Thailand 111, 113; and Timor-Leste 164; and Vietnam 122, 130; Western Pacific Regional Headquarters 216–217; Western Pacific Region Committee 39; *see also* Alma-Ata Declaration
World War I 7, 8, 89, 90, 94, 155, 192, 225–230, 288
World War II 3, 4, 6, 7, 9; and Australia 229–230, 232; and China 32–33; and Hong Kong 18, 21; and India 97; and Indonesia 140; and Japan 55, 61, 62–63, 70; and Korea 84; and Pacific Island states 277, 280, 289; and Papua New Guinea 259–261; and Thailand 109; and Timor-Leste 162, 155–156
Wuchereria Bancrofti 280, 303n
Wu Lien-teh 26, 28, 31

Xanana, Gusmão 165–166

yang-saeng 73
yaws: in Indonesia 150, 155, 156; in Pacific Island states 281, 288, 289, 291; in Papua New Guinea 254, 256, 258, 259, 261–262
yellow fever 172, 224
Yeoh Eng-kiong 42
Yersin, Alexandre 16
Yi Ik 74
Yi Kyu-kyung 74
Y.M.C.A. 18

Zhang Dejiang 44
Zheng Xiaoyu 44, 49n
Zoellick, Robert 40

For Product Safety Concerns and Information please contact our EU
representative GPSR@taylorandfrancis.com
Taylor & Francis Verlag GmbH, Kaufingerstraße 24, 80331 München, Germany

www.ingramcontent.com/pod-product-compliance
Lightning Source LLC
Chambersburg PA
CBHW070749020526
44115CB00032B/1553